MW00044009

LIGAND-BINDING ASSAYS

LIGAND-BINDING ASSAYS
DEVELOPMENT, VALIDATION, AND IMPLEMENTATION IN THE DRUG DEVELOPMENT ARENA

Edited by

Masood N. Khan
John W.A. Findlay

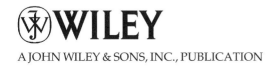

A JOHN WILEY & SONS, INC., PUBLICATION

Copyright © 2010 by John Wiley & Sons, Inc. All rights reserved.

Published by John Wiley & Sons, Inc., Hoboken, New Jersey
Published simultaneously in Canada

No part of this publication may be reproduced, stored in a retrieval system, or transmitted in any form or by any means, electronic, mechanical, photocopying, recording, scanning, or otherwise, except as permitted under Section 107 or 108 of the 1976 United States Copyright Act, without either the prior written permission of the Publisher, or authorization though payment of the appropriate per-copy fee to the Copyright Clearance Center, Inc., 222 Rosewood Drive, Danvers, MA 01923, (978) 750-8400, fax (978) 750-4470, or on the web at www.copyright.com. Requests to the Publisher for permission should be addressed to the Permissions Department, John Wiley & Sons, Inc., 111 River Street, Hoboken, NJ 07030, (201) 748-6011, fax (201) 748-6008, or online at http://www.wiley.com/go/permission.

Limit of Liability/Disclaimer of Warranty: While the publisher and authors have used their best efforts in preparing this book, they make no representations or warranties with respect to the accuracy or completeness of the contents of this book and specifically disclaim any implied warranties of merchantability or fitness for a particular purpose. No warranty may be created or extended by sales representatives or written sales materials. The advice and strategies contained herein may not be suitable for your situation. You should consult with a professional where appropriate. Neither the publisher nor authors shall be liable for any loss of profit or any other commercial damages, including but not limited to special, incidental, consequential, or other damages.

For general information on our other products and services or for technical support, please contact our Customer Care Department within the United States at (800) 762-2974, outside the United States at (3 17) 572-3993 or fax (317) 572-4002.

Wiley also publishes its books in a variety of electronic formats. Some content that appears in print may not be available in electronic formats. For more information about Wiley products, visit our web site at www.wiley.com.

Library of Congress Cataloging-in-Publication Data:

Ligand-binding assays : development, validation, and implementation in the
drug development arena / [edited by] Masood N. Khan, John W.A. Findlay.
       p. ; cm.
    ISBN 978-0-470-04138-3 (cloth)
    1. Radioligand assay. 2. Drug development.   I. Khan, Masood N.   II. Findlay,
John W. A.
    [DNLM: 1. Drug Design. 2. Immunoassay. 3. Ligands. 4. Protein Binding.
QV 744 L723 2009]
    RS425.L54 2009
    615′.19--dc22
                                                          2009036489

Printed in the United States of America

1 0 9 8 7 6 5 4 3 2 1

■ CONTENTS

13 Alternative and Emerging Methodologies in Ligand-Binding Assays **343**

Huifen F. Wang and John W.A. Findlay

Ligand-binding assays in the form of radioimmunoassay were first developed and applied to protein analysis about 50 years ago. This new technique was sensitive and was also characterized by the unique specificity conferred by the key antibody binding reagent. Since the development of this radioimmunoassay for insulin, ligand-binding assay methodology has undergone many cycles of evolution, primarily along two lines. The first of these is concerned with the technology for detection of the end point of the ligand-binding assay. Progress in this area included detection by enzyme activity assays, such as in enzyme-linked immunosorbent assays (ELISAs), by fluorescence and luminescence end points in many formats (including, most recently, electro-chemiluminescence), by surface plasmon resonance, and by immuno-polymerase chain reaction (IPCR). All of these approaches allow the user to be relieved of the hazards of working with radioactivity and the burden of radioactive waste disposal, while maintaining or improving on the sensitivity of radioactivity-based ligand-binding assays. The other line of progress relates to the key binding reagent employed in the assay. Polyclonal antibodies were initially, and are still, widely used in this role. However, the development of monoclonal antibody technology offered reagents of greater specificity (although sometimes of somewhat lower affinity). Receptors and transport proteins have also been used in these assays, but more intriguing has been the work done on molecularly imprinted polymers, also known as "synthetic antibodies" which offers the prospect of unlimited supply of a single batch of binding reagent for use in a large number of assays.

Although ligand-binding assays continue to be applied to the bioanalysis of some classes of low molecular weight molecules, such as some agricultural chemicals, screening of drugs of abuse, and clinical chemistry applications, the continued vitality of ligand-binding assays has been ensured by the burgeoning interest in research and development of biological macromolecules as potential therapeutics. A large number of macromolecules are currently in clinical evaluation in a number of therapeutic areas, with a major emphasis on oncology. Many of these drug candidates are proteins, such as monoclonal antibodies and fusion proteins, but they also include other macromolecules such as antisense and other oligonucleotides. The bioanalysis of such molecules in complex matrices, such as plasma and serum, can not yet be performed by the powerful mass spectrometry based methods that now dominate the bioanalysis of low molecular weight xenobiotics, and ligand-binding assays remain the cornerstone of support for pharmacokinetic and toxicokinetic studies of macro-molecules. Until advances in mass spectrometry based methods permit their typically high specificity and sensitivity to be applied to analyses of macromolecules in complex matrices, ligand-based assays will remain the methods of choice for the bioanalysis of biological macromolecules.

The idea for this book arose from conversations between the editors from time to time after they chaired a roundtable session on challenges in immunoassay validation at the 1998 AAPS Annual Meeting in San Francisco. Validation of bioanalytical methods in general had been a topic of increasing attention over the last decade, with the first Crystal City meeting in 1990 as a milestone. Ten years later, the second Crystal City meeting in 2000 reviewed progress in bioanalytical method validation and a separate meeting was also held on macromolecule bioanalysis. Finally, a third Crystal City meeting in 2006 addressed validation of chromatography-based and ligand-binding assays jointly, as well as in separate sessions. In early 2000 we, along with a number of coauthors, separately published a discussion of validation approaches for ligand-binding assays that provided a framework for the subsequent discussions and workshops.

Reflecting on all of these activities, we felt that there was no text currently available that presented the range of activities related to the development, validation, and implementation of ligand-binding assays in the context of drug development in a truly practical sense. We felt that such a volume would be of great help to practitioners in varied fields, both in the pharmaceutical and allied industries and in related contract research organizations and academic laboratories, and perhaps even in the field of diagnostics and clinical chemistry. To this end, we enrolled a group of authors highly skilled and experienced in the development and implementation of ligand-binding assays to contribute to this book.

The contents of the book cover a wide range of topics related to development, validation, and implementation of ligand-binding assays in the development of drug candidates. These include general discussion of challenges and proven approaches in the development of ligand-binding assays, as well as more detailed examination of characteristics of these assays when applied in support of pharmacokinetic and toxicokinetic studies of compounds at different stages in the discovery or development timeline. A concise, but detailed, discussion of validation of ligand-binding assays for macromolecules is included, as is a practical approach to "fit-for-purpose" validation of assays for biomarkers, those molecules receiving increased attention as potentially demonstrating that the target chosen in Discovery is being modulated by the candidate therapeutic, both in nonclinical and clinical studies. As expected, calibration curves and assay performance are supported by statistical treatments, and this topic is discussed in depth, covering both European and North American perspectives. Deployment of assays in high-throughput format requires automation of ligand-binding assays and, particularly in the current environment, internal capabilities are often reduced, accompanied by increased outsourcing of bioanalytical work. The critical aspects of both of these topics, including successful transfer of assays to a contract research organization, are reviewed in depth. As in most fields of science, technologies related to ligand-binding assays continue to advance. Consequently, newer and emerging ligand-binding assay technologies are reviewed. Given the continuing interest in the question of whether the efficacy or safety of a biological macromolecule may be compromised by antibodies elicited in response to treatment, assays for the detection and characterization of such antidrug antibodies in animals or humans (immunogenicity assays) are discussed in detail. In light of the critical role of calibration standards in ligand-binding assays, the importance of characterized reference standards in interpreting assay results is discussed. At various stages in the drug discovery and development process, some analyses may be conducted by the use of commercially available assay kits; some of the challenges in qualification or validation and implementation of such assay kits are presented. Finally, the importance of proper documentation of experimental bioanalytical findings in assay validation or study reports from a regulatory viewpoint is emphasized.

The editors are grateful for the energy and expertise of all of our contributors to this book. We trust that basic and applied research scientists will find this book valuable in further understanding and expanding the successful application of ligand-binding assays to bioanalysis of a variety of molecules in complex biological media.

JOHN W.A. FINDLAY
Durham, North Carolina

MASOOD N. KHAN
Rockville, Maryland

John L. Allinson, F.I.B.M.S., ICON Development Solutions, Manchester, UK

Bruno Boulanger, Ph.D., UCB Pharma SA, Braine-L'alleud, Belgium

Ronald R. Bowsher, Ph.D., Millipore, St. Charles, MO, USA

John D. Chappell, B.Sc., C.Chem., M.R.S.C., ICON Development Solutions, Oxford, UK

Proveen D. Dass, Ph.D., PhytoBio Solutions Inc., Raleigh, NC, USA

Binodh S. DeSilva, Ph.D., Amgen Inc., Thousand Oaks, CA, USA

Viswanath Devanarayan, Ph.D., Abbott Laboratories, Souderton, PA, USA

Walthère Dewé, M.Sc., GSK Biologicals, Rixensart, Belgium

Deborah Finco, M.S., Pfizer Inc., Groton, CT, USA

John W.A. Findlay, Ph.D., Gilead Sciences, Inc., Durham, NC, USA

Michele Gunsior, Ph.D., Covance Laboratories Inc., Chantilly, VA, USA

Howard Hill, Ph.D., M.R.S.C., Huntingdon Life Sciences, Alconbury, UK

Stephen Keller, Ph.D., Facet Biotech, Redwood City, CA, USA

Marian M. Kelley, M.A., MKelley Consulting LLC, West Chester, PA, USA

Masood N. Khan, Ph.D., GLP Solutions Inc., Rockville, MD, USA

Wolfgang Klump, Ph.D., SAFC Pharma, Carlsbad, CA, USA

Jean W. Lee, Ph.D., Amgen Inc., Thousand Oaks, CA, USA

John H. Leete, Ph.D., 640 Marquette Court, Frankfort, MI, USA

Marjorie A. Mohler, B.A., Ciencia Group, Yountville, CA, USA

Chris Morrow, B.A., Genentech, South San Francisco, CA, USA

Peter J. O'Brien, Ph.D., Pfizer Inc., San Diego, CA, USA

Jacqueline A. O'Shaughnessy, Ph.D., U.S. Food and Drug Administration, Silver Spring, MD, USA

Yang Pan, Ph.D., M.B.A., Amgen Inc., Seattle, WA, USA

Thomas H. Parish, M.S., Procter & Gamble Pharmaceuticals, Norwich, NY, USA

Marie T. Rock, Ph.D., Midwest BioResearch, Skokie, IL, USA

Chanchal Sadhu, Ph.D., Covance Laboratories Inc., Chantilly, VA, USA

Richard F. Schuman, Ph.D., BioReliance Corporation, Rockville, MD, USA

CT. Viswanathan, Ph.D., U.S. Food and Drug Administration, Silver Spring, MD, USA

Huifen F. Wang, Ph.D., Pfizer Inc., New London, CT, USA

Ren Xu, M.Sc., M.B.A., Amgen Inc., Seattle, WA, USA

Ligand-Binding Assays in Drug Development: Introduction and Historical Perspective

JOHN W.A. FINDLAY

Gilead Sciences, Inc., Durham, NC, USA

MASOOD N. KHAN

GLP Solutions Inc., Rockville, MD, USA

1.1 GENERAL

A ligand-binding assay (LBA) may be defined as an assay in which the key step is an equilibrium reaction between the ligand (analyte) and a binding molecule, most often a protein and, in many cases, a specific antibody or receptor directed against the ligand of interest. This reaction is governed by the law of mass action. The end point of the reaction reflects, either directly or inversely (depending on whether the assay format is competitive or noncompetitive), the concentration of the analyte present in the sample. Although this approach may be applied in a qualitative sense, ligand-binding assays are generally implemented as sensitive, quantitative analytical methods. These assays cover a broad scope. Binding molecules may include antibodies or antibody fragments, receptors, transport proteins, or oligonucleotides such as aptamers or spiegelmers. Detection and quantitation of the reaction end point may involve one of many technologies, including radioactivity or enzyme activity producing UV/visible-absorbing, fluorescent, luminescent, or chemiluminescent products. Ligand-binding assay formats may be competitive or noncompetitive, with solution- or solid-phase configurations.

This chapter will provide a brief history of the development of ligand-binding assays and their increasing and changing applicability to the determination of various types of molecules to provide context for more detailed discussions in subsequent

Ligand-Binding Assays: Development, Validation, and Implementation in the Drug Development Arena. Edited by Masood N. Khan and John W.A. Findlay
Copyright © 2010 John Wiley & Sons, Inc.

chapters. The formation of the Ligand-Binding Assay Bioanalytical Focus Group (LBABFG), sponsored by the American Association of Pharmaceutical Scientists (AAPS), has resulted in active promotion of consistent approaches to the development, validation, and implementation of ligand-binding assays for macromolecule therapeutics. The origins, activities, and numerous contributions of the LBABFG to the field of LBAs are also reviewed in this chapter.

1.2   HISTORICAL REVIEW

Approximately 50 years have passed since Yalow and Berson reported on the binding interaction between insulin and an insulin-binding antibody [1], followed by the first development and application of a ligand-binding assay in the form of a radioimmunoassay (RIA) for insulin [2]. This development marked a major advance in the sensitive and specific measurement of protein hormones in blood-based fluids, taking advantage of the competition between a limited mass of radiolabeled insulin and increasing concentrations of unlabeled insulin for insulin-binding sites on a limited amount of anti-insulin antibody molecules. The greater the amount of unlabeled insulin in the system, the smaller the amount of radiolabeled insulin detected in the antigen–antibody complex; this relationship between antibody-bound radiolabeled and unlabeled insulin concentrations formed the basis of the insulin assay calibration curve, from which insulin concentrations in study samples could be interpolated. The work of Yalow and Berson, who were subsequently awarded the Nobel Prize for Medicine, ushered in an era of widespread development and application of the new immunoassay methodology to many biomedical fields. Despite a subsequent general movement away from the use of radioactivity as an end point detection technology, application of RIA technology in several formats, such as solution-phase, solid-phase, competitive, and immunoradiometric assays, has continued to the present day due to case-specific advantages such as high sensitivity for the analyte compared to alternative immunoassay formats. The work of Landsteiner in 1945 [3] demonstrated that immunization of animals with hapten–protein conjugates, in addition to producing antibodies to the carrier protein, elicited antibodies in the animal against the small molecule hapten. This observation provided the foundation for the subsequent broad application of immunoassay technology to analysis of low molecular weight drugs and other small molecules. Thus, in the same time period as Yalow and Berson reported on assay applications for anti-insulin antibodies, Beiser and coworkers demonstrated that immunization with steroid–protein conjugates resulted in production of antisteroid antibodies [4], which led to widespread applications of radioimmunoassay in the field of steroid biochemistry. Several years passed before these assays were applied to the analysis of therapeutic drugs, initially for the quantitation of digitoxin [5] in biological fluids. Due to the advantages of high sensitivity, relatively good specificity, and high-throughput capabilities, there were extensive and rapid applications of immunoassay to drug analyses, as chronicled in several review articles [6–8]. The impressive potential specificity of antibodies, even in the recognition of very limited, defined molecular structural variations, was illustrated in the stereoselectivity of antibodies to, and immunoassays for, chiral small drug molecules, as reviewed by Got and

Schermann [9]. The other important applications of immunoassay have been in the determination of small molecules in agricultural applications for pesticide analysis [10], in the support of the development of genetically modified crops [11], and in the screening of drugs of abuse [12]. In the latter application, an immunoassay is typically used as a screening approach, often followed by specific identification of the drug involved and quantitation by liquid chromatography/mass spectrometry (LC/MS). Wu [13] and Lepage and Albert [14] have reviewed the major impact of ligand-binding assays, initially in manual and, more recently, automated formats, on rapid progress in the clinical and endocrinology laboratory environments, respectively. In the pharmaceutical industry, the application of immunoassay to determination of small molecules in biological matrices has declined sharply in recent years, being largely surpassed by the advent of highly sensitive and specific LC/MS-based analytical methods [15].

An ongoing migration to the use of nonradioactive immunoassay reaction end point detection started with the introduction of the solid-phase enzyme-linked immunosorbent assay (ELISA) by Engvall and Perlmann [16] and van Weemen and Schuurs [17] and the homogeneous enzyme-multiplied immunoassay technique (EMIT, [18]). Subsequently, nonisotopic detection technology applications such as time-resolved fluorescence [19], electrochemiluminescence [20], and other newer techniques were introduced, as discussed later in this book.

1.3 LBAs FOR MACROMOLECULES

The primary reason for the continued strong interest in ligand-binding assay development and application in the drug development arena is the recent upsurge in interest in the therapeutic potential and promise of various classes of biological macromolecules. Recent years have seen a remarkable increase in research and development of proteins, oligonucleotides (as aptamers and antisense compounds), and other macromolecular therapeutic drug candidates [21]. Macromolecules are in various stages of development in a wide range of therapeutic areas, most notably in oncology, buoyed by recent major clinical and commercial successes of a broad range of biotechnology products [22]. Although applications of various modes of mass spectrometry continue to be evaluated, mass spectrometric assays have not yet evolved to the point required for routine determination of proteins and other macromolecules in complex biological matrices, such as plasma. Thus, immunoassays and other binding assays (e.g., hybridization assays for quantitation of oligonucleotides) remain the mainstay techniques for the determination of these molecules due to their ability to detect macromolecules with high sensitivity and adequate specificity in highly complex biological matrices generally without separation of the analyte of interest prior to assay. Due to the increasing impact of biological macromolecules on therapy of many diseases, development and validation of LBAs for these have received increasing attention. Several workshops [23–26] and review articles [27–29] have discussed validation of these assays in considerable detail. With the increased research and development interest in macromolecules as potential therapeutics has come the need to monitor potential immune response to these large molecules, a situation that is generally rare with low molecular weight drugs. Detection of immunogenicity is important, since an antidrug antibody response to the potential therapeutic may result in loss of efficacy if the elicited antibodies neutralize the intended beneficial activity of the candidate therapeutic. In this situation, safety is also an important consideration, as exemplified by the case of antibodies elicited to recombinant erythropoietin, which neutralized the effects of the endogenous erythropoietin, resulting in the development of life-threatening pure red cell aplasia [30]. This need has generated a new class of LBAs related to detection of immunogenicity of macromolecular drugs, a topic discussed in detail later in this book.

1.4 ADVANTAGES AND LIMITATIONS OF LBAs

As will be discussed in detail in subsequent chapters, LBAs offer a number of advantages over other bioanalytical methods. Due to the high affinity of the key binding reagent, these assays generally have high sensitivity for the analyte, translating into low limits of quantitation (LLOQ). Thus, some immunoassays have been reported to have zeptomolar sensitivities. Depending on the specificity of the binding protein, LBAs can be highly specific for the analytes of interest. This is particularly true when the binding protein is an antibody carefully crafted against the analyte of interest, as exemplified by the stereospecificity of some small-molecule immunoassays. In such cases, the selectivity of the assay for the analyte of interest can be defined more clearly, due to extensive, accumulated knowledge of analyte metabolism and clearer knowledge of metabolite structures than is typically the case for macromolecule assays, where specific steps in biotransformation are largely unknown. Thus, in the former case, cross-reactivity and potential interference of available synthetic metabolite standards in the assay can be evaluated directly. Although the general pathways of protein anabolism by successive peptide bond hydrolysis leading, eventually, to amino acids are well known, the identity of the intermediary products (catabolites) generally remains unknown. Therefore, in the case of many macromolecule LBAs, the lack of this detailed knowledge means that caution is warranted in interpretation of generated data, since these data will reflect the interaction of all molecular species with affinity for the binding reagent used in the assay.

1.5 LIGAND-BINDING ASSAY BIOANALYTICAL FOCUS GROUP OF AAPS

In view of the increasing use of LBAs to support drug development programs, the inherent complexities of the technology, and the lack of specific regulatory guidance in this area, a group of interested scientists formed the Ligand-Binding Bioanalytical Focus Group of AAPS in 2000. The primary objectives of this group include addressing technical and regulatory issues related to LBAs, making genuine and concerted efforts to reach consensus on issues of general interest, publishing white papers, and providing continuing education and a platform for continuous exchange of ideas related to ligand-binding assays. It is, therefore, of historical interest to summarize here the sequence of events occurring before 2000 that led to the establishment of the LBABFG.

It is well known that, for years, the proceedings of the 1990 conference on bioanalytical method validation to support bioavailability, bioequivalence, and pharmacokinetic studies served as a *de facto* guidance for bioanalytical method validation in the pharmaceutical industry [23]. Although this report briefly acknowledged the need for some special considerations for nonchromatographic assays, including LBAs and microbiological assays, there was much to be addressed. In 1994, at the Bio-International-2 meeting in Munich, Germany, one of us (J.F.) brought the issues of LBA challenges to the public platform [31]. Around that period, the other of us (M.K.), while establishing an immunoanalytical laboratory at a then emerging contract research organization (CRO) (Phoenix International Life Science (PILS)) in Montreal, had experienced firsthand the difficulties encountered in validating and implementing LBAs in a GLP-compliant environment, and also had the opportunity to address the general deficiencies in approaches to handling and computing LBA-related parameters then practiced across the industry. LBA practitioners in the industry were trying to apply the same acceptance criteria and methods for the computation of validation parameters as were being used for chromatographic assay validation. For instance, computation procedures being used for between-run and within-run variability were particularly inappropriate for application to LBAs.

Typically, within-assay (intra-assay) evaluation was done by analyzing a large number (e.g., 10) of samples at each level of control in a single run. The standard deviation (SD) and percent coefficient of variation (%CV) would be calculated and used as measure of intra-assay (within-run) precision. On the other hand, for between-run variability computation, each control sample in duplicate would be assayed in a minimum of five independent assays and the data would be used to compute the inter-assay precision. However, due to the relatively large imprecision associated with LBAs, one may observe a small intra-assay CV (e.g., 5.2%) one day and a relatively large CV (e.g., 25%) the other day for the same assay, indicating that the estimation of intra-assay precision based on just one run may not depict the true picture. Therefore, it was thought that to obtain better estimates of within-run CV, one could analyze replicate controls (e.g., five aliquots of a control sample in duplicate) in multiple runs (e.g., five runs) preferably on different days. Using the data thus generated, pooled SD and corresponding CV could be calculated. Pooled intra-assay SD is the square root of the pooled intra-assay sample variance, which is just the arithmetic mean of the squared intra-assay standard deviations. Hence, the pooled SD and the corresponding CV should give a more realistic estimate of within-assay precision [32]. In this approach, the same data can also be used for the computation of between-run variability, obviating the need to perform a separate set of experiments. In collaboration with Bob Parks (a statistician colleague at PILS), an Excel worksheet was designed for the computation of pooled statistics for inter- and intra-assay precision and accuracy. This, essentially, marked the beginning of a different and more appropriate computation of the critical validation parameter of assay precision. This Excel worksheet provided a very useful and convenient tool to perform complex statistical calculations even by those lab analysts who were not well versed in statistics. Moreover, this could also be used to harmonize inter-laboratory practices for computation of accuracy and precision parameters for an easy comparison of interlaboratory performances of the method.

At the same time, accessory calibrators, outside the dynamic range of quantification, that were used to optimize the curve fit were being implemented in routine use at PILS. These accessory calibrators were also referred to by Findlay as "anchor points" [31]. Much of the work done with immunoassays till that time had been routinely conducted with data processing algorithms that attempted to linearize the calibration curve response–analyte concentration relationship. However, it is well recognized that LBA calibration curves are inherently nonlinear and best described by four-parameter or five-parameter logistic algorithms. Inclusion of high- and low-concentration anchor points beyond the declared range of the calibration curve often improves the fit of the calibration curve to these models, resulting in overall improved assay performance and data quality [31].

Arising from the uncertainty about optimal approaches to LBA validation, M.K. had in-depth discussions in 1997 with several leading LBA practitioners in the industry, in particular with Ron Bowsher (then at Eli Lilly), the late John Gilbert (then at Merck), and Nancy Hopkins (then at Pharmacia & Upjohn) related to the urgent need for a public platform to discuss and exchange ideas on the challenges faced in the LBA arena. In 1998, the current authors organized a roundtable on the topic of "Challenges of Immunoassay Validation and Implementation for GLP Studies" at the AAPS Annual Meeting in San Francisco. Perhaps, this was the first time LBA-specific challenges were discussed at length on a public platform [25,27,33]. Following the roundtable, in collaboration with the speakers at the event (Fig. 1.1), we published a

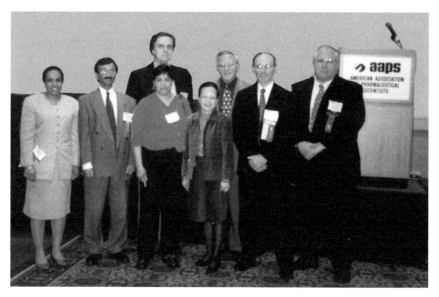

FIGURE 1.1 (From left to right) *First row*: Binodh DeSilva (P&G), Masood Khan (MedImmune), Ira Das (Searle), Jean Lee (MDS), Wendell Smith (Eli Lilly), and Ronald Bowsher (Eli Lilly); *second row*: Gerald Nordblom (Parke-Davis) and John Findlay (Searle).

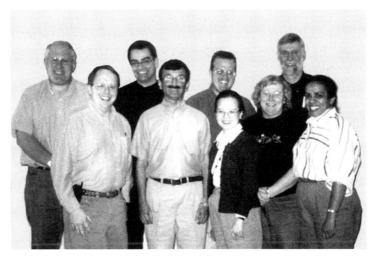

FIGURE 1.2 (From left to right) *First row*: Jeffrey Sailstad (GSK), Masood Khan (MedImmune), Jean Lee (MDS), Marian Kelley (J&J), Binodh DeSilva (P&G); *second row*: Ronald Bowsher (Eli Lilly), John Ferbas (Amgen), Russell Weiner (BMS), and Richard Tacey (PPD).

white paper on the industry perspective on LBA validation in 2000 [27]. This white paper directly influenced the discussions on LBA issues at the AAPS- and FDA-sponsored workshop on Bioanalytical Method Validation for Macromolecules, held in Crystal City, VA, in 2000. Later in 2000, a day before the 2000 AAPS Annual Meeting in Indianapolis, Ron Bowsher and his wife, Penny, graciously hosted a notable gathering of some very enthusiastic and concerned LBA scientists from the industry (Fig. 1.2). At this meeting, we discussed and formulated the basic framework and future directions for the focus group that was to be formally inaugurated at the AAPS Annual Meeting. Later, in a very lively e-mail contest, the name Ligand-Binding Assay Bioanalytical Focus Group was chosen for the newly formed focus group. The primary mandate of this focus group is to provide a forum to address LBA-specific issues and promote education on the bioanalysis of a broad range of analytes using this technology.

The LBABFG is an independent entity operating within the BIOTEC section of AAPS. It has an online newsletter and has also created an online forum for public discussion of LBA-related issues at the AAPS Web site. Over the past 8 years, the focus group has played a key role in organizing short courses, roundtables, symposia, and hot topic discussions and in increasing the LBA-related content in overall programming at the AAPS national meetings and workshops. In 2003, one of us (M.K.) organized the first short course on "GLP-Compliant Validation of Ligand-Binding Assays: A Practical and Rational Approach," at the AAPS Annual Meeting in Salt Lake City, Utah. Faculty members of this short course included Howard Hill, Jean Lee, Jeffrey Sailstad, Tony Mire-Sluis, and Wendell Smith. This short course was audio recorded for the AAPS Continuing Education Series. Three years later, in 2006, Ron Bowsher and colleagues redesigned the course as a 2-day course that has been offered every year since then. Faculty members of this course included Binodh DeSilva, Bonita Rup, Jeffrey Sailstad, Marie Rock, Ronald Bowsher, Viswanath Devanarayan, and Wendell Smith. LBABFG continues to provide training and developmental tools to the practitioners of ligand-binding assay technology.

Since the inception of the focus group, several subcommittees were formed that addressed unique issues related to the application of LBAs in various disciplines. These committees have published white papers related to the validation of LBAs for quantitative drug analysis [28], "fit-for-purpose" method validation of biomarkers [29], antidrug antibody assay method validation [34], and validation of assays for neutralizing antidrug antibodies [35].

1.6 SCOPE OF THE PRESENT VOLUME

Despite the current extensive work on the development of biologic macromolecules as potential therapeutics, there does not appear to be a broad-based text collating experience with LBAs, which are still the bioanalytical methods of choice for supporting the nonclinical and clinical development of these compounds. The editors hope that this book will prove a useful reference text for approaches to the development, validation, implementation, and documentation of LBAs in the context of drug development to personnel from laboratory analysts to managers in the pharmaceutical and biotechnology, contract research, diagnostic and related industries, as well as in academic and hospital laboratories. The scope of the book is broad, and practical situations and examples of challenges likely to be encountered are presented.

In Chapter 2, the authors review the characteristics of ligand-binding assays intended for supporting the pharmacokinetic or toxicokinetic studies of biological macromolecules. These are put in the context of a discussion of the differences in assay methods for small-molecule xenobiotics and macromolecules, as well as the marked differences in the pharmacokinetic disposition of these two general categories of drugs. Pharmacokinetics of low molecular weight xenobiotic drugs is generally more clearly defined than in the case of macromolecules. In the former case, metabolite pathways are relatively easily defined and specificity of LBAs for these compounds is more readily identifiable. Protein macromolecules are catabolized by peptide hydrolytic pathways, with the possibility of unidentified intermediate products that may interfere with the LBA by cross-reactivity with key binding reagents. The role of the Brambell receptor in the clearance of IgG-based antibody drugs is also discussed. This chapter describes the requirements for a successful LBA for supporting pharmacokinetic studies in the context of these complexities. The chapter also addresses critical ligand-binding assay considerations at different stages of the research and development process.

To have an assay to validate, a robust assay must be developed. Chapter 3 discusses, in a systematic and pragmatic way, the approaches to the development of LBAs. This discussion focuses on the practical aspects of LBA development for use in the GLP-compliant environment. A structured strategy for the development of a validatable LBA that would withstand the rigor of prestudy and in-study method validation processes is presented. The application of the analyst's tools and the assay components are reviewed in depth, and the optimization of the assay is also discussed. In the latter section of the chapter, all major steps for successful optimization of the assay are discussed, including evaluation of such characteristics as specificity and selectivity, plate coating for multiwell assays, and evaluation of any prozone effects. LBAs "act up" in practice as often, or even more frequently than, do chromatographic assays. Chapter 3 also provides an in-depth discussion on troubleshooting LBAs.

Validation of bioanalytical assays in general and LBAs in particular has been the subject of intensive debate for the past 18 years or more. Chapter 4 focuses on the key agreements on a phased approach to the validation of LBAs, including evaluation of all critical validation parameters prior to implementation of the method to the analysis of any study samples (prestudy validation) as well as in-study validation to assure high performance of the assay during analysis of actual study samples. Also covered in this chapter are the topics of when and how to conduct full validations, partial validations, and cross-validation.

Chapter 5 discusses in depth the statistical considerations related to LBA development and validation. In addition to the most appropriate algorithms for describing the nonlinear calibration curves typically found in LBAs, the authors also provide further insight into the performance characteristics to be evaluated during assay validation, including the concepts of total error in prestudy validation and the use of the "4-6-X rule." The decision rules at the prestudy validation and routine assay implementation stages are also discussed in some detail in Chapter 5.

Identification of biomarkers for animal models of diseases has become crucial in demonstrating the proposed mechanisms of pharmacological action preclinically, in making decisions on whether to allow the progress of a compound from discovery to development, and in providing mechanistic data in support of the desired beneficial effect of the agent in clinical trials in the disease population. Demonstration of the desired effect on a biomarker of disease in early clinical trials is important to the development of the molecule in clinical testing or to the decision to terminate the development prior to large investments in pivotal trials that may fail to demonstrate the desired efficacy in disease patient populations. Chapter 6 addresses the development and validation of assays for these biomarkers, including the considerations in the development and validation of LBAs for biomarkers. The subcategories of biomarker assays (definitive quantitative, relative quantitative, quasi quantitative, and qualitative) are discussed in terms of the degree to which they may be characterized with calibration standards of defined content and the degree to which they may be validated as quantitative assays. The concept of an LBA being "fit for purpose" is also discussed.

A significant amount of LBA work, particularly in diagnostics and the burgeoning field of biomarker assays, employs LBAs in the form of manufacturer's kits. Chapter 7 focuses on considerations for the correct application of these kit assays, including the proper level of validation needed to support specific applications.

Treatment of animals or humans with macromolecular drug candidates may result in an immune response to the macromolecule, most frequently happening upon repeated dosing. This is most often seen with protein molecules, but experience with other macromolecules, such as oligonucleotides, may not yet be sufficient to be conclusive about the potential immunogenicity of these molecules. It is important to reliably demonstrate the presence or absence of these antidrug antibodies and characterize those detected, because of their potential to antagonize the beneficial therapeutic effects of the macromolecule or, in some cases, to cross-react with endogenous analogues of the new therapeutic. Since the latter situation has been shown to result in serious toxicity in some cases, it is critical to develop assays to reliably detect these antibodies. Chapter 8 deals in detail with the assays for the detection and characterization of antibodies elicited in response to treatment with biological macromolecules as therapeutics or therapeutic candidates. Both LBA and supporting competitive neutralizing and cell-based neutralizing assays are discussed in detail.

Reference standards for macromolecule LBAs are inherently heterogeneous and complex, in contrast to the homogeneity of low molecular weight drugs. This subject is elaborated in Chapter 9, accompanied by a number of illustrative examples. Characterization of USP and non-USP standards is discussed in this chapter in terms of such parameters as purity, potency, and stability. Case studies illustrate the assay effects of variability in reference standard quality.

Outsourcing of bioanalytical work to CROs is widely practiced in the pharmaceutical industry and, indeed, has grown markedly in recent years. The work at the CRO may involve *de novo* assay development, validation, and implementation on behalf of the client company or, more frequently, may involve transfer of an existing assay from a client, followed by its validation and implementation. Transfer of assays between clients and CROs is a challenging process but, because of the current extensive outsourcing of bioanalytical work by pharmaceutical and biotechnology companies, is vital for the continuity of many preclinical and clinical development programs. The challenges involved in the interaction between sponsors and CROs and recommendations for success in this exercise are presented in Chapter 10.

One of the significant advantages of LBAs is their potential for high-throughput sample analysis. To take full advantage of this potential, LBAs may be coupled with automated sample processing and assay systems. Automation of LBAs brings a fresh set of challenges that are discussed in Chapter 11. Logical phased implementation of automation projects is discussed, as are specific automated instrumentation units, including full robotic systems.

In a regulated environment, proper documentation to support both data and reports is of paramount importance; responsibilities for documentation and appropriate documentation practices to support the validation and implementation of LBAs in this regulatory environment are discussed in Chapter 12.

Assay methods, formats, and technologies continue to change, with some newer LBA technologies possessing remarkable sensitivities. Another feature of newer assays is the attempt to miniaturize and automate assays, leading toward the goal of an assay on a chip or compact disk. Chapter 13 discusses some of these newer assay methods (including DELFIA, ELISPOT, immuno-PCR, ECLIA, hybridization-ELISA, SPR, applications of molecularly imprinted polymers, and coupled chromatography–LBA methods). These authors also offer a glimpse of possible future directions for LBA development.

REFERENCES

1. Berson, S.A., and Yalow, R.S. (1959) Quantitative aspects of reaction between insulin and insulin-binding antibody. *Journal of Clinical Investigation*, **38**, 1996–2006.

2. Yalow, R.S., and Berson, S.A. (1960) Immunoassay of endogenous plasma insulin in man. *Journal of Clinical Investigation*, **39**, 1157–1175.

3. Landsteiner, K. (1945) *The Specificity of Serological Reactions*. Harvard University Press, Boston, MA (reprinted by Dover, New York, 1962).

4. Beiser, S.M., Erlanger, B.F., Agate, F.J., and Lieberman, S. (1959) Antigenicity of steroid–protein conjugates. *Science*, **129**, 564–565.

5. Oliver, G.C., Parker, B.M., Brasfield, D.L., and Parker, C.W. (1968) The measurement of digitoxin in human serum by radioimmunoassay. *Journal of Clinical Investigation*, **47**, 1035–1042.

6. Landon, J., and Moffat, A.C. (1976) The radioimmunoassay of drugs: a review. *Analyst*, **101**, 225–243.

7. Butler, V.P. (1978) The immunological assay of drugs. *Pharmacological Reviews*, **29**, 103–184.

8. Findlay, J.W.A. (1987) Applications of immunoassay methods to drug disposition studies. *Drug Metabolism Reviews*, **18**, 83–129.

9. Got, P.A., and Schermann, J.-M. (1997) Stereoselectivity of antibodies for the bioanalysis of chiral drugs. *Pharmaceutical Research*, **14**, 1516–1523.

10. Kaufman, B.M., and Clower, M. (1995) Immunoassay of pesticides: an update. *Journal of AOAC International*, **78**, 1079–1090.

11. Grothaus, G.D., Bandia, M., Currier, T., Giroux, R., Jenkins, G.R., Lipp, M., Shan, G., Stave, J.W., and Pantella, V. (2006) Immunoassay as an analytical tool in agricultural biotechnology. *Journal of AOAC International*, **89**, 913–928.

12. Eskridge, K.D., and Guthrie, S.K. (1997) Clinical issues associated with urine testing of substances of abuse. *Pharmacotherapy*, **17**, 497–510.

13. Wu, A.H.W. (2006) A selected history and future of immunoassay development and applications in clinical chemistry. *Clinica Chimica Acta*, **369**, 119–124.

14. Lepage, R., and Albert, C. (2006) Fifty years of development in the endocrinology laboratory. *Clinical Biochemistry*, **39**, 542–557.

15. Xu, R.N., Fan, L., Reiser, M.J., and El-Shourbagy, T.A. (2007) Recent advances in high-throughput quantitative bioanalysis by LC–MS/MS. *Journal of Pharmaceutical and Biomedical Analysis*, **44**, 342–355.

16. Engvall, E., and Perlmann, P. (1971) Enzyme-linked immunosorbent assay (ELISA). Quantitative assay of immunoglobulin G. *Immunochemistry*, **8**, 871–874.

17. van Weemen, B.K., and Schuurs, A.H.W.M. (1971) Immunoassay using antigen–enzyme conjugates. *FEBS Letters*, **15**, 232–236.

18. Rubinstein, K.E., Schneider, R.S., and Ullman, E.F. (1972) "Homogeneous" enzyme immunoassay. *Biochemical and Biophysical Research Communications*, **47**, 846–851.

19. Dickson, E.F.G., Pollak, A., and Diamandis, E.P. (1995) Time-resolved detection of lanthanide luminescence for ultrasensitive bioanalytical assays. *Journal of Photochemistry and Photobiology B*, **27**, 3–19.

20. Beaver, D.R. (1995) A new non-isotopic detection system for immunoassays. *Nature*, **377**, 758–760.

21. 2008 PhRMA Report, Medicines in Development Biotechnology. Available at http://www.phrma.org/files/Biotech%202008.pdf. Accessed December 24, 2008.

22. Lawrence, S. (2007) Pipelines turn to biotech. *Nature Biotechnology*, **25**, 1342.

23. Shah, V.P., Midha, K.K., Dighe, S., McGilveray, I.J., Skelly, J.P., Yacobi, A., Layloff, T., Viswanathan, C.T., Cook, C.E., McDowall, R.D., Pittman, K.A., and Spector, S. (1992) Conference report—analytical methods validation: bioavailability, bioequivalence and pharmacokinetic studies. *Pharmaceutical Research*, **9**, 588–592.

24. Shah, V.P., Midha, K.K., Findlay, J.W.A., Hill, H.M., Hulse, J.D., McGilveray, I.J., McKay, G., Miller, K.J., Patnaik, R.N., Powell, M.L., Tonnelli, A., Viswanathan, C.T., and Yacobi, A. (2000) Bioanalytical method validation: a revisit with a decade of progress. *Pharmaceutical Research*, **17**, 1551–1557.

25. Miller, K.J., Bowsher, R.R., Celniker, A., Gibbons, J., Gupta, S., Lee, J.W., Swanson, S.J., Smith, W.C., and Weiner, R.S. (2001) Workshop on bioanalytical methods validation for macromolecules: summary report. *Pharmaceutical Research*, **18**, 1373–1383.

26. Lee, J.W., Weiner, R.S., Sailstad, J.M., Bowsher, R.R., Knuth, D.W., O'Brien, P.J., Fourcroy, J.L., Dixit, R., Pandite, L., Pietrusko, R.G., Soares, H.D., Quarmby, V., Vesterqvist, O.L., Potter, D.M., Wiliff, J.L., Ftitche, H.A., O'Leary, T., Perlee, L., Kadam, S., and Wagner, J.A. (2005) Method validation and measurement of biomarkers in nonclinical and clinical samples in drug development: a conference report. *Pharmaceutical Research*, **22**, 499–511.

27. Findlay, J.W.A., Smith, W.C., Lee, J.W., Nordblom, G.D., Das, I., DeSilva, B.S., Khan, M.N., and Bowsher, R.R. (2000) Validation of immunoassays for bioanalysis: a pharmaceutical industry perspective. *Journal of Pharmaceutical and Biomedical Analysis*, **21**, 1249–1273.

28. DeSilva, B., Smith, W., Wiener, R., Kelley, M., Smolec, J., Lee, B., Khan, M., Tacey, R., Hill, H., and Celniker, A. (2003) Recommendations for the bioanalytical method validation of ligand-binding assays to support pharmacokinetic assessments of macromolecules. *Pharmaceutical Research*, **20**, 1885–1900.

29. Lee, J.W., Devanarayan, V., Barrett, Y.C., Weiner, R., Allinson, J., Fountain, S., Keller, S., Weinryb, I., Green, M., Duan, L., Rogers, J.A., Millham, R., O'Brien, P.J., Sailstad, J., Khan, M., Ray, C., and Wagner, J.A. (2006) Fit-for-purpose method development and validation for successful biomarker measurement. *Pharmaceutical Research*, **23**, 312–328.

30. Casdevall, N., Nataf, J., Viron, B., Kolta, A., Kiladjian, J.J., Martin-Dupont, P., Michaud, P., Papo, T., Ugo, V., Teyssandier, I., Varet, B., and Mayeux, P. (2002) Pure red cell aplasia and anti-erythropoietin antibodies against human erythropoietin in patients treated with recombinant erythropoietin. *New England Journal of Medicine*, **346**, 469–475.

31. Findlay, J.W.A. (1995) In: Blume, H.H., and Midha, K.K. (eds), *Bio-International: Bioavailability, Bioequivalence and Pharmacokinetic Studies*, Vol. 2. Medpharm Scientific Publishers, Stuttgart, pp. 361–370.

32. Garrett, P.E., and Krouwer, J.S. (1985) Method evaluation II: precision and sensitivity considerations. *Journal of Clinical Immunoassay*, **8**, 165–168.

33. The AAPS Ligand Binding Assay Bioanalytical Focus Group (2005) *AAPS Newsmagazine*, **8**, 20–25.

34. Shanker, G., Devanarayan, V., Amravadi, L., Barrett, Y.-C., Bowsher, R., Finco-Kent, D., Foscella, M., Gorovits, B., Kirschner, S., Moxness, M., Parish, T., Quarmby, V., Smith, H., Smith, W., Zukerman, L., and Koren, E. (2008) Recommendations for the validation of immunoassays used for detection of host antibodies against biotechnology products. *Journal of Pharmaceutical and Biomedical Analysis*, doi: 10.1016/j.jpba.2008.09.020.

35. Gupta, S., Indelicato, S.R., Jetwa, V., Kawabata, T., Kelley, M., Mire-Sluis, A.R., Richards, S.M., Rup, B., Shores, E., Swanson, S.J., and Wakshull, E. (2007) Recommendations for the design, optimization, and qualification of cell-based assays used for the detection of neutralizing antibody responses elicited to biological therapeutics. *Journal of Immunological Methods*, **321**, 1–18.

CHAPTER 2

Ligand-Binding Assays to Support Disposition Studies of Macromolecular Therapeutics

MARIAN M. KELLEY

MKelley Consulting LLC, West Chester, PA, USA

MARJORIE A. MOHLER

Ciencia Group, Yountville, CA, USA

JOHN W.A. FINDLAY

Gilead Sciences, Inc., Durham, NC, USA

2.1 INTRODUCTION

Ligand-binding assays (LBAs) have been applied in support of pharmacokinetic (PK) studies for both low molecular weight and macromolecular drug candidates [1,2]. However, bioanalytical methods of choice for small molecules are now concentrated on liquid chromatography with mass spectrometric (LC/MS) detection, while LBAs remain the preferred bioanalytical method for macromolecule determination in biological matrices. Current broad interest in the development of macromolecules for treatment of serious diseases across a number of therapeutic areas [3] ensures that LBAs will be widely applied in support of these drug candidates for the foreseeable future. Thus, the focus of this chapter is on those characteristics of LBAs for macromolecules that are critical to enable their application to support disposition studies of these molecules. An understanding of the pharmacology, pharmacokinetics, absorption, distribution, metabolism, and excretion (PD/PK/ADME) and immunogenic potential of large-molecule biologics is needed to interpret any individual set of bioanalytical data for the compound of interest in biological media. Such knowledge will facilitate interpretation of any unexpected and apparently confounding

Ligand-Binding Assays: Development, Validation, and Implementation in the Drug Development Arena. Edited by Masood N. Khan and John W.A. Findlay
Copyright © 2010 John Wiley & Sons, Inc.

bioanalytical or PK data arising from individual studies and clarify the degree of assay validation needed to support measurement of the therapeutic agent at different stages of the discovery and development process.

This chapter will discuss characterization or validation considerations for LBAs applied in support of nonclinical or clinical PK studies of macromolecular biotherapeutic agents. LBAs will be discussed in the context of the assay need; that is, the assay is reliable for its intended purpose [4,5]. This "fit-for-purpose" approach [6,7] proposes that the performance characteristics and the extent of validation of the assay should be sufficient to support the particular application of the assay. It is important that both the assay development scientists and their collaborators, perhaps working in a Drug Metabolism, Pharmacology, Toxicology, or Clinical Department, understand the performance characteristics and limitations of a particular LBA and the data generated by it, so that expectations of all interested parties are met. To promote the most efficient and effective development of truly important new therapeutic agents, scientists in different disciplines within the same organization or working in a team with an outside CRO should collaborate to identify the intended application of an assay and, through regular communication, understand its performance and limitations during ongoing assay development, improvements, and validation. This open communication will facilitate understanding of how best to apply a particular assay and interpret results generated from its use.

2.2   DIFFERENCES BETWEEN LOW MOLECULAR WEIGHT MOLECULES AND MACROMOLECULES

To facilitate the understanding of the specific applications and interpretation of validation parameters for LBAs, it is useful to consider first some important differences between low molecular weight compounds and macromolecules, especially differences in the *in vivo* disposition of these two classes of molecules and between the chromatographic assays and LBAs used for their respective quantitation.

2.2.1   Assay Methods for Low Molecular Weight Compounds and Macromolecules

To date, the majority of new drugs have been low molecular weight compounds, and much of the focus of the pharmaceutical industry has been directed at understanding the chemistry, biology, and bioanalysis of those molecules. Assays for the quantification of small molecules evolved from gas chromatography to basic HPLC to the hyphenated LC technologies, typically based on mass spectrometric detection and quantitation [8]. These new technology platforms permitted a combination of chemical properties and specific mass spectral fragmentation patterns to uniquely and specifically identify and quantify the parent molecule (or metabolite) of interest. Efficient automation technologies have made it possible to support even the largest Phase III trials in a relatively short time frame, without losing the required selectivity and specificity. With the addition of the analyte labeled with a stable isotope (such as deuterium or ^{13}C) as an internal standard, the target molecule can be measured by eliminating potentially interfering matrix elements. In these methods, detector response is directly related to concentration in the sample under analysis. In contrast, biologics must be quantified by indirect methods based on the ability of an antibody, or other binding reagent, to bind to the therapeutic agent of interest and, consequently, these methods do not provide a unique identification of the analyte under evaluation.

2.2.1.1   Calibration Curves   Calibration curves for chromatography-based methods are typically linear, frequently in several orders of magnitude. Antibody-based assays give rise to nonlinear calibration curves (typically sigmoidal in shape). This leads to the need to define the "best fit" experimentally, often a four- or five-parameter logistic algorithm, with or without the need for weighting [1,2,9]. The calibration range for these methods is often defined over only one to two orders of magnitude.

2.2.1.2   Reference Standards and Certificates of Analysis   In any discussion of the differences between technologies for quantification of small and large molecules, it is important to consider reference standards. Low molecular weight reference standards for xenobiotics are typically homogenous in nature and produced in well-defined conditions by organic synthesis. A well-controlled and narrowly defined Certificate of Analysis (COA) is expected to accompany the reference standard used to prepare the calibrations standards that define the standard curve to support sample analysis. Unlike those for small molecules, the standards produced for biologics are heterogeneous by virtue of their preparation methods using living cells. Since the tests used for identifying macromolecule reference standards are themselves variable and include biological potency assays, their COAs are, by necessity, not so narrowly and clearly defined as for low molecular weight compounds. Preparation of these critical reagents demands rigorous and documented control over production. This topic of reference standards is discussed in more depth in Chapter 9.

2.2.1.3   Specificity   LC/MS-based bioanalytical methods for low molecular weight compounds typically include extraction of the analyte of interest from the biological matrix. Specificity can generally be achieved for these assays by a combination of chromatographic separation and selective ion monitoring, which greatly reduce the probability of interference from metabolites or related structures. Following demonstration of specificity, these methods, in general, need only to demonstrate acceptable intra- and interday precision and accuracy of the calibration and quality control or validation standards prior to being applied to study sample analysis. In contrast, the analyte cannot readily be extracted from the matrix prior to sample analysis in macromolecule LBAs and, consequently, there may be interferences by a variety of endogenous or exogenous molecules, resulting in numerous and significant challenges in demonstrating specificity for the analyte of interest. For small-molecule LBAs, this challenge may be alleviated by appropriate comparison of the LBA results with data derived by an LC/MS method [10,11]. In the case of macromolecule LBAs, assay developers frequently rely on diluting the sample to reduce the effects of nonspecific interferences on the assay. Yet this solution impacts the sensitivity of the assay directly, and this strategy is limited, especially in some first-in-human (FIH) trials where initial doses are very low. This approach also does not remove potential interferences in the assay; it merely reduces them to an acceptably low level relative to the signal from the analyte of interest (see discussion of specificity under Section 2.3.2).

2.2.1.4   General Considerations   Because the end point detection methods of LBAs are indirect, it is important to compile as much information as possible to understand how the method is working. Orthogonal methods that help further clarify the interpretation of the data are all too frequently overlooked in the push to initiate sample analysis. Although studies of low molecular weight xenobiotics have historically relied on *in vivo* studies with a radiolabeled molecule to clarify the compound's disposition [12], such studies are applied relatively infrequently to macromolecules. The use of radiolabeled proteins in disposition studies is advisable, in conjunction with LBAs, to avoid drawing unwarranted conclusions from LBA results alone, especially during the research and early drug development stages when the disposition of the macromolecule is poorly understood. While technology allows a much clearer picture of small-molecule xenobiotic metabolism to be developed, important knowledge of macromolecule disposition may be gained from well-designed *in vivo* studies with radiolabeled macromolecules. Such experiments may yield important knowledge about a role for binding proteins, immunogenicity, tissue distribution, and even unexpected metabolism or aggregation [13]. However, it is important to design these studies thoughtfully, acknowledge the limitations of data from such studies, and ensure that erroneous conclusions regarding parent molecule disposition are not drawn from total radioactivity data [14]. Additional understanding of the LBA method may be gained by comparing data from a related bioassay for the drug of interest to a ligand-binding assay [15], to assess whether biological activity and LBA binding activity agree or diverge over time after *in vivo* dosing, lending more or less significance or credence to the LBA data.

Taken together, the similarities and differences between the technologies supporting the quantification of small or large molecules require specific approaches on a case-by-case basis. A "fit-for-purpose" validation implies that continued progress of the drug through development would be supported by increased validation of the method and an increased knowledge about the protein drug itself over time.

2.2.2   Differences in the Disposition of Low Molecular Weight Compounds and Macromolecules

2.2.2.1   Disposition of Low Molecular Weight Compounds   To help understand more fully the different characteristics of assays used to study the disposition of these two classes of molecules, some discussion of the differences in their PK/ADME is warranted. Generally speaking, the disposition of small molecules can be elucidated relatively easily. As discussed above, modern LC/MS methods allow the quantitation of parent molecule and metabolites specifically and sensitively in a broad array of biological fluids and tissues. Studies with molecules radiolabeled at specific sites in the molecule, supported by appropriate chromatographic and spectrometric methods, allow clear statements to be made about the distribution of these compounds in the body, by which routes they are metabolized and eliminated, what the chemical structures of any biotransformation products are, and the enzymes and processes involved in their formation from the parent molecule. *In vitro* studies with tissue preparations (e.g., liver or other tissue homogenates, hepatocytes, etc.) are routinely used to elucidate or predict the likely extent of metabolism and the pathways of metabolism in nonclinical species and humans. Other cell-based systems are used to predict probable extents of absorption and interaction with uptake or efflux transporter molecules. These data are also evaluated to draw preliminary conclusions on the likelihood of the molecule interacting with other drugs being given concomitantly to the intended patient population. Similarly, data on binding of small-molecule compounds to plasma proteins are relatively easy to derive from well-defined *in vitro* experiments. Thus, for the typical low molecular weight xenobiotic molecule, extensive data on disposition can be derived from this range of, now relatively routine, experiments, which typically provide clear-cut information at an early or intermediate stage of development [12].

2.2.2.2 *Disposition of Macromolecules*

Although PK/ADME properties cannot be readily demonstrated with such relative clarity for macromolecules, some consistent parameters of disposition have been reported for these molecules. These properties need to be considered when applying LBAs for quantitation of macromolecules, as many (such as the possibility of protein-bound forms of the macromolecule cross-reacting with the LBA capture reagent or potential differences in relative cross-reactivity of glycosylated and nonglycosylated forms of the molecule) may have impact on LBA performance. The complexities of the pharmacokinetics and pharmacodynamics of biologic macromolecules have been reviewed recently [16–18]. For macromolecules, different clearance mechanisms often come into play than for low molecular weight drugs [19]. Macromolecules, such as proteins and oligonucleotides, suffer from low oral bioavailability [17] and are most frequently given by intravenous, intramuscular, or subcutaneous injection. While absorption directly into the blood stream may occur following intramuscular administration, the lymphatic system appears to play a significant role in the absorption of monoclonal antibodies and oligonucleotides dosed subcutaneously [20,21]. Absorption from subcutaneous or intramuscular sites may be slow, perhaps because of a depot effect at the site of injection or the slow diffusion of these large molecules through capillary pores. Some alternative routes of administration for proteins, such as inhalation [22] and intranasal [23] and transdermal administration [24], have shown some promise. There are continuing efforts to deliver macromolecules by the oral route, including evaluation of absorption, encapsulation in microparticles or nanoparticles, and chemical modification of the macromolecule to improve resistance to enzymatic degradation in the gut [17]. The effects of route of administration of macromolecules on the relative proportions of parent molecule and catabolites/metabolites reaching the systemic circulation have not been reported, although it is likely, for example, that more extensive biodegradation of a macromolecule may occur at the site of subcutaneous injection, prior to absorption than following intramuscular administration into highly perfused tissue or intravenous injection.

In contrast to many small-molecule drugs, the volume of distribution of macromolecular drugs appears to be limited to the extracellular space [25,26] due, in part, to their limited mobility through biomembranes. For some peptides and proteins, such as atrial natriuretic peptide [27], the volume of distribution may be substantially higher, due to active uptake into tissues or binding to intra- or extravascular proteins. Although generally less thoroughly studied than is the case for small-molecule drug candidates, binding of therapeutic macromolecules, particularly recombinant analogues of endogenous molecules, to endogenous transport proteins may also limit their distribution from the central vasculature. Examples include human growth hormone [14], human DNase [28], human insulin-like growth factor [29], and human vascular endothelial growth factor [30]. Binding to these or other types of binding proteins, such as antibodies, may result in either decreased or accelerated clearance of the therapeutic biologic and reduction in efficacy, or a paradoxical enhancement of biological activity through a depot effect in the circulation [31]. Other factors influencing distribution include binding of the biologic to a cell membrane disease target receptor, with subsequent endocytosis and uptake into target tissue (the so-called target-mediated clearance).

Pharmacokinetics of macromolecules that are predominantly cleared by target-mediated clearance at low doses frequently exhibits nonlinearity with increasing dose (i.e., pharmacokinetics is dose dependent). For these molecules, clearance decreases with dose, as binding of the macromolecule to its target or receptor becomes saturated [32]. Elimination half-lives of macromolecular drugs vary widely, from hours to as high as tens of days in the case of a humanized monoclonal antibody directed against respiratory syncytial virus [33]. Proteins and peptides are generally metabolized by the same proteolytic enzymes that catabolize endogenous proteins, with product amino acids being reutilized for *de novo* synthesis of natural proteins. However, the identities (and potential cross-reactivities in LBAs) of intermediary products in this general process are unknown, and this has significant implications for the true specificity of LBAs. Proteolytic enzymes are widely distributed in the body, so that metabolism of biologic molecules may occur in many tissues, including blood. However, the principal sites of metabolism of proteins are the liver, kidney, and gastrointestinal tract. In most cases, renal or biliary excretion of intact proteins is negligible due to their large size.

The particular complexities of antibody pharmacokinetics and their relationship to pharmacodynamics have been thoroughly reviewed by Lobo and coworkers [16]. Many of the characteristics discussed above for macromolecules in general also apply in the case of antibodies. Thus, absorption following subcutaneous or intramuscular administration may be slow, with involvement of lymphatic transport, and attainment of peak blood concentrations may take days. Although absorption of antibodies from the gastrointestinal tract following oral administration to adult humans is very limited, absorption of IgG from the gastrointestinal tract of neonates of several species has been demonstrated [34]. This absorption occurs via interaction with the neonatal receptor for the Fc portion of the immunoglobulin molecule (FcRn) present in the gastrointestinal epithelium, but is generally active only in the first short period of neonatal life (a few weeks only in the case of rodents). This mechanism is responsible for the transmission of protective IgG from mother's milk to the newborn. Other unique influences of the FcRn receptor, also known as the Brambell receptor [34], on antibody pharmacokinetics will be discussed below. Absolute bioavailabilities of antibodies and fusion proteins appear to range generally from about 50% to 100% following subcutaneous or intramuscular administration [35–38], probably being affected by, among other things, variable extent of proteolytic degradation at the site of administration.

As discussed above, the tissue distribution of macromolecules appears to be quite limited. However, it has been pointed out [16] that typical pharmacokinetic calculation methods may underestimate the steady-state volume of distribution (and, hence, tissue distribution and tissue loading) of antibodies, due to some erroneous assumptions. In particular, the common pharmacokinetic assumption that the site of elimination of the molecule is in rapid equilibrium with plasma (i.e., it is in the central compartment) may not apply for antibodies, since catabolism of these molecules can occur in a wide variety of tissues. Thus, in cases of high-capacity, high-affinity binding of antibody to tissue receptors and where the rate of antibody distribution from blood to tissue is considerably slower than the rate of catabolism in that tissue, the steady-state volume of distribution may be erroneously concluded to be as low as the plasma volume. In these cases, direct determination of tissue concentrations of antibodies provides more reliable data for estimation of volume of distribution [16]. Antibodies may enter tissue cells by pinocytosis, mediated through binding to Fcγ receptors or by direct binding to a target molecule on the exterior of the cell membrane. Following endocytosis, IgG molecules may be protected from degradation by binding to the Brambell receptor (see below) and released intact into the interstitial fluid of tissues or back into blood.

The role of the FcRn receptor in protecting IgG from rapid elimination and prolonging its half-life in humans merits some additional discussion. It was known that the elimination half-life of IgG was concentration dependent, decreasing with increasing serum concentration [39]. Brambell and coworkers [40] hypothesized that IgG may be a substrate for a protective transport protein that may become saturated at higher concentrations, resulting in increased elimination rates. This receptor for IgG has been cloned and has been shown to be specific for IgG and to be the receptor responsible for absorption of IgG from the gastrointestinal tract of neonatal mice and rats [41]. Major changes in elimination rates of IgG have been observed in FcRn knockout mice with no change in kinetics of IgA. The FcRn receptor has been shown to be present in a wide variety of tissues in human adults, including endothelial cells of kidney, liver, lung, hepatocyte, intestinal macrophage, peripheral blood monocyte, and dendritic cell [16]. By virtue of its protection of IgG from degradation, this receptor contributes significantly to the disposition of IgG molecules, in particular to their long elimination half-lives. It has also been shown that serum half-lives of IgG molecules are directly related to their binding affinity for the FcRn receptor [42,43]. Following internalization of IgG molecules to cells via pinocytosis as discussed above, the FcRn has low affinity for IgG in the relatively neutral pH environment.

However, as the pH in the endosome decreases, the affinity of binding of IgG to FcRn increases. While unbound IgG is taken up by the lysosome and catabolized, FcRn-bound IgG is returned intact to the central compartment for recirculation. The capacity of the FcRn system is large, as evidenced by the large body load of endogenous IgG, estimated to be 50–100 g by Lobo et al. [16]. Thus, administration of relatively small additional doses of potent antibody therapeutics is unlikely to disturb the pharmacokinetics of endogenous IgG. Attempts have been made to modulate the pharmacokinetics of candidate antibody therapeutics by engineering changes into the Fc region to alter FcRn affinity [44].

The production of endogenous antibodies against an administered biologic (immunogenicity) may also play an important role in its pharmacokinetics. The immunogenic potential of protein drugs appears to depend on a number of factors, including the route and frequency of administration, degree of aggregation of the molecule in the administered formulation, presence of degradation products, and the degree of foreignness of the molecule to the administered host. However, the extent of immune response generated by a biologic in animal species is, generally, a poor predictor for potential immunogenicity in humans [45]. Administration by the subcutaneous route is more often associated with the development of an immune response than intravenous administration [46], and immunogenicity in humans generally decreases with increasing degree of "humanization" of an antibody [47]. Appearance of an immune response to a monoclonal antibody typically appears to develop over approximately 7–10 days and may require repeated administrations. Immunogenicity may affect pharmacokinetics and/or pharmacodynamics of the administered biologic [16]. The magnitude of these effects may depend on whether the antibodies generated against the biologic of interest bind to the biologic without blocking its pharmacologic effects or neutralize its biological activity as a consequence of binding. Considerable efforts have been expended in recent years [48] to develop assays to characterize antibodies elicited by administration of biologic macromolecules to humans. Although the effects of endogenously generated antibodies on the pharmacokinetics and pharmacodynamics of biologics vary from slowing to accelerating their elimination [16], the greater concern is that such antibodies will accelerate elimination of the molecule and reduce its efficacy on repeated administration. The presence of antibodies directed against the administered biologic in matrix samples to be analyzed in pharmacokinetic studies creates special challenges for ligand-binding assays, as discussed below.

The pharmacokinetics of biologics may vary with the degree of glycosylation of the molecule [49]. In addition, molecular modifications to slow elimination of biologic macromolecules have included pegylation [50], reported to prolong the elimination half-life and, possibly, reduce immunogenicity, and covalent coupling of smaller biologics to large, hydrophilic carrier proteins such as albumin that are eliminated more slowly [51]. Such approaches often result in molecules with reduced intrinsic potency, which is compensated for by reduced elimination rates and prolonged higher circulating concentrations. These modifications to the original protein all raise assay challenges for the bioanalyst, particularly around questions of assay specificity for the modified protein relative to the original molecule.

2.3 LBA ASSAY CONSIDERATIONS RELATIVE TO RESEARCH AND DEVELOPMENT STAGE

Considerations of assay performance characteristics, extent of characterization, and thoroughness of validation in the discovery and development environments should be aligned with the "fit-for-purpose" philosophy discussed above. Recommendations consistent with application of this approach at various stages of the research and development continuum are summarized in Table 2.1 and discussed in the sections below.

2.3.1 Research Stage Assay Considerations

At the earliest stages of discovery, the likelihood that the molecule under evaluation will not move forward into development is high. Consequently, investment of extensive time, personnel, and capital resources into development of a highly refined assay cannot be justified. At this stage, rapid turnaround times for data are important, to allow the next set of discovery biology or pharmacology experiments to proceed on an informed basis. Carefully selected key reagents for assay optimization may not be available, and the data to permit rational selection of such reagents may not have been generated. Yet, credible information is needed even in this uncertain environment. Relevant questions to be answered may include the following: (a) Can the molecule be quantified with the required degree of accuracy and precision in the relevant nonclinical pharmacology model? (b) Is there evidence that the activity of the intended target is modulated by the molecule under investigation or of efficacy in the chosen nonclinical model? (c) Is there a correlation of drug concentration with relevant biomarkers or efficacy? Consequently, it is not necessary to have a fully developed and validated quantification method in hand at this stage. Credible data are needed to help support the proposed mechanism of action (pharmacodynamics), define the pharmacokinetics in the *in vivo* animal model(s), and identify which compound to move forward. Once adequate reagents are available, a method can usually be formatted in buffer fairly quickly following some fundamental method development experiments. A basic requirement to produce credible bioanalytical data is some defined level of method characterization that provides the required degree of confidence in the data generated with the LBA. The effect of the matrix on the assay compared to the initial assay set up in buffer should be investigated early in assay development. At least one quality control sample should be prepared in undiluted matrix. While there is no requirement for acceptance criteria at this stage, one should at least understand the accuracy the method provides by performing three assay runs and reviewing the accuracy and precision of the control sample prepared in matrix. If interference in the assay is observed, this will require some thoughtful investigation over time as the drug moves forward. Immediately, however, the method should be characterized in terms of its ability to recover a known amount of drug in matrix.

At the discovery stage, assay performance requirements are less onerous, since nonclinical studies with one or more species may be intended primarily for internal

TABLE 2.1 Validation Recommendations for Different Research and Development Stages

Parameter	Discovery	Preclinical Development	Clinical Development
Reagents and reference materials	• Likely will change but should have some documentation on early characterization • Continue to screen for optimal reagents • Lot no. and history (notebook reference)	• Evaluate different reagents and identify critical reagents • Determine if sufficient quantities are available and their stability for later bioanalytical needs • Include C of A for reference materials in assay validation documents • Keep records of source and lot no.	• Use optimized capture/detection reagents • Use characterized reference standard from final manufacturing process with C of A • Record all lot nos. and sources
QCs	• Use at least one individually prepared QC in matrix	• Prepare batches (three concentrations) in matrix and run in validation runs and in-study runs • Refine acceptance criteria	• Run assay routinely with three QCs across established calibration range • Establish acceptance criteria

TABLE 2.1 *(Continued)*

Parameter	Discovery	Preclinical Development	Clinical Development
Precision and accuracy	• With method established perform three runs	• Perform at least six runs • Apply appropriate statistics • Evaluate reproducibility of incurred samples in each toxicology species	• Clearly defined and acceptable • Evaluate reproducibility of incurred samples in key studies
Stability	• Complete sample analysis ASAP due to lack of stability data	• Determine short and long-term stability for critical reagents and QCs in matrix	• Determine short and long-term stability for critical reagents and QCs in human matrix
Dilutional linearity	• Demonstrate that high-concentration samples can be diluted into range with no hook effect	• Demonstrate low- and high-concentration samples can be diluted into range with acceptable accuracy and precision	• Demonstrate low- and high-concentration samples can be diluted into range with acceptable accuracy and precision
Documentation	• Maintain complete records	• Method is documented in an SOP • Validation documents are GLP compliant • Amend master validation report as needed	• Method is documented in an SOP • Validation documents are GLP compliant • Amend master validation report as needed

decision-making purposes only, for instance, to optimize selection of a drug candidate for entry into the development stage. Such data may never be included in a regulatory submission, since most molecules studied will not progress into development. In that case, understanding assay performance may be all that is required. It is sufficient to demonstrate that the accuracy and precision of an assay are adequate for the intended application (fit for purpose) rather than to meet the exacting validation requirements to support regulated nonclinical and clinical studies later in development. Nevertheless, it is important that the characteristics of the assay are well understood so that misinterpretations of data are avoided. Thus, the biologist needs to appreciate, for example, that assay accuracy of ±30–50% may be adequate to answer some basic pharmacokinetic questions and to realize that use of a nonspecific antibody as capture reagent in an immunoassay limits potential conclusions on the data as representing only the parent molecule. Both of these, somewhat loose, assay performance characteristics may be quite acceptable in the discovery setting, depending on the questions being addressed at that stage. For example, if the discovery program is targeted at an antibody with a potentially decreased elimination rate, derived by point mutation changes in the IgG Fc portion of the molecule [44], the assay employed to determine the resulting PK profiles of the altered molecules should only require sufficient accuracy, precision, and specificity to provide confidence that the desired increase in elimination half-life can be reliably observed. Generic, lower specificity assays may be acceptable for generation of data on a family of molecules in discovery [52], with subsequent refinement of the assay through development of optimized key assay reagents (e.g., binding reagents) for the molecule chosen to enter development. Analysts and colleagues working in discovery should understand, for example, that specific assays are not always required, but if it is imperative that a critical interfering cross-reactivity be avoided, it is important to demonstrate before the critical experiments begin that the assay has that capability. Other areas that should be fully understood, and not assumed, include demonstrating that high-concentration samples can be diluted into the range of the curve with no "hook effect" (i.e., the paradoxical situation in which low and high analyte concentrations give the same signal response in the assay). Since little, if any, stability data are normally available at this stage, it is recommended that sample analysis be conducted soon after sample collection to reduce any effects of storage conditions on analyte stability and recovery. Finally, while full validation reports are not typically written at this stage, some clear and inclusive record keeping is important. Determining and following these purpose-driven recommendations for method characterization will ensure that credible data are provided to support the goals of the discovery work.

2.3.2 Preclinical Development Stage Assay Considerations

When a macromolecule moves into development, early toxicokinetic (TK) protocols (e.g., dose range finding) and ADME studies will require bioanalytical assay support. At this time, better characterized reference standard should be available, along with more mature critical reagents. The assay developer continues to gain knowledge of the assay performance by continuing characterization studies and initiating validation experiments. Based on information gleaned from assay performance in discovery, appropriate quality control samples spiked with the macromolecule at three concentrations can be incorporated routinely into assays conducted for sample analysis. Since the earliest toxicology range-finding studies may not be required to be conducted under GLP regulations, there is still some leniency in method performance characteristics compared to those defined for full validation to support the pivotal GLP studies [53,54].

Quality control samples used during the conduct of the validation are, in reality, surrogates prepared by adding known amounts of the therapeutic into the matrix of interest. As such, they can only help define the validity of a method to a limited extent. The assay developer must look to additional investigations to understand the impact of possible catabolites/metabolites, patient sera components, concomitant medications, and so on. Therefore, to ensure that the assay method is fit to quantify the therapeutic drug in the presence of possible interferences, key validation parameters must be more thoroughly investigated, including specificity and selectivity; both of these, in turn, affect the sensitivity of the method for intact parent macromolecule. While it is feasible to design some exploratory experiments to characterize these parameters, technology today generally does not allow a fully rigorous, or absolute, definition of specificity for the parent molecule alone. Assay developers have been content until now to assume that protein macromolecules, for example, are biotransformed by successive proteolytic degradation to amino acids that may then be reutilized in endogenous pathways of synthesis to new protein molecules. Hence, to address specificity, the assay developer investigates the impact of unrelated antibodies, concomitant medications, or other exogenous compounds on the accuracy of the LBA for measuring the parent macromolecule [55]. However, to truly test the specificity and selectivity of the method, the assay developer should understand the metabolism of the therapeutic agent and the actual specificity of the reagents used to detect the analyte [56]. That is to say, the analyst should determine whether the capture reagent (e.g., an antibody) solely binds to the intact molecule, or whether possible intermediary catabolites/metabolites could cross-react with the capture reagent used in the assay, resulting in an impact on the reported assay results. One possible approach to elucidating some of these unknowns, albeit labor intensive, would be to apply orthogonal assays such as bioassays or *in vivo* studies with the radiolabeled macromolecule to help more fully characterize the ligand-binding assay of interest.

As discussed in Section 2.2, for low molecular weight drugs, some factors affecting pharmacokinetics such as rates of absorption, rates and routes of metabolism, routes and extent of excretion, extent of tissue distribution, and plasma protein binding may be well established. For the majority of macromolecular biologics, few of these parameters have been clearly defined for a given molecule, even by the time that the molecule is at an advanced stage of development or, indeed, is marketed. Such data for macromolecules are generally much more difficult to determine than for small-molecule drugs, in large part due to the lack of suitable routine technologies.

An additional bioanalytical parameter of great current interest [54] is reproducibility of analysis of samples from dosed subjects (the so-called incurred samples). Whether such analyses are to be conducted in all species or most appropriately in relevant human matrices (from normal, healthy subjects, disease populations, etc.) is a cause of much debate and must be defined on a case-by-case basis. To design such studies, one must decide *a priori* the number and selection of samples and the acceptable accuracy based on the method's intrinsic variability. Since the entire study may be called into question if the reanalysis fails, one should plan an immediate event investigation if repeat analysis criteria are not achieved.

From the point of view of method performance, the transition from discovery to preclinical to clinical development support should be viewed as a continuum of meeting increasingly rigorous assay validation criteria. This continuous improvement of the assay should reflect application of all of the information gleaned along the way concerning TK/ADME and pharmacology of the compound in the species under study, with resulting key reagent selection, based on observations of assay specificity changes with changes in key reagents (e.g., capture and detection antibodies).

As the chosen molecule moves further into development, the performance characteristics required of the assay may change. In early drug development, nonclinical safety studies provide an understanding of toxicokinetics that relates systemic exposure of the new drug candidate to the observed safety of the molecule prior to its first dose to humans. Increasingly higher doses and systemic exposures are evaluated in animals to define the safety margin for the FIH trial. IND-enabling and subsequent toxicity studies are typically conducted under GLP regulations and employ fully validated assays to support these studies, as required by regulatory agencies [53]. Thus, assay parameters such as accuracy and precision need to be defined and meet standard criteria. The specificity of the method, including matrix interference effects, should be defined to the extent possible with the available technology (see discussion above); there should certainly be a demonstration that the known matrix interferences are surmountable or minimized. Toxicology evaluations begin with single-dose (dose range finding) studies in one or more species (rodent and/or nonrodent) and, given a demonstrated level of safety, progress through chronic studies in one or both species. The choice of species in some cases is driven by the extent of their pharmacological responsiveness to the biologic compared to that expected for humans. Thus, for many biologics, toxicologic evaluation is conducted only in monkeys, since the pharmacological target either does not exist in rodents or is poorly cross-reactive, while in monkeys, there is often cross-reactivity with the human target molecule or receptor. Potential approaches to toxicological assessment of such biologics in both rodent and nonrodent species include development of a transgenic rodent model bearing the human target [57] or evaluation of the toxicology of a macromolecule directed against the equivalent rodent target [57]. Neither of these solutions is perfect, while both have the limitations of being time consuming and expensive and, in the latter case, involve evaluation of a different molecule than the proposed therapeutic. Such approaches have obvious implications for bioanalytical support and performance characteristics of assays to support them; in the latter case, a new assay for the rodent-specific macromolecule will need to be developed and validated. The primary intent of bioanalytical support of these studies is to demonstrate exposure of the animals to the macromolecule of interest through the duration of the study. Given the typically high doses administered to animals in these studies (designed to determine clinical and target organ toxicities), high assay sensitivity is not typically required, except in cases of very high potency macromolecules administered at low doses in toxicology studies. In addition, high assay specificity should not be critical as long as there is reasonable confidence that ligand-binding assay data and biological data are not diverging too dramatically over time after dosing. For example, if there is suspicion that the molecule is rapidly and extensively breaking down *in vivo* to immunoreactive, but biologically inactive products, efforts should be made to develop a capture antibody with better specificity for the parent macromolecule and lower cross-reactivity with biologically inactive breakdown products.

Repeated-dose toxicology studies provide an opportunity to establish whether treatment of the particular species evokes an immune response to the macromolecule. This may be manifested in the bioanalytical data as a decline (sometimes precipitous) in apparent plasma concentrations of the macromolecule [58,59]; however, in some cases, there appears to be prolongation of apparent plasma concentrations through a depot-like effect of binding of macromolecule to the evoked antibody and subsequent release [60]. Pharmacokinetic data from these studies must be considered estimates only, since assay formats frequently employed are subject to interference from competition for binding of the macromolecule between the capture antibody (or antigen) employed in the assay and the antimacromolecule antibody present in the sample. To properly evaluate this potential interference with the PK data, the presence of an anti-drug antibody should be demonstrated definitively in blood samples collected at times sufficiently late after drug administration to ensure that the administered macromolecule has been eliminated from the circulation, thus avoiding the assay ambiguity discussed above. These challenges are discussed in more detail in Chapter 8, which describes assays for detection and characterization of antidrug antibodies. The point is that detection of any immune response should be noted, as well as concomitant effects on the LBA used to measure the macromolecule and on the pharmacokinetic parameters of the administered macromolecule determined by use of the LBA.

2.3.3 Clinical Development Stage Assay Considerations

As the macromolecule moves forward into human evaluation, the assay performance characteristics become more stringent and knowledge of the assay's limitations should be well understood. During the FIH trial, low doses are initially given to humans, dose and systemic exposure thereafter being slowly and judiciously increased as safety is monitored. Later in the development process, dose–response and other clinical trials define the therapeutic dose and route of administration and determine the dosage strength and composition of the final marketed drug formulation(s). Concomitant with each phase of the drug discovery and development process, some assay requirements will differ. Nonetheless, since methods that support pharmacokinetic studies are quantitative, and the one consistent purpose from early development to submission for approval to market the drug is safety, a high standard of validation and documentation of the assay supporting these clinical studies is expected, to assure the quality of the data through this stage of development. As the clinical trials continue, it is important to constantly monitor the bioanalytical method for reproducibility. To that point, the sponsors of the Crystal City III workshop [54], including representatives from the FDA, have added a new facet to assay validation. They have recommended that some standard procedures be adopted to employ incurred sample reanalysis in an attempt to assure assay reproducibility[61]. Other authors have also recently expressed opinions on approaches to incurred sample reanalysis [62–64]. Thus, validation parameters are continually being reevaluated and it is important for assay developers to stay abreast of the latest thought to ensure the credibility and reliability of their data throughout the drug development process.

2.4 CRITICAL FUTURE CHALLENGES FOR LIGAND-BINDING ASSAYS

Given the foregoing discussion of some of the unique characteristics of macromolecules that lead to clear differences in their pharmacokinetics compared to those typical of small-molecule drugs, there is a subset of the entire group of bioanalytical assay validation parameters that are of key importance in support of pharmacokinetics of candidate macromolecular therapeutics. Assuming demonstration of accuracy and precision of sufficient quality for the intended application of the assay (e.g., non-GLP discovery support or GLP toxicokinetic support, as discussed above), the most important characteristics of a given assay in support of pharmacokinetic studies are likely to be selectivity, specificity, and reproducibility for analysis of incurred samples. These are all related to the ability of the LBA to detect and quantitate solely, or as closely as possible to solely, the analyte of interest.

Evaluation of these parameters is less challenging for LBAs for small-molecule xenobiotics than for assays for protein-based or other macromolecules, since specificity and selectivity for a small-molecule LBA can be more readily evaluated. For example, at progressive stages of discovery and development, data will probably be developed on the structural identity of metabolites of the small molecule. These compounds can be synthesized and evaluated, along with any relevant, concomitantly administered medications, for interference (cross-reactivity) in the LBA for the parent molecule. For small molecules, there is also a reasonable probability that a validated chromatographic assay, such as an LC/MS method, may be available to cross-validate the LBA by an agreed protocol [10,11]. However, for macromolecules, although catabolism is known to occur by repeated peptide bond hydrolysis by proteases ultimately to yield amino acids, knowledge of intermediate anabolic or metabolic products is generally much less clearly defined, and the cross-reactivities of these compounds in LBAs for the parent molecule cannot, generally, be readily determined. The potential for assay interference from concomitant, macromolecular medications has also been discussed and illustrated recently by Lee and Ma [65]. Generally, protein molecules are degraded by typical proteolytic processes, while monoclonal antibodies are cleared by recycling via the neonatal Fc receptor [34,40] and, in some cases, by specific target-mediated mechanisms [32]. Oligonucleotide biologics are typically metabolized from the $3'$- and/or $5'$-ends by single-nucleotide cleavages by exonucleases [66]. In many cases, particularly in the case of therapeutic proteins, the identity of these catabolic or metabolic products of biologics is unknown, and reference standards are not readily available for evaluation of cross-reactivity in LBAs for the parent molecules. There are some exceptions in which limited information is available on the structures of precursor proteins, anabolites, or oligonucleotide metabolites. Generally, for macromolecules, the results from LBAs reflect an aggregate interaction of those molecules with sufficient intact epitope or other molecular structures to allow recognition by the binding site on the key capture reagent. Theoretically, this could include multiple biochemical degradation products of administered parent macromolecule, some of which may retain the desired biological activity and some of which may not, as long as sufficient molecular structure to interact with the capture reagent is retained. In the worst-case scenario, an LBA for a biologic may provide highly misleading pharmacokinetic data, reporting apparent concentrations of the molecule of interest, while truly only representing those molecules capable of binding to the binding reagent used in the assay, which may have little relationship with biological activity or with circulating concentrations of the intact parent molecule of interest [67]. Until technology and scientific knowledge advance to the point of designing truly specific LBAs for macromolecules, results from these assays should, therefore, be viewed with caution and considered to be "immunoequivalent" concentrations or "binding equivalent" concentrations rather than concentrations of only the molecule of interest.

The field of oligonucleotide research provides some relevant examples of the potential interference of metabolite or degradation products in ligand-binding assays. Assays for these molecules typically depend on capture of the oligonucleotide of interest by a complementary oligonucleotide probe immobilized on the surface of a multiwell plate, followed by an ELISA-like step to provide the final readout (the so-called hybridization-ELISA assay). These molecules are generally metabolized by nucleases by base deletions from either, or both, of the $3'$- or $5'$-ends of the molecule. Therefore, the extent of cross-reactivity of these metabolites in the LBA will directly affect the specificity of the assay for the parent molecule. For a scintillation proximity competitive hybridization assay for a 15-base antisense oligonucleotide, de Serres and coworkers [68] showed that loss of three bases from either end of the molecules resulted in greatly reduced cross-reactivity in the assay, while loss of four bases from either end resulted in negligible interference. Since loss of one or two bases resulted in appreciable cross-reactivity, the application of this assay in support of a nonclinical toxicology study probably produced approximate toxicokinetic data, as the metabolic profile of the parent molecule in the monkey was not yet defined and circulating concentrations of these potential metabolites were unknown. In the case of another antisense oligonucleotide [69], a competitive hybridization ELISA was shown to suffer no more than 1% cross-reactivity from potential metabolites. This assay was applied to determination of pharmacokinetics of the parent molecule in a Phase I trial.

The true specificity of LBAs for macromolecules is rarely addressed in depth, primarily for the reason that breakdown products of the macromolecule (metabolites and catabolites) are rarely available as reference standards for inclusion in cross-reactivity studies. Where possible, attempts are made to derive some data to support specificity, although this may not provide any information on the relative "trueness" of the pharmacokinetic data reported for the parent molecule. For example, Weiner et al. [55] reported the lack of cross-reactivity of murine CTLA4Ig in an EIA for human CTLA4Ig in support of a pharmacokinetic study of human CTLA4Ig in the mouse. While demonstrating the specificity of the assay for the human version of this fusion protein over the mouse analogue, these data provided no information on the accuracy of the pharmacokinetic data for unchanged human CTLA4Ig relative to potentially cross-reacting metabolites *in vivo*.

2.5 CONCLUSIONS

It is clear that assays to support both GLP studies and pivotal clinical studies, such as bioequivalence studies, are expected to be conducted using rigorously validated assays. However, the degree of characterization of assays needed to support earlier studies is not as clearly defined. "Fit for purpose" is a prudent approach to help define the necessary characterization of those assays. Thus, the stage of development and the final use of the data should determine the extent of validation needed. This chapter has also presented some of the differences between small and large molecules from the perspective of their pharmacokinetics and the assay methods developed to support disposition studies of each of these categories. Unique aspects of the disposition of macromolecules have important implications for assays developed to measure them in biological matrices. The sigmoidal LBA calibration curve, effects of matrix, dependence of reported concentrations on an indirect signal, and lack of internal standard, for instance, are challenges that the macromolecule LBA analyst must take into consideration when setting up and validating these methods. The potential impact of these factors on the correct interpretation of data generated by the LBA should not be ignored. The complex and ill-defined metabolism of proteins and other macro-molecules, as compared to small molecules, taken together with the above-noted challenges associated with the LBA format, may lead to potential inaccuracies in the study data reported. Since it is very difficult to fully define the true specificity and selectivity of the critical LBA binding reagent(s), supportive experiments (e.g., radiolabeled studies) may be beneficially employed to further understand the performance and capabilities of the method.

REFERENCES

1. Findlay, J.W.A., Smith, W.C., Lee, J.W., Nordblom, G.D., Das, I., DeSilva, B.S., Khan, M.N., and Bowsher, R.R. (2000) Validation of immunoassays for bioanalysis: a pharmaceutical industry perspective. *Journal of Pharmaceutical and Biomedical Analysis*, **21**, 1249–1273.
2. DeSilva, B., Smith, W., Wiener, R., Kelley, M., Smolec, J., Lee, B., Khan, M., Tacey, R., Hill, H., and Celniker, A. (2003) Recommendations for the bioanalytical method validation of ligand-binding assays to support pharmacokinetic assessments of macromolecules. *Pharmaceutical Research*, **20**, 1885–1900.

3. 2008 PhRMA Report, Medicines in Development Biotechnology. Available at http://www. phrma.org/files/Biotech%202008.pdf. Accessed December 24, 2008.

4. Shah, V.P., Midha, K.K., Dighe, S., McGilveray, I.J., Skelly, J.P., Yacobi, A., Layloff, T., Viswanathan, CT., Cook, C.E., McDowall, R.D., Pittman, K.A., and Spector, S. (1992) Analytical methods validation: bioavailability, bioequivalence and pharmacokinetic studies. *Pharmaceutical Research*, **9**, 588–592.

5. Shah, V.P., Midha, K.K., Findlay, J.W.A., Hill, H.M., Hulse, J.D., McGilveray, I.J., McKay, G., Miller, K.J., Patnaik, R.N., Powell, M.L., Tonnelli, A., Viswanathan, CT., and Yacobi, A. (2000) Bioanalytical method validation: a revisit with a decade of progress. *Pharmaceutical Research*, **17**, 1551–1557.

6. Lee, J.W., Devanarayan, V., Barrett, Y.C., Weiner, R., Allinson, J., Fountain, S., Keller, S., Weinryb, I., Green, M., Duan, L., Rogers, J.A., Millham, R., O'Brien, P.J., Sailstad, J., Khan, M., Ray, C., and Wagner, J.A. (2006) Fit-for-purpose method development and validation for successful biomarker measurement. *Pharmaceutical Research*, **23**, 312–328.

7. Lee, J.W., Weiner, R.S., Sailstad, J.M., Bowsher, R.R., Knuth, D.W., O'Brien, P.J., Fourcroy, J.L., Dixit, R., Pandite, L., Pietrusko, R.G., Soares, H.D., Quarmby, V., Vesterqvist, O.L., Potter, D.M., Witliff, J.L., Fritche, H.A., O'Leary, T., Perlee, L., Kadam, S., and Wagner, J.A. (2005) Method validation and measurement of biomarkers in nonclinical and clinical samples in drug development: a conference report. *Pharmaceutical Research*, **22**, 499–511.

8. Xu, R.N., Fan, L., Rieser, M.J., and El-Shourbagy, T.A. (2007) Recent advances in high-throughput quantitative bioanalysis by LC–MS/MS. *Journal of Pharmaceutical and Biomedical Analysis*, **44**, 342–355.

9. Findlay, J.W.A., and Dillard, R.F. (2007) Appropriate calibration curve fitting in ligand binding assays. *The AAPS Journal*, **9**, E260–E267.

10. Ellis, J.D., Hand, E.L., and Gilbert, J.D. (1997) Use of LC–MS/MS to cross-validate a radioimmunoassay for the fibrinogen receptor antagonist, Aggrastat (tirofiban hydrochloride) in human plasma. *Journal of Pharmaceutical and Biomedical Analysis*, **15**, 561–569.

11. Gilbert, J.D., Greber, T.F., Ellis, J.D., Barrish, A., Olah, T.V., Fernandez-Metzler, C., Yuan, A.S., and Burke, C.J. (1995) The development and cross-validation of methods based on radioimmunoassay and LC/MS–MS for the quantification of the Class III antiarrythmic agent, MK-0499, in human plasma and urine. *Journal of Pharmaceutical and Biomedical Analysis*, **13**, 937–950.

12. Borchardt, R.T., Smith, P.L., and Wilson, G. (eds) (1996) *Models for Assessing Drug Absorption and Metabolism*, 1st edition. Springer, New York.

13. Ferraiolo, B.L., and Mohler, M.A. (1992) Goals and analytical methodologies for protein disposition studies. In: Ferraiolo, B.L., Mohler, M.A., and Gloff, C.A. (eds), *Protein Pharmacokinetics and Metabolism*. Plenum Press, New York, pp. 1–21.

14. Toon, S. (1996) The relevance of pharmacokinetics in the development of biotechnology products. *European Journal of Drug Metabolism and Pharmacokinetics*, **21**, 93–103.

15. Wills, R.J., and Ferraiolo, B.L. (1992) The role of pharmacokinetics in the development of biotechnologically derived agents. *Clinical Pharmacokinetics*, **23**, 406–414.

16. Lobo, E.D., Hansen, R.J., and Balthasar, J.P. (2004) Antibody pharmacokinetics and pharmacodynamics. *Journal of Pharmaceutical Sciences*, **93**, 2645–2668.

17. Tang, L., Persky, A.M., Hochhaus, G., and Meibohm B. (2004) Pharmacokinetic aspects of biotechnology products. *Journal of Pharmaceutical Sciences*, **93**, 2184–2204.

18. Mahmood, I., and Green, M.D. (2005) Pharmacokinetic and pharmacodynamic considerations in the development of therapeutic proteins. *Clinical Pharmacokinetics*, **44**, 331–347.

19. Baumann, G., Shaw, M.A., and Buchanan, T.A. (1988) *In vivo* kinetics of a covalent growth hormone-binding protein complex. *Metabolism*, **38**, 330–333.

20. Porter, C.J., and Charman, S.A. (2000) Lymphatic transport of proteins after subcutaneous administration. *Journal of Pharmaceutical Sciences*, **89**, 297–310.

21. Supersaxo, A., Hein, W., Gallati, H., and Steffen, H. (1988) Recombinant human interferon alpha-2a: delivery to lymphoid tissue by selected modes of application. *Pharmaceutical Research*, **5**, 472–476.

22. Adjei, A.L., and Gupta, P.K. (eds) (1997) *Inhalation Delivery of Therapeutic Peptides and Proteins*, 1st edition. Informa Healthcare, New York.

23. Kydronieus, A.F. (ed.) (1992) *Treatise on Controlled Drug Delivery*, 1st edition. Informa Healthcare, New York.

24. Amsden, B.G., and Goosen, M.F.A. (1995) Transdermal delivery of peptide and protein drugs: an overview. *American Institute for Chemical Engineers Journal*, **41**, 1972–1997.

25. Reilly, R.M., Sandhu, J., Alvarez-Diez, T.M., Gallinger, S., Kirsh, J., and Stern, H. (1995) Problems of delivery of monoclonal antibodies: pharmaceutical and pharmacokinetic solutions. *Clinical Pharmacokinetics*, **28**, 126–142.

26. Zito, S.W. (1997) *Pharmaceutical Biotechnology: A Programmed Text*. Technomic Publishing Company, Lancaster, PA.

27. Tan, A.C.I.T.L., Russel, F.G.M., Thien, T., and Benraad, T.J. (1993) Atrial natriuretic peptide: an overview of clinical pharmacology and pharmacokinetics. *Clinical Pharmacokinetics*, **24**, 28–45.

28. Mohler, M., Cook, J., Lewis, D., Moore, J., Sinicropi, D., Championsmith, A., Ferraiolo, B., and Mordenti, J. (1993) Altered pharmacokinetics of recombinant human deoxyribonuclease in rats due to the presence of a binding protein. *Drug Metabolism and Disposition*, **21**, 71–75.

29. Baxter, R.C. (2000) Insulin-like growth factor (IGF)-binding proteins: interactions with IGFs and intrinsic bioactivities. *American Journal of Physiology, Endocrinology and Metabolism*, **278**, E967–E976.

30. Eppler, S.M., Combs, D.L., Henry, T.D., Lopez, J.J., Ellis, S.G., Yi, J.-H., Annex, B.H., McCluskey, E.R., and Zioncheck, T.F. (2002) A target-mediated model to describe the pharmacokinetics and hemodynamic effects of recombinant human vascular endothelial growth factor in humans. *Clinical Pharmacology and Therapeutics*, **72**, 20–32.

31. Piscitelli, S.C., Reiss, W.G., Figg, W.D., and Petros, W.P. (1997) Pharmacokinetic studies with recombinant cytokines: scientific issues and practical considerations. *Clinical Pharmacokinetics*, **32**, 368–381.

32. Mager, D.E., and Jusko, W.J. (2001) General pharmacokinetic model for drugs exhibiting target-mediated drug disposition. *Journal of Pharmacokinetics and Pharmacodynamics*, **28**, 507–532.

33. Meissner, H.C., Groothuis, J.R., Rodriguez, W.J., Welliver, R.C., Hogg, G., Gray, P.H., Loh, R., Simoes, F.A.F., Sly, P., Miller, A.K., Nichols, A.I., Jorkasky, D.K., Everitt, D.E., and Thompson, K.A. (1999) Safety and pharmacokinetics of an intramuscular monoclonal antibody (SB209763) against respiratory syncytial virus (RSV) in infants and young children at risk for severe RSV disease. *Antimicrobial Agents and Chemotherapy*, **43**, 1183–1188.

34. Junghans, R.P. (1997) Finally! The Brambell receptor (FcRB). Mediator of transmission of immunity and protection from catabolism for IgG. *Immunological Research*, **16**, 29–57.

35. Lin, Y.S., Nguyen, C., Mendoza, J.-L., Escandon, E., Fei, D., Meng, Y.G., and Modi, N.B. (1999) Preclinical pharmacokinetics, interspecies scaling, and tissue distribution of a humanized monoclonal antibody against vascular endothelial growth factor. *Journal of Pharmacology and Experimental Therapeutics*, **288**, 371–378.

36. Pepin, S., Lutsch, C., Grandgeorge, M., and Scherrmann, J.M. (1997) Snake F(ab′)2 antivenom from hyperimmunized horse: pharmacokinetics following intravenous and intramuscular administration in rabbits. *Pharmaceutical Research*, **12**, 1470–1473.

37. Lebsack, M.E., Hanna, R.K., Lange, M.A., Newman, A., Ji, W., and Korth-Bradley, J.M. (1997) Absolute bioavailability of TNF receptor fusion protein following subcutaneous injection in healthy volunteers. *Pharmacotherapy*, **17**, 1118–1119.

38. Vaishnaw, A.K., and TenHoor, C.N. (2002) Pharmacokinetics, biologic activity, and tolerability of alefacept by intravenous and intramuscular administration. *Journal of Pharmacokinetics and Pharmacodynamics*, **29**, 415–426.

39. Waldmann, T.A., and Strober, W. (1969) Metabolism of immunoglobulins. *Progress in Allergy*, **13**, 1–110.

40. Brambell, F.W.R., Hemmings, A., and Morris, I.G. (1964) A theoretical model of gamma-globulin catabolism. *Nature*, **203**, 1352–1355.

41. Junghans, R.P., and Anderson, C.L. (1996) The protection receptor for IgG catabolism is the beta2-microgolulin-containing neonatal intestinal transport receptor. *Proceedings of the National Academy of Sciences of the United States of America*, **55**, 5512–5516.

42. Ghetie, V., Popov, S., Borvak, J., Radu, C., Matesoi, D., Mendesan, C., Ober, R.J., and Ward, E.S. (1997) Increasing the serum persistence of an IgG fragment by random mutagenesis. *Nature Biotechnology*, **15**, 637–640.

43. Dell'Acqua, W.F., Woods, R.M., Ward, E.S., Palaszynski, S.R., Patel, N.K., Brewah, Y.A., Wu, H., Kiener, P.A., and Langermann, S. (2002) Increasing the affinity of a human IgG1 for the neonatal Fc receptor: biological consequences. *Journal of Immunology*, **169**, 5171–5180.

44. Hinton, P.R., Johlfs, M.G., Xiong, J.M., Hanestad, K., Ong, K.C., Bullock, C., Keller, S., Tang, M.T., Tso, J.Y., Vasquez, M., and Tsurushita, N. (2004) Engineered human IgG antibodies with longer serum half-lives in primates. *Journal of Biological Chemistry*, **279**, 6213–6216.

45. Bugelski, P.J., and Treacy, G. (2004) Predictive power of preclinical studies in animals for the immunogenicity of recombinant therapeutic proteins in humans. *Current Opinion in Molecular Therapeutics*, **6**, 10–16.

46. Schellekens, H. (2002) Immunogenicity of therapeutic proteins: clinical implications and future prospects. *Clinical Therapeutics*, **24**, 1720–1740.

47. Rebello, P.R.U.B., Hale, G., Friend, P.J., Cobbold, S.P., and Waldmann, H. (1999) Anti-globulin responses to rat and humanized CAMPATH-1 monoclonal antibody used to treat transplant rejection. *Transplantation*, **68**, 1417–1419.

48. Mire-Sluis, A.R., Barrett, Y.C., Devanarayan, V., Koren, E., Liu, H., Maia, M., Parish, T., Scott, G., Shankar, G., Shores, E., Swanson, S.J., Taniguchi, G., Wierda, D., and Zuckerman, L.A. (2004) Recommendations for the design and optimization of immunoassays used in the detection of host antibodies against biotechnology products. *Journal of Immunological Methods*, **289**, 1–16.

49. Drickamer, K., and Taylor, M.E. (1998) Evolving views of protein glycosylation. *Trends in Biochemical Sciences*, **23**, 321–324.

50. Koslowski, A., Charles, S.A., and Harris, J.M. (2001) Development of pegylated interferons for the treatment of chronic hepatitis C. *Biodrugs*, **15**, 419–429.

51. Osborn, B.L., Sekut, L., Corcoran, M., Poortman, C., Sturm, B., Chen, G., Mather, D., Lin, H.L., and Parry, T.J. (2002) Albutropin: a growth hormone–albumin fusion with improved pharmacokinetics and pharmacodynamics in rats and monkeys. *European Journal of Pharmacology*, **456**, 149–158.

52. Kanarek, A.D. (ed.) (2004) *A Guide to Good Laboratory Practice for Start-up and Growing Laboratories in Industry and Academia*, 1st edition. International Business Communications Inc., New York.

53. Food and Drug Administration (2001) *Guidance for Industry: Bioanalytical Method Validation*. U.S. Department of Health and Human Services, Food and Drug Administration, Center for Drug Evaluation and Research, Rockville, MD.

54. Viswanathan, C.T., Bansal, S., Booth, B., DeStefano, A.J., Rose, M.J., Sailstad, J., Shah, V.P., Skelly, J.P., Swann, P.G., and Weiner, R. (2007) Workshop/conference report—quantitative bioanalytical methods validation and implementation: best practices for chromatographic and ligand binding assays. *The AAPS Journal*, **9**, E30–E42.

55. Weiner, R.S., Srinivas, N.R., Calore, J.D., Fadrowski, C.G., Shyu, W.C., and Tay, L.K. (1997) A sensitive enzyme immunoassay for the quantitation of human CTLA4Ig fusion protein in mouse serum: pharmacokinetic application to optimizing cell line selection. *Journal of Pharmaceutical and Biomedical Analysis*, **15**, 571–579.

56. Blasco, H., Lalmanach, G., Godat, E., Maurel, M.C., Canepa, S., Belghazi, M., Paintaud, G., Degenne, D., Chatelut, E., Cartron, G., and Guellec, C.L. (2007) Evaluation of a peptide ELISA for the detection of rituximab in serum. *Journal of Immunological Methods*, **325**, 127–139.

57. Wei, L.N. (1997) Transgenic animals as new approaches in pharmacological studies. *Annual Review of Pharmacology and Toxicology*, **37**, 119–141.

58. Queseda, J.R., and Gutterman, J.U. (1983) Clinical study of recombinant DNA-produced leukocyte interferon (clone A) in an intermittent schedule in cancer patients. *Journal of the National Cancer Institute*, **70**, 1041–1046.

59. Queseda, J.R., Rios, A., Swanson, D., Trown, P., and Gutterman, J.U. (1985) Antitumor activity of recombinant-derived interferon alpha in metastatic renal carcinoma. *Journal of Clinical Oncology*, **3**, 1522–1528.

60. Rosenblum, M.G., Unger, B.W., Gutterman, J.U., Hersh, E.M., David, G.S., and Frincke, J.M. (1985) Modification of human leukocyte interferon pharmacology with a monoclonal antibody. *Cancer Research*, **45**, 2421–2424.

61. Fast, D.M., Kelley, M., Viswanathan, CT., O'Shaughnessy, J., King, S.P., Chaudhary, A., Weiner, R., DeStefano, A.J., and Tang, D. (2009) Workshop report and follow-up—AAPS workshop on current topics in GLP bioanalysis: assay reproducibility for incurred samples—implications of Crystal City recommendations. *The AAPS Journal*, **11**, 238–241.

62. Rocci, M.L., Devanarayan, V., Haughey, D.B., and Jardieu, P. (2007) Confirmatory reanalysis of incurred bioanalytical samples. *The AAPS Journal*, **9**, E336–E343.

63. Findlay, J.W.A. (2009) Specificity and accuracy data for ligand-binding assays for macromolecules should be interpreted with caution. *The AAPS Journal*, **10**, 433–434.

64. Findlay, J.W.A. (2008) Some important considerations for validation of ligand-binding assays. *Journal of Chromatography B*, **877**, 2191–2197.

65. Lee, J., and Ma, H. (2007) Specificity and selectivity evaluations of ligand binding assay of protein therapeutics against concomitant drugs and related endogenous peptides. *The AAPS Journal*, **9**, E164–E170.

66. Temsamani, J., Roskey, A., Chaix, C., and Agrawal, S. (1997) *In vivo* metabolic profile of a phosphorothioate oligodeoxyribonucleotide. *Antisense and Nucleic Acid Drug Development*, **7**, 159–165.

67. Matsuyama, H., Ruhmann-Wennhold, A., Johnson, L.R., and Nelson, D.H. (1972) Disappearance rates of exogenous and endogenous ACTH from rat plasma measured by bioassay and radioimmunoassay. *Metabolism*, **21**, 30–35.

68. de Serres, M., McNulty, M.J., Christensen, L., Zon, G., and Findlay, J.W.A. (1996) Development of a novel scintillation proximity competitive hybridization assay for the determination of phosphorothioate antisense oligonucleotide plasma concentrations in a toxicokinetic study. *Analytical Biochemistry*, **233**, 228–233.

69. Sewell, K.L., Geary, R.S., Baker, B.F., Glover, J.M., Mant, T.G.K., Yu, R.S., Tami, J.A., and Dorr, F.A. (2002) Phase I trial of ISIS 104838, a 2′-methoxyethyl modified antisense oligonucleotide targeting tumor necrosis factor-α. *Journal of Pharmacology and Experimental Therapeutics*, **303**, 1334–1343.

CHAPTER 3

Development of Ligand-Binding Assays for Drug Development Support

MASOOD N. KHAN

GLP Solutions Inc., Rockville, MD, USA

PROVEEN D. DASS

PhytoBio Solutions Inc., Raleigh, NC, USA

JOHN H. LEETE

640 Marquette Court, Frankfort, MI, USA

RICHARD F. SCHUMAN

BioReliance Corporation, Rockville, MD, USA

MICHELE GUNSIOR and CHANCHAL SADHU

Covance Laboratories Inc., Chantilly, VA, USA

3.1 INTRODUCTION

The number of large molecule biotherapeutics such as recombinant proteins and monoclonal antibodies has steadily increased over the past three decades in proportion to our deepened understanding of mammalian biological systems. The current emphasis on macromolecule drug development programs within biotechnology and pharmaceutical companies will augment those biotherapeutics now on the market. A necessary requirement in any macromolecule drug program is a comprehensive bioanalytical characterization that includes quantification of the candidate molecule in pharmacokinetics and bioequivalence studies [1,2], detection of antidrug antibodies (ADA) in immunogenicity assessments [3–5], and estimation of the level of relevant biomarkers in pharmacodynamic evaluations [6]. The size and intricate nature of macromolecules render conventional chromatography-based

Ligand-Binding Assays: Development, Validation, and Implementation in the Drug Development Arena. Edited by Masood N. Khan and John W.A. Findlay
Copyright © 2010 John Wiley & Sons, Inc.

methods (e.g., LC–MS/MS, GC, GC–MS) typically used for small-molecule drug candidates inadequate for their larger counterparts [1,7]. The inherent dissimilarities between small and large molecules require an alternate approach, and with this in mind, a strong emphasis has been placed on the development of ligand-binding assays (LBAs) with high specificity, selectivity, and sensitivity for quantification of macromolecules.

Scientists face a challenging task in developing a robust LBA especially in a GLP-compliant environment. The effects of molecule instability, biological interactions in a heterogeneous matrix, and the possible presence of endogenous or structurally similar compounds with varying binding affinities are just a few of the many aspects they must consider in assay construction. In this chapter, we describe a systematic approach for the development of quantitative immunoassays that can withstand both the GLP-compliant prestudy validation process and the demanding environment of nonclinical and clinical sample analyses. We focus on LBAs that quantify the level of drug itself, emphasizing more the practical aspects of the development process and include a comprehensive section on assay troubleshooting. Most of the examples and discussions of LBAs provided in this chapter originate from immunoassays; thus, we use the two terms interchangeably. Development and validation of assays applicable to the evaluation of biomarkers and antidrug antibodies (immunogenicity) are described in Chapters 6 and 8, respectively.

3.1.1 Ligand-Binding Assay Defined

A ligand-binding assay exploits specific interactions between two molecules, for example, a receptor, antibody, or binding protein and its corresponding ligand, to quantify the analyte of interest. The term LBA is most commonly associated with immunoassays, which utilize antibodies that are highly specific to the given analyte; the analyte is then quantified using a detector molecule. Immunoassays have several variations (Table 3.1): (1) Enzyme-linked immunosorbent assay (ELISA) in which the detector molecule is an enzyme, generally horseradish peroxidase (HRP), alkaline phosphatase (AP), or β-galactosidase. Addition of substrate (e.g., p-nitrophenylphosphate for AP) results in conversion of a colorless substrate to a colored product, the intensity of which is directly proportional to the concentration of the captured analyte on the microtiter plate (Fig. 3.1). (2) Radioimmunoassays (RIAs) use radiolabeled reagents such as ^{125}I to detect the bound analyte. RIAs, however, require a skilled individual trained in handling, cleanup, and disposal of radiolabeled materials. (3) Electrochemiluminescence (ECL) format such as that marketed by Meso Scale Discovery (MSD). The detector molecule in this case is a ruthenium chelate that emits photons when an electrical charge is applied to the plate. Other available systems include Luminex and Gyros, which are both bead based and outside the scope of this chapter.

Sandwich immunoassays, such as those described above, often use two antibodies that recognize different epitopes on the analyte being quantified. The first antibody (capture antibody) is immobilized in the wells of an assay plate and binds the analyte of interest. A second anti-analyte antibody (detection molecule) binds to the captured

TABLE 3.1   **Common Signal Readout in Ligand-Binding Assays**

Format	Label or Tag	Example of Substrate	Signal or Readout	Detection Instrument
RIA/IRMA	Radioisotope			
	^{125}I	None	CPM	Gamma-counter
	^{3}H or ^{14}C	None	CPM	Beta-counter
ELISA/EIA	Enzyme-label			
	Horseradish peroxidase	TMB	Absorbance	Microplate reader with appropriate detection mechanism
		HPA	Fluorescence	
		AMPPD	Luminescence	
	Alkaline phosphatase	p-NPP	Absorbance	
		4-MUP	Fluorescence	
	Beta-galactosidase	ONPG	Absorbance	
		MUG	Fluorescence	
		AMPGD	Luminescence	
ECL-based	Ruthenium	None	Electrochemilu-minescence	ECL reader (sector imager)

For each type of assay, the label or tag involved is listed along with typical substrates, type of absorbance, and type of instrument required. RIA: radioimmunoassay; IRMA: immunoradiometric assay; CPM: counts per minute; ELISA: enzyme-linked immunosorbent assay; EIA: enzyme immunoassay; TMB: 5,5′-tetramethylbenzidine; HPA: p-hydroxyphenylacetic acid; AMPPD: 4-methoxy-4-(3-phosphatephenyl) spiro(1,2-dioxetane)-3,2′-adamantane; p-NPP: p-nitrophenyl phosphate; 4-MUP: 4-methylumbelliferyl phosphate; ONPG: o-nitrophenyl-β-galactopyranoside; MUG: 4-methylumbelliferyl β-D-galactopyrano-side; AMPGD: 3-(4-methoxyspiro(1,2-dioxetane-3,2′-tricyclo(3.3.1.1(3,7))decan-4-yl)phenylgalacto-pyranoside; ECL: electrochemiluminescence.

analyte and generates signal in subsequent steps. The detector antibody may be directly labeled with a signal-generating entity or tagged with a molecule such as biotin for detection by a streptavidin-labeled enzyme or protein, further extending the assay versatility. Since this approach makes use of two distinct epitopes on the analyte as shown in Fig. 3.1, it is also referred to as a "two-site ELISA." The relative ease of generation and availability of antibodies as well as the flexible assay format provides a cost-effective and high-throughput method that can be used extensively in drug discovery programs to screen numerous potential therapeutics.

3.1.2   An Overview of Assay Formats

Immunoassays can be designed in two formats: competitive assays, preferable for quantification of small molecules such as steroid hormones and prostaglandins, and noncompetitive, or sandwich, assays restricted almost exclusively to large molecules

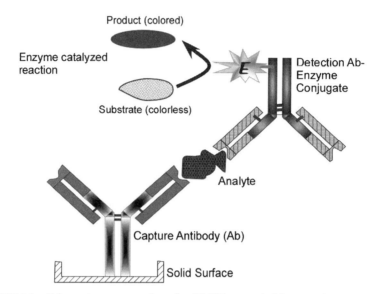

FIGURE 3.1 Schematic representation of an ELISA or sandwich assay. A capture antibody coated on the microplate binds to analyte; an enzyme-labeled detection antibody binds to a separate epitope on the analyte. Addition of substrate results in the formation of a colored product that can be detected spectrophotometrically.

such as proteins and antibodies. Both formats are heterogeneous; they require separation of the captured (or bound) analyte from the free analyte (usually accomplished with a wash step). For the sake of brevity, a comparison of the two immunoassay formats is provided in Table 3.2. The reader desiring an in-depth review of the theoretical aspects of various immunoassay formats and detection platforms is urged to consult one of several excellent books available on the subject [8–10].

3.2 INHERENT COMPLEXITIES OF IMMUNOASSAY DEVELOPMENT

A casual overview of a typical immunoassay gives the impression of a simple and easily developed method. However, in reality, this is a complex system influenced by a variety of internal and external factors. Some of the more challenging aspects of this system are summarized below.

1. The analyte in an immunoassay is detected indirectly through an antibody–analyte interaction. A sandwich assay utilizes the inherent ability of an antibody to bind specifically to the analyte/of interest that is then quantified indirectly through the binding of a second antibody conjugated to an enzyme or other labeling molecule. These indirect measurements in immunoassays yield less precise results than those of the chromatographic assays that directly detect the analyte itself. The resulting dose–response relationship in immunoassays is generally nonlinear; thus, selection of an optimum curve-fit model is of utmost importance, since a nonoptimal

TABLE 3.2 Typical Features of Competitive and Noncompetitive Ligand-Binding Assays

	Competitive	Noncompetitive
Typical examples	RIA Competitive ELISA	Two-site IRMA Sandwich ELISA
Analyte	One or more epitopes, usually small molecule	At least two distinct epitopes, large molecule
Analyte-specific antibody	One	At least two
Analyte-specific Ab concentration	Limited amount of high avidity antibody	In excess
Labeled component concentration	Limited	In excess
Analyte + labeled component incubation	Typically simultaneous	Simultaneous or sequential
Sensitivity	Affinity of Ab for analyte is critical for sensitivity	Dictated by NSB and specific activity of labeled Ab
Precision	Best precision in middle region of dose–response curve	Relatively high variability at the low end of the dose–response curve
Accuracy	Relatively high variability at both ends of curve	Relatively higher variability at the lower end mainly because of the low signal
Specificity	One Ab determines specificity	Enhanced by use of two antibodies specific to distinct epitopes on the analyte
Speed	Longer time to reach equilibrium (e.g., overnight or longer incubation)	Nonequilibrium assay (e.g., minutes to hours)

curve model can adversely affect the precision and accuracy of analyte quantification, particularly toward the extreme ends of the curve.

2. Immunoassay critical reagents such as the capture or detector antibodies and the enzymes used as labels are of biological origin, and thus may be subject to considerable lot-to-lot variation. For large molecule therapeutics, the lot-dependent differences in purity and heterogeneity of the reference standard also play a significant role in assay performance over time. Stability of these critical reagents can be greatly influenced by storage and handling conditions, further impacting reproducibility of the results.

3. In contrast to the chromatographic techniques where the analyte is extracted from the biological samples and reconstituted into a well-defined matrix prior to assay injection, immunoassay samples are usually analyzed without any

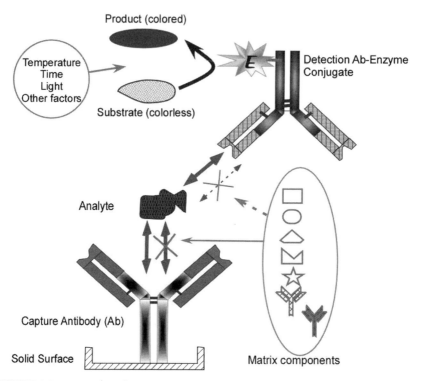

FIGURE 3.2   ELISA interference. Matrix components such as proteolytic enzymes, binding proteins, comedication, or heterophilic antibodies may cause interference through interaction with the analyte and/or the antibodies used in the system. Incubation time, temperature, and light among other factors can affect the formation of colored product.

pretreatment. As a result, numerous matrix components such as proteolytic enzymes, binding proteins, comedication, or heterophilic antibodies (i.e., antianimal antibodies) could interfere in assay performance through their interaction with the analyte and/or the antibodies used in the system (Fig. 3.2).

4. Finally, environmental conditions such as incubation time, temperature, exposure to light, humidity, and so forth may affect some steps of the immunoassay and therefore the overall performance.

The preceding factors make the development of a sensitive, specific, and robust immunoassay a challenging and more time-consuming undertaking than the development of a conventional chromatography-based assay. Careful attention to the details of each parameter is crucial for reproducible assay performance over time. A well thought out work plan, which factors in not only the above considerations (as well as those discussed in the following sections) but also the ultimate assay goal, minimizes potential setbacks in immunoassay development. The FDA's initiative to utilize "incurred sample reanalysis" for monitoring bioanalytical method reproducibility has further intensified the need to develop robust assays [11].

3.3   STEPS IN THE DEVELOPMENT OF A VALIDATABLE IMMUNOASSAY

This section elucidates some of the practical aspects that should be considered while developing an immunoassay. Although written with an emphasis on the sandwich assay format, and more specifically ELISAs over RIAs and ECL assays, it also applies to the competitive assay format. A systematic approach for immunoassay method development may consist of the steps shown in Fig. 3.3.

3.3.1   Define the Method Scope

The scope of the method development activity will depend on its intended use; necessary information includes (1) the type of studies the method would support (e.g., preclinical or clinical), (2) the sample matrix (e.g., serum, plasma, urine, cerebrospinal fluid, etc.), (3) the expected range of analyte concentration in the samples, (4) the presence of potential interfering compounds in the study samples (e.g., rheumatoid factor, binding proteins, antibodies), and (5) the acceptable level of variability in the results. This information, combined with the availability of critical reagents and the technology platform to be implemented, plays a critical role in selecting the assay type and format.

3.3.2   Assay Development Tools

Prior to initiating assay development, one should define all necessary assay components, instruments, and software and confirm their availability for the project. Essential elements include critical reagents, assay buffers, multichannel pipettes, microtiter plates, plate reader, plate washer, and appropriate software for data acquisition and processing. Freezers and refrigerators used to store samples and reagents, and instruments used to gather data must be calibrated, validated, and monitored during the lifetime of the assay. All equipment and instruments should be routinely maintained, and all maintenance, calibration, and validation records must be traceable and accessible. It should, however, be noted that the extensive instrument calibration and validation may not be practical in the drug discovery support labs. An assay that is totally or partially automated through the use of robotic systems requires special considerations as outlined in Chapter 11.

3.3.3   Assay Components

To generate a high-quality assay, the components, including critical reagents, microtiter plates, and assay buffers, must be qualified for use. Whenever feasible, a single batch of each critical reagent should be obtained in quantities sufficient for the life of the study. Since this may not always be practical, any introduction of new reagent lots requires that the comparability of the new lot must be confirmed. Each reagent should have a certificate of analysis (CoA) and a material safety data sheet (MSDS). A CoA should define the identity, activity, purity, and composition of the reagent and usually

① **Defining the scope of the method**
- Support for PK/PD/other studies
- Desired sensitivity
- Matrix of study samples
- Sample collection and storage conditions
- Assay format/technology platform

② **Assuring access to assay development tools**
- Production/sourcing of capture and detector antibodies
- Characterized material for calibrators and controls
- Critical reagents with proper documentation
- Microplate reader and washer
- Data reduction software

③ **Selection of blank matrix using prototype assay**
(Typically a prototype assay transferred from other lab)
- Assay setup in defined matrix (assay buffer)
- Curve fit model selected
- Screen biological matrix for low background
- Uniform analyte recovery

④ **Method development and optimization**
- Assay in biological matrix
- Calibrators and controls in biological matrix
- Selectivity and specificity
- Minimal required dilution (MRD)
- Range of quantification
- Preliminary analyte stability in biological matrix
- Parallelism/dilutional linearity
- Robustness and ruggedness

⑤ **Method transfer for pre-Study validation**
- Method development summary report
- Data table showing acceptable method performance
- Method is ready for pre-study validation

FIGURE 3.3   Steps in method development. A systematic approach for defining and developing a method is shown from the initial steps of determining the method scope to evaluation of reagents, method development, and optimization, and finally, transfer to prestudy validation.

includes the lot number, storage conditions, instructions for reconstitution, expiry date, and method of production. Reagents should be reconstituted, stored, and handled in accordance with the information provided in the CoA and MSDS and should not be used after the expiry dates, unless retested and found to be satisfactory. For new biological therapeutics, CoA and MSDS may not be available at an early stage of development.

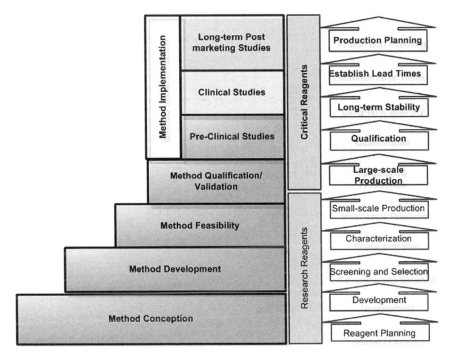

FIGURE 3.4   Management process of ligand-binding reagents during different phases of the assay life cycle.

3.3.3.1 Antibodies   Antibodies are the key components of an immunoassay and should be selected with care. The ideal candidate has a high affinity for the analyte of interest and minimal cross-reactivity with structurally similar molecules, such that they can even discriminate between isoforms of the analyte. Critical reagents must be procured, or developed, and selected soon after the method is conceptualized. Research grade reagents can be utilized during the development phase [12]. However, before the method is validated, one should produce the critical reagents in large enough quantities to cover pre-clinical, clinical, and long-term post-marketing studies (Fig. 3.4).

Purified antibodies are used almost exclusively in quantitative assays. The most common methods of antibody purification are Protein A-, Protein G-, ion exchange-, or analyte-specific affinity chromatography. Except for analyte-specific affinity chromatography, these techniques often copurify other immunoglobulins (Igs) present in the source material. Furthermore, both Protein A and Protein G can leach from the column during antibody elution creating a possible source of interference in subsequent assays. For this reason, affinity chromatography using a specific ligand is the method of choice to reduce or eliminate nonspecific Igs and other interfering molecules. This underscores the necessity for a CoA as well as verification of antibody purity by suitable analytical techniques.

Generally, antibodies that are used as a secondary reagent are available commercially, but analyte-specific antibodies are often custom produced. The use of commercial antibodies from reputable suppliers has several advantages including the availability of a CoA, MSDS, and cross-reactivity data. Antibodies produced in-house should be similarly characterized, and the information should be documented to comply with appropriate regulatory requirements.

Selection of antibodies is strongly influenced by the assay format to be used, and vice versa. If the second analyte-specific antibody is labeled with a reporter (such as HRP) or conjugated with a tag such as biotin, it is used directly as the 'detection' antibody. Such an antibody when practical, should not be of the same species as the coating antibody. However, if an unlabeled antianalyte antibody is used, requiring a secondary antibody–label conjugate (such as anti-rabbit IgG-HRP) for quantification of the binding complex, two precautions must be taken: (1) the unlabeled antibody must be of a different species of origin from that of the coating antibody and (2) the secondary antibody–label conjugate should show no cross-reactivity to the coating antibody or the analyte itself.

In sandwich LBAs, both polyclonal antibodies (PAbs) and monoclonal antibodies (MAbs) are used as capture–detector antibody pairs in various combinations. As MAbs recognize only a single epitope, they provide higher specificity than PAbs and are consequently more expensive to produce. Conversely, immunization of a single goat or sheep may provide a supply of PAbs sufficient for the execution of multiple studies over several years. PAbs can also provide higher sensitivity due to the presence of multiple antibodies binding to different epitope on the analyte molecule.

PAbs may show extensive batch-to-batch variation as there is no guarantee that a second animal will produce antibodies with the same specificity and titer, or even that the same animal will do so over time. Thus, for each new batch one should obtain cross-reactivity and titer information prior to use, and also keep in mind that any change in batch could result in considerable redevelopment work to match the original assay sensitivity and selectivity. Batch-to-batch variability of MAbs is less of a problem although information on critical characteristics such as specificity, affinity, and isoelectric point should be obtained for each batch.

Affinity and Avidity   Antibody strength of binding and specificity are the main determinants of the sensitivity and ruggedness of any immunoassay. Strength of binding reflects both affinity and avidity, which are described in more detail below and summarized in Table 3.3. Understanding these antibody characteristics will help in the appropriate selection of antibodies for assay development. A variety of methods for determining the affinity constant [13] and avidity index [14,15] have been reported.

Affinity, expressed as K_a, is a thermodynamic property determined by the rate of formation of an antibody–antigen complex relative to the rate of complex dissociation. It measures the strength of monovalent interactions between binding partners; a good fit between an antibody and antigen results in more noncovalent bonds (high affinity) than a poor fit (low affinity). Affinity of IgGs for their antigens can vary from micromolar to subnanomolar range. In general, the higher the affinity the

TABLE 3.3   Features of Antibody Affinity and Avidity of Antibody

Affinity

- Affinity denotes the strength of monovalent interactions between analyte and antibody.
- Affinity is expressed as the affinity constant K_a, which is the ratio between the rate constants for binding and dissociation of antibody and antigen.
- $K_a = \frac{[Ab-Analyte]}{[Ab][Analyte]} = \frac{1}{K_d}$, where K_a = affinity or equilibrium association constant; K_d = equilibrium dissociation constant; [Ab] = free Ab concentrations in mol/L; [Analyte] = free analyte concentration, in mol/L; [Ab–Analyte] = antibody–analyte complex concentration in mol/L.
- Typical values of $K_a = 10^5$–10^9 L/mol.
- High affinity antibody binds the analyte in a shorter period of time.
- Influenced by temperature, pH, and solution composition.
- K_a can be calculated by Scatchard analysis and other methods [13].

Avidity

- Avidity is the sum total of the strength of binding of two molecules to one another at multiple sites.
- Avidity denotes the stability of interactions between antibody and analyte as a whole. The total binding strength represents the sum strength of all the affinity bonds.
- Antibody avidity is a measure of the functional affinity of antibody to bind to antigen. It is also called as "functional affinity."
- Binding occurs because the shape and chemical natures of the molecular surfaces are complementary.
- In the immunization process with subsequent boosts of immunogen, as the affinity of IgG increases, the avidity of IgG increases.
- A variety of methods are used to determine avidity. Typically, an IgG titration assay is done in the absence and in the presence of denaturant and avidity is computed as the shift in the IgG titration curve in presence of a defined concentration of denaturant [14,15].

greater the method specificity and sensitivity. Antibody affinity contributes to the method sensitivity in several ways. Compared to the antibodies with lower affinity, more of the higher affinity antibodies remain bound to their cognate epitopes during assay incubation and wash steps, thereby enhancing the assay signal. High affinity antibodies are also less sensitive to interference from matrix components; this in turn reduces the minimum required dilution (MRD) of the test matrix, further enhancing the assay sensitivity. Antibody affinity can be determined empirically by comparing multiple antibody preparations in the same assay to establish which best meets the assay criteria. The antibody with the highest affinity is selected for further use.

Avidity represents the strength of all binding events that occur in an antibody–antigen interaction. It is not simply the sum of all affinities in a PAb antibody preparation, it also depends on the valencies of the antibody and antigen. IgG is a bivalent molecule, whereas IgM is decavalent, and the antigen can be multivalent as well if there is a multiplication of epitope within the molecule or the presence of multiple epitopes recognized by different antibodies. Conformational changes to antibody or antigen during binding of multiple sites and dilution of a heterogeneous antibody preparation also impact avidity. Since a PAb is not a homogeneous population, it is very complicated to estimate avidity. When comparing whole IgGs resulting from a MAb preparation, the affinity of the antibody becomes the key property as the population is identical and thus each molecule contributes equally to avidity.

Theoretically, any of the different antibody subclasses and isotypes may be used in an immunoassay. IgMs possess higher avidity due to their decavalent structure but have particular issues with their production, purification, stability, and specificity. IgGs are favored both as reagents and as therapeutics due to their high affinity, ease of manipulation at the molecular level, and large-scale production.

Specificity   Specificity of an antibody refers to its ability to bind the cognate antigen in the presence of structurally similar molecules. A highly specific antibody has low cross-reactivity and as a result dictates the specificity of an immunoassay. Knowledge of the antibody's cross-reactivity characteristics greatly assists in the selection of a suitable reagent. Cross-reactivity may be evaluated by assessing antibody binding to compounds structurally related to the analyte or compounds that could be present in the study samples. In a competitive assay format, the assessment of cross-reactivity can be performed by serial dilution of potential cross-reactants, or test compounds, in parallel with serial dilution of the analyte [9]. The concentrations corresponding to 50% of the maximum response (displacement of the labeled analyte) are used to calculate the degree of cross-reactivity using the following formula:

$$\% \text{ Cross-reactivity (using 50\% displacement method)}$$
$$= \frac{\text{Concentration of analyte at 50\% of maximum response}}{\text{Concentration of test compound at 50\% of maximum response}} \times 100$$

Figure 3.5a illustrates a cross-reactivity evaluation of an antidesmopressin antibody using a competitive assay. The antibody was raised against 8-vasopressin (DAVP), a nine-amino acid peptide, conjugated to KLH. Cross-reactivity was evaluated with two structurally close molecules: arginine-vasopressin (AVP) in which D-arginine is replaced by its L-isomer, and lysine-vasopressin (LVP) in which arginine is replaced by lysine. Cross-reactivities relative to DAVP (100%) were 0.29% and 0.04% for AVP and LVP, respectively, demonstrating that the antibody is highly specific to DAVP and suitable for use in DAVP quantification.

One can use a slightly different approach for determination of antibody cross-reactivity in a noncompetitive sandwich assay. In this approach, dose–response curves may be generated separately for the analyte and the test compounds. By using the responses to a preselected level of the analyte, generally the concentration in the middle of the dose–response curve, the degree of cross-reactivity can be determined. Figure 3.5b provides an example of this approach. The cross-reactivity of the anti-CVA151 antibody was evaluated at the CVA151 concentration of 200 pM. The absorbance at 200 pM of CVA151 was 1.10. In a separate dose–response curve, the concentration of the test compound, MWI704, at 1.10 OD was found to be 1718.4 pM.

The degree of cross-reactivity can be calculated using the formula

$$\% \text{ Cross-reactivity}$$
$$= \frac{\text{Concentration of analyte for which level of signal is computed}}{\text{Concentration of test compound corresponding to computed signal}} \times 100$$

Substituting with the above data,

$$\% \text{ Cross-reactivity} = \frac{200}{1718.4} \times 100 = 11.6$$

The cross-reactivity of MWI704 was found to be 11.6% relative to 100% cross-reactivity with CVA151. The other compound (MWI537) did not show any measurable cross-reactivity.

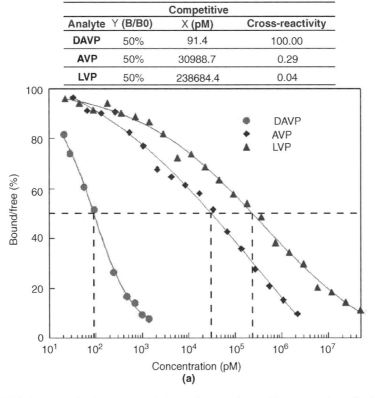

| Analyte | Competitive | | Cross-reactivity |
	Y (B/B0)	X (pM)	
DAVP	50%	91.4	100.00
AVP	50%	30988.7	0.29
LVP	50%	238684.4	0.04

FIGURE 3.5   (a) Antibody cross-reactivity evaluation of an antidesmopressin antibody using a competitive assay. A serial dilution of each test compound was incubated in parallel with labeled 8-vasopressin (DAVP, also desmopressin). The concentration at 50% of the maximum response is used to calculate the % cross-reactivity. Unlabeled DAVP as a test compound has 100% cross-reactivity. AVP, arginine-vasopressin; LVP, lysine-vasopressin.

Noncompetitive		
Analyte X (pM)	Y (Absorbance)	Cross-reactivity
CVA151 200.0	1.10	100.0
MWI704 1718.4	1.10	11.6
MWI537 ND	1.10	ND

ND = Not detectable

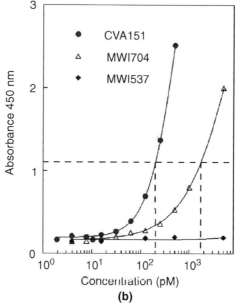

(b)

FIGURE 3.5 (*Continued*) (b) Antibody cross-reactivity evaluation of anti-CVA151 antibody using noncompetitive assay. Dose–response curves are generated separately for the analyte, CVA151, and test compounds, MWI704 and MWI537. The concentration of test compound at a preselected OD (corresponding to middle of the analyte dose–response curve) is used to determine cross-reactivity.

Other potential interferences, such as those due to comedication and related test compounds, can be evaluated simply by determining the ability of the method to measure the analyte concentration in the presence of such compounds. Typically, samples are prepared by spiking the analyte at two levels (concentrations corresponding to the middle and upper regions of the calibration curve). Analyte concentration is then determined in the presence of various concentrations of the test compound. The difference in analyte recovery (or signal) in the presence of the test compound relative to that in its absence indicates the extent of interference by the test compound and the method's tolerance of the test compound. It should be noted that metabolites of many peptides and most proteins are unidentified, so "test compounds" are not readily available for LBAs and the overall specificity profiles are both unknown and cannot be determined using another method, such as LC/MS. Therefore, the specificity of LBA data for samples from dosed animals or humans must be viewed with circumspection.

3.3.3.2 Microtiter Plates The flat-bottom 96-well plate is the most frequently used solid surface for immunoassays, and a variety of plates are available from a large number of vendors including BD Biosciences, Cayman Chemical, Corning Costar, Greiner Bio-One, and Nalgene/Nunc. Plates made of polystyrene are preferred for ELISA development due to their low background absorbance, uniform optical surfaces, and high capacity that easily adsorbs proteins and peptides [16]. The plates vary in well size, protein-binding capacity, and may also come "precoated" with streptavidin. Medium-binding plates are suitable for molecules with predominantly hydrophobic domains, while high-binding plates work well with molecules that contain mixed hydrophobic and hydrophilic domains. A vast amount of product information is available on the web sites of plate manufacturers.

3.3.3.3 Assay Buffers and Solutions Besides critical reagents and microtiter plates, the third major component of an ELISA method comprises assay buffers and solutions, including coating buffer, blocking solution, assay diluents, wash buffer, enzyme and substrate, and stop solution.

Coating Buffer The first step in an ELISA is immobilization of the analyte anti-analyte antibody on the microtiter plate. Immobilization occurs passively through van der Waals forces and hydrophobic interactions between the protein and the plastic surface. Proteins have minimum net charge and maximum hydrophobicity near their isoelectric points (IEPs); thus, a coating buffer with a pH close to the IEP of the protein aids in its adsorption to the plate. Unfortunately, information about the IEP of the protein may not be available. In such situations, one should evaluate the suitability of commonly used coating buffers such as 100 mM bicarbonate–carbonate buffer (pH 8–10), 50 mM PBS (pH ~7.4), or 50 mM acetate buffer (pH 5) [17,18].

Blocking Solution Coating microtiter plates with a protein is a nonspecific process except when using streptavidin plates and biotin-labeled reagent. Depending upon the concentration of the coating material, only a fraction of binding sites on the plastic surface may be occupied by the coating material, leaving open the possibility of a large number of unoccupied binding sites available to other components of the assay. These sites must be blocked to minimize nonspecific binding (NSB) of other assay components that may result in a high background signal. A suitable blocking agent saturates the unoccupied binding sites and minimizes or prevents NSB. Characteristics of the microtiter plate, the type of molecule used for coating, and the method of detection influence the selection of blocking reagent. Ideally, the blocking agent should inhibit NSB of assay components to the solid surface, have no interaction with the assay components, stabilize the coating material by minimizing denaturation, and exhibit lot-to-lot consistency. The majority of blocking agents used in ELISAs consist of proteins and/or detergents.

Proteins are routinely used as blockers as they not only occupy any available binding sites but also help to stabilize the biomolecule bound to the surface of the plate, thereby reducing steric hindrance and denaturation issues. However, unlike detergents, proteins are natural products with inherent lot-to-lot variability. The variety of commercially available proprietary blockers represents a convenient option where lot-to-lot consistency is maintained.

Predominant protein blockers include bovine serum albumin (BSA), nonfat dry milk (NFDM), casein, and fish gelatin. NFDM, used at 0.1–0.5%, is inexpensive but preparations vary in quality. Some NFDM preparations contain histones that interfere with anti-DNA determinations or inhibitors of the biotin–(strept)avidin interaction such as biotin itself. Casein is a chief component of NFDM and is often used alone as a blocking agent.

BSA is typically used in a blocking solution at 1–3% (w/v) solution and is often included in assay buffers and assay diluents. However, BSA exhibits lot-to-lot variability and cross-reactivity with antibodies prepared against BSA-conjugated immunogens. If the antibody preparation possesses activity toward BSA, the assay is likely to exhibit unacceptably high background signal, a phenomenon regularly observed with polyclonal sera. Additionally, BSA should be avoided if the particular analyte also binds to BSA. For example, high background is observed with BSA in assays analyzing the level or activity of CD11b and CD11c integrins [19]. Whenever BSA is suspected as the cause of high background, alternative blocking agents should be explored. Substitution of BSA with human serum albumin (HSA) is one way to alleviate these high background issues.

Detergents, unlike proteins, do not permanently inhibit binding of molecules to the solid surface as they can be removed by washing with aqueous solutions and are thus considered temporary blockers. Nonionic detergents such as Tween-20 and Triton X-100 are used as blockers of NSB in assay diluents, buffers (except for the coating buffer), and wash solutions. They must be used at concentrations greater than their critical micelle concentration value (between 0.01% and 0.10% for Tween-20). Detergents are inexpensive, very stable, and can be stored at room temperature for months without losing their blocking activity. The potential drawbacks of detergents are disruption of noncovalent bonds, residual detergent interference with peroxidase activity, and competition with lipopolysaccharides for surface space. However, these disadvantages are minimized at low concentrations. Zwitterionic detergents are extremely poor blocking agents and should not be used [20].

Assay Diluents   As the noncovalent interactions between antibody and analyte are influenced by pH, ionic strength, and temperature, typical assay buffers are isotonic solutions at or near neutral pH. Assay buffer and diluent formulations should not only promote analyte–antibody interactions but also minimize the nonspecific interactions between the critical reagents and the variety of biomolecules in the sample matrix. Components such as BSA, HSA, and nonionic detergents are often included in assay buffers. Phosphate buffered saline (PBS) or 10 mM Tris-HCl solutions (both near pH 7.4) containing 1% BSA and 0.05% Tween-20 are common buffers that can also be used for dilution of test samples and detection reagents, as well as wash buffers. When wash buffers are used in large quantities and stored at room temperature, preservatives such as sodium azide or thimerasol are often added to increase their shelf life. It should be noted, however, that some components of the wash buffer may have adverse effects on the assay system; for example, sodium azide and phosphate ions (in PBS) may have inhibitory effects on the peroxidase or alkaline phosphatase enzyme activities, respectively. Thus, caution should be exercised in selection of wash buffers to avoid negative effects on the assay performance.

Enzyme Labels and Substrate   Key properties of an ideal enzyme label for ELISA include the presence of reactive groups for covalent linkage, purity and ease of preparation, easily detectable activity, high stability in conjugated form, a low K_m (i.e., high affinity) for substrate but a high K_m (i.e., low affinity) for product, and compatibility with assay conditions including pH and ionic strength. High sensitivity requires an enzyme with a high turnover number. Immunoassays often use AP, HRP, and, less commonly, β-galactosidase as enzyme labels, and HRP- and AP-conjugated detection antibodies are available from multiple commercial suppliers. Polymerized enzymes, such as streptavidin-poly-HRP, which has multiple molecules of HRP conjugated to a streptavidin molecule, can enhance assay sensitivity [21]. Differences in the antibodies themselves or in the conjugation procedures among suppliers necessitate that the detection reagents from several manufacturers be evaluated prior to validation of an assay.

After selection of a suitable enzyme conjugate, one must then choose an appropriate chromogenic substrate at a concentration that will provide the best response over the assay range. An ideal chromogenic substrate for use in ELISA has these properties:

- Water soluble, stable, odorless, colorless, nonmutagenic, and nontoxic.
- High binding constant for the enzyme (low K_m value).
- Generation of a product with high molar extinction coefficient.
- Linearity between color intensity of the product and enzyme concentration over a wide range.

Enzymes used for labeling, their substrates, and the type of signal generated are summarized in Table 3.1.

Since the enzyme activity is pH and temperature dependent, these factors must be controlled during assay development and sample analysis. Activity strongly decreases outside the pH optima; thus, buffer pH is especially important during the enzymatic reaction. Although commercially prepared buffers are optimized for the activity of the detection enzyme, it is nonetheless important to understand the pH requirement. For example, the AP from *Escherichia coli* is optimally active at approximately pH 8, whereas AP from calf intestine is most active at approximately pH 10. HRP is active within the pH range of 4–8 with an optimum at approximately pH 7.0 [8].

Stop Solution   Once the enzymatic reaction has progressed to the desired extent, the activity of the enzyme should be stopped so that the color intensity of the reaction mixture remains within the quantification range of the plate reader. This can be achieved by acidifying the reaction mixture with a dilute solution of sulfuric or hydrochloric acid, or by the addition of commercially available substrate-specific stop solutions.

3.3.3.4 Instruments Microplate readers are essential components in a laboratory where ELISAs are performed. The nature of the signal generated in the assay dictates the type of microplate reader needed. Currently, 96-well plates and spectrophotometric signal output (e.g., chromogenic end point) are standard features of most ELISA methods; however, plate readers able to measure fluorescence, luminescence, and 384-well plates are also available. We have had satisfactory experiences with the SpectraMax line of readers from Molecular Devices (Sunnyvale, CA) for absorbance readout; Wallac 1420 VICTOR^2™, a multilabel, multitask plate reader by PerkinElmer (Waltham, MA) for luminescence- and fluorescence-based assays; and the SECTOR™ Imager 6000 from MSD (Gaithersburg, MD) for ECL-based assays. Without endorsing a particular instrument or vendor, we note our experience to provide starting points for those seeking to procure equipment.

As for plate washers, we have had success using the ELx 400 series of plate washers from BioTek Instruments (Winooski, VT) and the PW384 Plate Washer from TECAN (Durham, NC).

It is recommended that all instruments (including microplate readers and washers) undergo validation, calibration, and routine maintenance programs established and documented to meet regulatory requirements. This eliminates instruments as a cause of poor assay performance and streamlines the assay troubleshooting process.

3.3.3.5 Data Processing Software The software package used for data reduction should contain a variety of curve-fitting methods including linear, semi-log, log-logit, four-parameter, and five-parameter logistic functions. The five-parameter logistic function is especially important if an ECL format has been chosen. Extra features of the software allowing data transfer to other programs are a plus, and an intuitive interface enhances software usability. Each software system must be 21 CFR Part 11 compliant, capable of tracking changes made after data accumulation. Finally, the functionality to interface with a laboratory information management system (LIMS) is essential for the analysis of thousands of samples. Although several are available [22], two software packages preferred in the pharmaceutical industry are SoftMax Pro® from Molecular Devices (Sunnyvale, CA) and StatLIA® Quantum from Brendan Technologies (Carlsbad, CA).

3.3.4 ELISA versus ECL-Based Assay

An immunoassay is inherently the same whether run in an ELISA with chromogenic substrate or in an ECL format; however, the ECL format has some advantages over traditional ELISAs. This section focuses specifically on the MSD platform as we have had success with the instrument and platform.

ECL involves the use of a specific tag that emits light when electrochemically stimulated [23]. The tag is a stable ruthenium tris-bipyridine [Ru(bpy)$_3$] moiety that can be linked to the entity of choice through NHS ester or other coupling chemistry. Application of a charge in the presence of Ru(bpy)$_3$ and tripropylamine emits light (signal) that is then captured by a charge-coupled device (CCD) camera. Multiple cycles of excitation enhance the signal and improve sensitivity. Only those molecules near the carbon-based electrode at the bottom of the well are stimulated and emit energy allowing for the use of unwashed formats as well as smaller sample volumes (as little as 20 µL on a 96-well plate can be used significantly reducing the amount of sample needed). The background signals are also reduced relative to ELISAs because the stimulation process is decoupled from signal emission (and instrument noise is minimal—on the order of 10 counts for a 96-well single-spot plate). The end result is an assay that is sensitive, has a large dynamic range (approximately six orders of magnitude, up to 2 million counts), and is versatile.

Background signals may be further reduced by specific labeling of the detection antibody with SULFO-TAG as opposed to a SULFO-TAG-labeled antispecies detection or SULFO-TAG-labeled streptavidin. The labeling process is no different than any NHS-ester conjugation to primary amines; the biologic to be labeled must be free of interfering molecules such as gelatin and BSA (which would also be labeled with SULFO-TAG) and amine-containing molecules such as Tris buffers, sodium azide, and EDTA, in addition to protein stabilizers like glycine. If these molecules are present, the solution should be buffer exchanged and interfering molecules removed before labeling. The optimal ratio of SULFO-TAG to biologic depends upon the specific application, but good results can be obtained with a SULFO-TAG:protein molar incorporation ratio of 2 : 1 to 10 : 1. Molar ratios of 6 : 1, 12 : 1, and 20 : 1 SULFO-TAG:protein are commonly used, and the specific choice depends on the size of the protein and the number of available lysines. For example, to label a peptide with numerous lysines it may be desirable to use a lower ratio so that the label is evenly distributed along the peptide and no one potential epitope is masked. However, in larger molecules, increasing the number of incorporated SULFO-TAG molecules can increase the sensitivity of the assay. One should also be aware that a high labeling ratio may lead to masked epitopes and increased NSB. The SULFO-TAG labeling works best for molecules >10,000 Da, and subsequent to purification, the labeled molecule may have a yellowish-orange color.

There are a variety of plate options available for use in MSD format from standard to Hi-bind bare plates, as well as plates coated with strept(avidin), GST, and antispecies antibody. The carbon spot allows for passive adsorption of desired biological material whether cells, proteins, or antibodies. The biologic may be spot or solution coated on the plate under a variety of conditions varying pH and matrix components. One must be careful while using bare plates as these are hydrophobic surfaces and the addition of detergent is necessary. Coated plates or Hi-bind plates are treated surfaces and, as a result, are hydrophilic. Another significant advantage of the ECL-based assay over ELISAs is the ability to multiplex assays; kits are available that allow the user to measure 4, 7, or 10 analytes such as biomarkers, cytokines, and phosphoproteins in a single sample. However, a multispot plate cannot be coated by the user.

There are a few precautions to be taken while using ECL: (1) the plate is read at a fixed focal length, which for a 96-well plate means 150 µL of read buffer should be added to the well, although slightly more or less volume may not have a large effect; (2) it is best to use a "reverse-pipetting" technique when adding read buffer to avoid introduction of bubbles, which may reduce the precision and accuracy of the results; and (3) once a plate is read, it cannot be reread. The application of a voltage to the electrode essentially reduces the biologics to char, and a second read gives data of poor quality.

Disadvantages of the system include the need for a labeled detection reagent (the labeling of which may potentially alter binding sites), the cost of plates, and a single source supplier. Very often, these disadvantages are outweighed by the versatility of the format, the sensitivity, dynamic range (reducing the number of dilution repeats), the ability to decrease the number of wash steps thereby increasing the probability of detecting low affinity antibodies, the tolerance to different types of matrices and buffers, even those containing small amounts of ionic detergents such as SDS (up to 0.1%) and denaturing reagents such as urea, and tolerance to free drug.

3.4 DEVELOPMENT AND OPTIMIZATION OF AN IMMUNOASSAY

The ultimate goal of a development scientist is to design an assay that accurately and reproducibly measures the desired analyte under the rigor of prestudy and in-study method validation. The selection and procurement of critical reagents, buffers, instruments, and other materials for the assay completes the first stage of method development. To achieve the above stated goal, the scientist evaluates the following: (1) selection and procurement of the matrix, (2) uniformity of plate coating, (3) calibration curve-fit model, (4) method specificity, (5) selectivity, (6) minimal required dilution, (7) dilutional linearity, and (8) analyte stability in the biological matrix. We will address the basic concepts of these steps and other considerations below. Detailed instructions on how to develop a variety of immunoassays can be found elsewhere [8–10]. Precision and accuracy evaluations, a critical step used in validation of any LBA, are described in Chapter 4 and in the literature provided in Ref. [1,2].

3.4.1 Selection of Blank Matrix Using Prototype Assay

The analyte may be present in a variety of matrices such as plasma, serum, cerebrospinal fluid (CSF), urine, or other biological fluid, all of which contain a multitude of interfering factors that can impact the method's performance. As mentioned earlier in the chapter, LBA samples are not pretreated prior to analysis, thus calibrators and quality control (QC) samples should also be prepared in the study matrix to best mimic these samples and ensure accurate measurements. The ideal matrix (1) has low background signal in the assay (OD ≤ 0.1 for chromogenic end points), (2) has minimal or no analyte-like activity, (3) is devoid of interfering factors, and (4) demonstrates a response that is proportional to the concentration of the spiked analyte. Access to a prototype method using an assay buffer of defined composition as a reference helps to identify an appropriate matrix.

A prototype method can be obtained from a pharmaceutical company's QC or discovery group, an academic institution, or some other source, although often the scientist may need to design and develop such a method. Checkerboard experiments [8,10] define the optimal concentration of coating material, detector antibody concentration, and approximate range of the calibration curve. A calibration curve generated in assay buffer serves as a reference to assess the suitability of blank matrix for spiking calibrators and QC samples.

Initially, 15–20 individual blank matrix samples should be screened as described below. The samples are obtained in small aliquots (5-mL size) from a commercial supplier instructed to reserve and store larger quantities of the same matrix until notified otherwise. Each matrix sample is assayed in the prototype method with and without spiking the analyte (at approximately $3\times$ the provisional lower limit of quantification level) to identify matrices with low background signals and a uniform level of analyte recovery. The analyte recovery may not meet the standard criteria associated with selectivity evaluation experiments (80–120% of nominal concentration) as the standard calibrators at this stage are in a different matrix from that of the test sample. In cases where matrix gives significantly high signal or poor analyte recovery, the matrix should be reassayed at multiple dilutions as detailed in Section 3.4.4. Matrix samples with acceptable background and a consistent spike recovery ($\geq75\%$) are obtained in larger quantities, pooled, retested, and used for spiking the calibrators and QC samples. An assay in which the calibrators and the QC samples are in the relevant biological matrix will constitute the first functional assay that should undergo further optimization before prestudy validation.

3.4.1.1 Interference in Immunoassays Since the samples in an LBA are tested in their biological matrix, interference due to the matrix components may pose a substantial challenge in the development of a robust method. In particular, heterophilic antibodies and autoantibodies bear significant consideration in the preparation of serum and plasma matrix pools. As the name implies, autoantibodies are antibodies against self proteins such as insulin, present in the patient serum. Heterophilic antibodies are preexisting antibodies often originating from the administration of an antigen similar to the test analyte that may cross-react with any of the assay components (for a review, see Ref. [24]). With increasing use of recombinant antibodies as therapeutics, human antimurine antibodies (HAMA) tend to be the most commonly observed heterophilic antibodies. As heterophilic antibodies recognize a large variety of epitopes with a range of affinities, they may alter the assay signal, as shown in Fig. 3.6a and b. In fact, a survey of immunoassays on 74 analytes in 66 laboratories indicated that 8.7% of the 3445 results examined might be classified false positive for the presence of analyte [25].

The nature of interference by heterophilic antibodies and the impact on assay performance is unique for each study subject, adding difficulty to predicting their frequency in a particular study. A correctly designed assay format minimizes possible interference from heterophilic antibodies resulting in an assay with low baseline signal over a very large number of subjects and an extended study timeline. Low and steady baseline results are valuable in reliably measuring the drug concentration in study samples, even when concentration in the subjects' blood is minimal. Data generated with such assays are of immense importance in accurate pharmacokinetic (PK) profiling of the drug and in bioequivalence studies.

3.4.2 Plate Coating

Plate coating, the first step of an ELISA, is influenced by the concentration and nature of the coating molecule, the pH and ionic strength of the coating buffer, and the time and temperature of incubation [26]. A sandwich immunoassay requires an excess of coating agent while only a limited amount is used in a competitive ELISA. Parameters

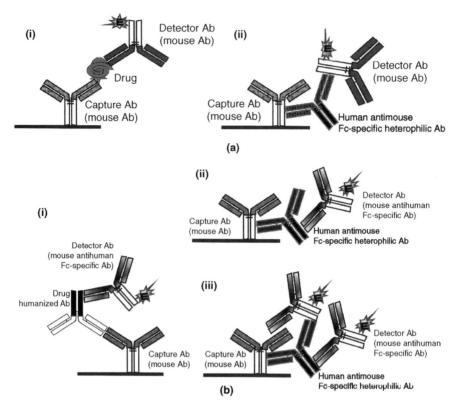

FIGURE 3.6 (a) Example of interference due to heterophilic antibody in an assay where a protein drug is quantified by a two-site ELISA. Although both the capture and the detector Abs are of mouse origin, they have distinct specificities. Diagram (i) illustrates an interaction between drug and reagent antibodies in the absence of heterophilic antibodies; this produces a true-positive signal. In diagram (ii), heterophilic antibodies in the test sample recognize the constant regions of the mouse Ab reagents and cross-link the detector and capture Ab, which leads to the generation of a false-positive signal.

(b) Example of heterophilic Ab interference in a bridging assay where the drug is a humanized Ab. The mouse monoclonal capture Ab recognizes the variable domain of the drug, while the detector Ab (also of mouse origin) binds the constant region of the drug. Diagram (i) represents an interaction between the drug and the reagent antibodies in the absence of any heterophilic antibody generating a true-positive signal. (ii) Binding of a heterophilic human antimouse antibody (HAMA) that recognizes the constant region of mouse Abs. Since the detector Ab binds the constant domain of the humanized drug, it will also bind the constant region of the heterophilic Ab, which is of human origin. Such an interaction leads to the generation of a false-positive signal. (iii) Signal amplification as a result of two detector Ab molecules bound to the Capture Ab via one heterophilic Ab molecule.

can be optimized for each coating reagent by varying first pH, then temperature and time of incubation followed by analysis using multiple sets of a single calibration curve. Alternately, plates are coated overnight in bicarbonate buffer or PBS at 4°C unless otherwise suggested by experimental observations.

When the coating agent is an antibody, typical conditions do not guarantee correct orientation on the plate. However, orientation can be dictated first by coating the plate with an antispecies Fc antibody (the species of coating antibody), followed by the coating antibody itself. For example, a goat–antirabbit Fc-IgG can be used for precoating when a rabbit antidrug IgG is used as the coating (i.e., capture) antibody. This strategy introduces additional reagents and steps, but leads to reproducible orientation of the capture antibody.

Coating uniformity across the entire plate is another essential feature for any ELISA. Although most of the high binding capacity flat-bottom plates are adequate, a prudent scientist should test for any systemic or random well-to-well variations in the chosen plate [16,26] during the early stages, since a defective lot or particular brand of plate could significantly impact assay performance. The adverse effects manifest in relatively high variation of signal in adjacent duplicate wells or random variation throughout the plate. The uniformity of plate coating should be evaluated at the first sign of high and unexplainable variability in the performance of QC samples or calibrators. The case study described below depicts a typical experimental design for evaluating the uniformity of the plate coating.

Case Study: During the initial stages of an ELISA development, unacceptably high analytical recovery (%AR) was repeatedly observed for QC samples, persisting across runs and analysts. In an initial troubleshooting experiment, the signal of a single QC sample was assessed over the entire plate. Analysis of the resulting data indicated a very small overall CV (3.5%) of the signal as shown in Fig. 3.7a. Furthermore, mean OD values for each row and column (0.488–0.520) were within one standard deviation of the all-well mean value with corresponding CV values under 5.0%, reflecting a narrow range of response from individual wells. This seemingly normal plate coating performance failed to provide clues to the original issue. The same data set was then analyzed as if resulting from a typical experiment in which duplicate controls and/or samples occupy adjacent wells. The analysis now identified relatively higher CV values in localized areas on the plate (Fig. 3.7b). When %CV values between duplicate wells were plotted graphically in 3D as shown in Fig. 3.7c, the pattern becomes glaringly apparent and corresponds to the plate region where abnormal recoveries of analytes were observed. The pattern was reproducible in multiple plates, and continued investigation revealed that the entire plate lot was defective. The case study demonstrates that a detailed analysis taking into account the average signal of adjacent wells (pairwise analysis) is more insightful than an overall analysis of the signal response across the plate. Analysis aimed at a pattern-specific evaluation (as opposed to the numerical values of CVs) proved more informative in detecting nonuniform coating.

3.4.3 Calibrator Standards and Limits of Quantification

The FDA bioanalytical guidance document [27] recommends a minimum of six nonzero calibrators for immunoassay standard curves. The 3rd AAPS/FDA

Bioanalytical Workshop (Arlington, VA, May 1–3, 2006) recommended at least 75% of the calibrator standards in the range of quantification should be within the acceptable performance criteria set *a priori* [11]. Therefore, the number of calibrator levels within the range of quantification should not be less than eight, providing flexibility to mask up to two levels with unacceptable %CV or %AR and still meet the minimum criteria set by the FDA and AAPS.

During method development, considerable work may be required to make a judicious choice for the lower limit of quantification (LLOQ). To obtain an initial

(i)

Rows

	A	B	C	D	E	F	G	H	Mean	%CV
1	0.522	0.511	0.555	0.497	0.497	0.512	0.509	0.497	0.512	3.74
2	0.520	0.524	0.528	0.506	0.504	0.513	0.511	0.492	0.512	2.28
3	0.513	0.504	0.507	0.507	0.508	0.518	0.517	0.491	0.508	1.71
4	0.509	0.495	0.491	0.500	0.547	0.487	0.507	0.496	0.504	3.73
5	0.517	0.511	0.508	0.554	0.551	0.531	0.490	0.482	0.518	5.02
6	0.520	0.508	0.513	0.554	0.535	0.530	0.504	0.485	0.519	4.10
7	0.509	0.509	0.534	0.514	0.508	0.478	0.488	0.493	0.504	3.42
8	0.506	0.534	0.523	0.518	0.514	0.526	0.488	0.480	0.511	3.69
9	0.501	0.486	0.525	0.501	0.535	0.505	0.501	0.513	0.508	3.05
10	0.503	0.500	0.496	0.479	0.513	0.509	0.494	0.482	0.497	2.40
11	0.499	0.502	0.471	0.489	0.507	0.519	0.504	0.472	0.495	3.45
12	0.492	0.497	0.496	0.498	0.521	0.503	0.502	0.472	0.498	2.76
									All Wells	
Mean	0.509	0.507	0.512	0.510	0.520	0.511	0.502	0.488	Mean	0.507
%CV	1.83	2.54	4.38	4.52	3.40	3.17	1.89	2.38	%CV	3.53

Columns

(ii)

Rows

		A	B	C	D	E	F	G	H
1		0.522	0.511	0.555	0.497	0.497	0.512	0.509	0.497
2		0.520	0.524	0.528	0.506	0.504	0.513	0.511	0.492
	Mean	0.521	0.517	0.541	0.502	0.501	0.512	0.510	0.494
	%CV	0.28	1.78	3.41	1.31	1.05	0.09	0.29	0.76
3		0.513	0.504	0.507	0.507	0.508	0.518	0.517	0.491
4		0.509	0.495	0.491	0.500	0.547	0.487	0.507	0.496
	Mean	0.511	0.499	0.499	0.504	0.527	0.503	0.512	0.493
	%CV	0.62	1.21	2.19	0.97	5.18	4.38	1.39	0.63
5		0.517	0.511	0.508	0.554	0.551	0.531	0.490	0.482
6		0.520	0.508	0.513	0.554	0.535	0.530	0.504	0.485
	Mean	0.519	0.510	0.510	0.554	0.543	0.531	0.497	0.484
	%CV	0.31	0.30	0.66	0.01	2.02	0.19	1.99	0.35
7		0.509	0.509	0.534	0.514	0.508	0.478	0.488	0.493
8		0.506	0.534	0.523	0.518	0.514	0.526	0.488	0.480
	Mean	0.508	0.522	0.528	0.516	0.511	0.502	0.488	0.487
	%CV	0.36	3.40	1.44	0.61	0.89	6.82	0.10	1.88
9		0.501	0.486	0.525	0.501	0.535	0.505	0.501	0.513
10		0.503	0.500	0.496	0.479	0.513	0.509	0.494	0.482
	Mean	0.502	0.493	0.511	0.490	0.524	0.507	0.498	0.497
	%CV	0.00	0.01	0.01	0.01	0.01	0.00	0.00	0.01
11		0.499	0.502	0.471	0.489	0.507	0.519	0.504	0.472
12		0.492	0.497	0.496	0.498	0.521	0.503	0.502	0.472
	Mean	0.496	0.500	0.483	0.494	0.514	0.511	0.503	0.472
	%CV	0.00	0.00	0.01	0.00	0.01	0.01	0.00	0.00

Columns

(a)

FIGURE 3.7   Plate coating uniformity test. (a) (i) Signal resulting from a single QC level added to the plate. The mean and %CV for each row and column as well as the entire plate was calculated showing overall good reproducibility. (a) (ii) The same data set analyzed as if resulting from typical experiment with replicates in adjacent wells. This pairwise analysis reveals localized area of high %CV. (b) Graphical illustration of %CV values between duplicate wells showing uneven plate coating. The root cause was determined to be a defective plate lot.

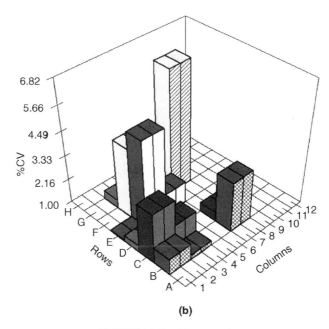

(b)

FIGURE 3.7   (*Continued*)

estimate of the lower and upper limits of quantification (ULOQ) a precision profile can be constructed using 12 or more calibrator levels and the experimental design shown in Fig. 3.8a, in which one predefined set of calibrators fits the calibration curve and the three remaining calibrator sets are treated as test samples. The %CV of the measured concentration is plotted against nominal concentration to construct a precision profile (Fig. 3.8b). If a horizontal line is drawn at the intended level of precision, the intersection points of this line with the precision curve provides an estimate of LLOQ and ULOQ. A tighter limit of acceptable precision should be used at this stage ($\pm 15\%$ rather than $\pm 20\%$) as the resulting CV data obtained at the method development stage often underestimate the overall assay imprecision observed during prestudy or in-study method validation.

A high LLOQ results in decreased assay sensitivity, but an apparently sensitive assay with low LLOQ runs the risk of frequent overlap with the blank matrix response, requiring change in LLOQ from assay to assay. Therefore, in addition to the CV-based approach described above, one may need to take into account the absolute blank matrix response as well. For example, if the OD corresponding to the chosen LLOQ is close to that obtained for matrix blank, then one should consider an upward revision of the LLOQ even when the %AR and %CV criteria defined above are met. Once the limits of quantifications are approximated, the positions of low, mid, and high QC samples can be set following recommendations provided in the FDA guidance document [27], white papers [1,2], conference reports [11,28], and in Chapter 4.

Selection of an appropriate model to fit the calibration curve is critical for the accuracy of the method. The four-parameter logistic (4PL) model is applied

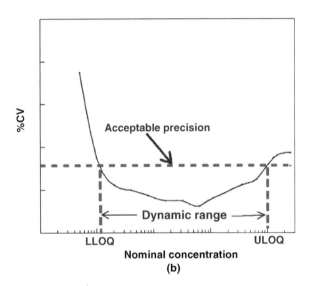

	1	2	3	4	5	6	7	8	9	10	11	12	
A	STD-1	STD-2	STD-3	STD-4	STD-5	STD-6	STD-7	STD-8	STD-9	STD-10	STD-11	STD-12	Calibrators
B	STD-1	STD-2	STD-3	STD-4	STD-5	STD-6	STD-7	STD-8	STD-9	STD-10	STD-11	STD-12	
C	STD-1	STD-2	STD-3	STD-4	STD-5	STD-6	STD-7	STD-8	STD-9	STD-10	STD-11	STD 12	Test samples (Set-1)
D	STD-1	STD-2	STD-3	STD-4	STD-5	STD-6	STD-7	STD-8	STD-9	STD-10	STD-11	STD-12	
E	STD-1	STD-2	STD-3	STD-4	STD-5	STD-6	STD-7	STD-8	STD-9	STD-10	STD-11	STD-12	Test samples (Set-2)
F	STD-1	STD-2	STD-3	STD-4	STD-5	STD-6	STD-7	STD-8	STD-9	STD-10	STD-11	STD-12	
G	STD-1	STD-2	STD-3	STD-4	STD-5	STD-6	STD-7	STD-8	STD-9	STD-10	STD-11	STD-12	Test samples (Set-3)
H	STD-1	STD-2	STD-3	STD-4	STD-5	STD-6	STD-7	STD-8	STD-9	STD-10	STD-11	STD-12	

(a)

(b)

FIGURE 3.8 (a) Precision profile plate map. Four sets of 12 calibrator levels are assayed; one predefined set is used to fit a calibration curve, and the remaining sets are treated as samples. (b) Precision profile plot. The %CV of "calibrators as samples" is plotted versus nominal concentration to give a precision profile. The concentrations at which a certain precision level is met, for example, 15% CV, define the preliminary lower and upper levels of quantification (LLOQ and ULOQ).

extensively in fitting immunoassay data [29,30]; however, since the 4PL model assumes symmetry of response over the entire calibration curve range, the five-parameter logistic (5PL) model was created for asymmetrical data [31]. Gottschalk and Dunn [31] compared the two models and determined that the 5PL provides substantial improvements in accuracy estimates. In contrast, Findlay and Dillard [28] conclude that the 4PL model demonstrates excellent curve fitting for ELISA data, and they recommend the use of 5PL model "with reluctance." When using an ECL format, the 5PL model employing a weighted fit is preferred because of the asymmetry generally observed over the large dynamic range. For any data set, the simplest model that accurately describes the system provides the best curve fit.

Dilution Fold	Serum-1	Serum-2	Serum-3	Serum-4	Serum-5	NHS	Mean	%CV
			%Analytical recovery					
2.5	42.9	72.4	30.8	39.0	86.7	90.2	60.3	43.0
5	74.1	78.4	46.0	61.8	83.7	88.1	72.0	21.7
10	94.5	95.6	79.0	86.0	93.3	102.2	91.8	8.9
15	114.0	91.2	93.0	111.7	89.9	97.6	99.6	10.7

FIGURE 3.9 Evaluation of minimal required dilution. Individual and pooled normal human serum samples are analyzed at multiple dilutions. The matrix dilution at which spike recovery falls within an acceptable range (80–120%) in at least 80% of the samples indicates the MRD.

3.4.4 Minimal Required Dilution of Sample

Biological matrices often exhibit a high background signal or poor analyte recovery necessitating some dilution of the samples to reduce or eliminate these effects. Minimum required dilution (MRD) is determined by testing individual matrix samples at multiple dilutions, each spiked with the same concentration of analyte. The matrix dilution at which spike recovery falls within an acceptable range (80–120%) in at least 80% of the samples indicates the MRD. Interference may not be observed in some matrices, for example, a normal human serum (NHS) pool, so it is crucial to evaluate several individual samples as shown in Fig. 3.9. In this case, a 10-fold dilution of matrix results in four of five test sera meeting the above criteria. Note that increasing the dilution of the matrix decreases the assay detection limit. For example, if the LLOQ is 5 ng/mL, a sample diluted 10-fold for use in the assay must have at least 50 ng/mL analyte to be quantified.

An alternate method of determining the MRD is to assess the effect of matrix on the entire curve. A blank matrix pool is spiked with analyte such that the final analyte concentration is consistent across various dilutions of matrix. An example of this approach in the MSD system is shown in Fig. 3.10. The highest calibrator, 500 ng/mL, has a greatly depressed signal in 25% matrix versus 0.01% matrix, although at each dilution the analyte recovery is within 80–120% of nominal. The dynamic range in terms of electrochemiluminescence units increases with decreasing percent matrix; in addition, increasing matrix dilution aids %AR at the lower calibration levels. The final matrix dilution chosen was 1%, for an MRD of 1:100. The absolute difference in electrochemiluminescence units for 1% and 0.01% matrix was similar, but a matrix dilution of 0.01% greatly decreases the sensitivity of the assay.

3.4.5 Method Specificity

Method specificity is based on the ability of the selected antibodies to interact exclusively with the analyte, without demonstrable reactivity to other molecules present in the matrix. Specificity is also, in part, dependent on the expected concentrations of cross-reactants in the study sample. For example, an antibody with low cross-reactivity (<1%) to a compound is unsuitable if the concentration of

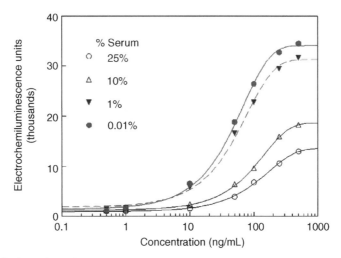

FIGURE 3.10 Effect of matrix dilution on calibration curve. A blank matrix is spiked with analyte such that the final concentration is consistent over all dilutions. Comparison of the dose–response curves resulting from each matrix dilution illustrates the effect of matrix over the assay dynamic range. In this example, the analytical recoveries of each calibrator level was within 80–120% of nominal concentration over all dilutions, but a final matrix concentration of 25% results in a greatly reduced dynamic range.

cross-reactant in the sample is very high relative to the analyte. In such cases, a sample cleanup method is required to remove the cross-reactant prior to analysis. In contrast, an antibody with 20% cross-reactivity with another molecule could be acceptable for use if the analyte is expected to be in great excess (and thus the concentration of cross-reactant relatively lower). Procedures to test the specificity of an antibody are discussed earlier in this chapter.

3.4.6 Method Selectivity

Method selectivity, the ability of a method to measure an analyte in the presence of unknown matrix components [1,2,11,27], is a formalized extension of the blank matrix evaluation and is determined by testing multiple individual matrix samples from normal subjects or the untreated disease population under assay conditions. The choice of matrix should reflect the target treatment population; if a treatment is gender specific, the matrix samples should also be gender specific. Similarly, if the target population has a specific disease state, such as arthritis, then the matrix samples should be representative of that population.

For selectivity determination, individual matrices are tested with and without analyte spiked at one or more concentrations between the LLOQ and LQC levels. A selective method has the targeted analytical recovery (typically within 100 ± 20–25% of the nominal spiking concentration) in $\geq 80\%$ of the samples. During the development phase, method selectivity can be evaluated using a small number of individual matrices; however, during validation, 30–50 samples should be tested.

3.4.7 Dilutional Linearity

Most LBAs require some level of sample dilution prior to analysis due to either the assay MRD or high analyte concentrations in the study samples. It is imperative to demonstrate during method development that the analyte, when present in levels above the ULOQ, can be diluted to concentrations within the quantitative range. This may be accomplished by illustrating that the analytical recovery of an ultrahigh matrix spike ($\sim$100–1000 times ULOQ), diluted serially in assay matrix, remains acceptable over a wide concentration range (when corrected for the dilution factor). Dilutional linearity experiments often reveal the presence of a prozone or Hook effect, which is discussed in the next section.

Parallelism is another assay parameter that is conceptually similar to dilutional linearity, but unlike dilutional linearity that is assessed using spiked analyte, parallelism is demonstrated using incurred samples. Tests of parallelism show that the dose response of analyte in study samples is similar to that generated with analyte spiked into naïve matrix. Moreover, parallelism demonstrates that all components in the actual study sample dilute (cross-react with the antibody) in a similar way to that of the calibrator. However, deviations from the ideal situation may occur for a variety of reasons; for example, the structure of the study sample analyte could be different from that of the analyte used as a calibrator standard. Similarly, nonparallelism may demonstrate nonparallel cross-reactivity, which can mean that the study sample may not generate reproducible results through the entire range of quantification. In practice, plotting the responses produced by diluted incurred samples against the calibration curve gives a visual impression of parallelism. Multiple approaches to the analysis of parallelism have been described in the referenced literature [6,32].

3.4.8 Prozone or Hook Effect

The presence of high analyte levels in samples can suppress the signal resulting in a gross underestimation of analyte concentration as shown in Fig. 3.11. This phenomenon, known as the prozone or "high-dose Hook effect" (HDHE), is particularly common in one-step sandwich immunoassays in which analyte is incubated simultaneously with both the capture and detection antibodies [33]. If the analyte concentration is higher than the maximum capacity of the capture antibody, the free analyte molecules bind the detection antibody, preventing it from binding the captured analyte. Any detection antibody bound to free analyte is washed away, yielding a reduction in response. Increasing the concentration of both capture and detection antibodies can increase the analyte concentration at which the HDHE occurs (Fig. 3.12).

HDHE, if present in a one-step sandwich immunoassay, can be eliminated in the two-step immunoassay by washing the plate (thereby removing free analyte) prior to the addition of the detection antibody (Fig. 3.12). The two-step immunoassay format is not entirely free from the Hook effect; a polyclonal antibody with varying affinity or a monoclonal antibody with low affinity may be ineffective capture reagents, releasing the analyte during incubation with detection antibody and again decreasing signal.

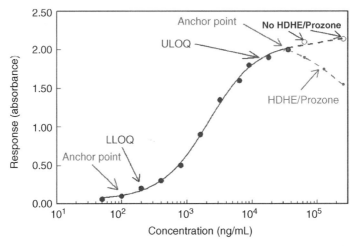

FIGURE 3.11 Graphical representation of a high-dose Hook effect (HDHE). High levels of analyte can result in the suppression of signal (dotted line with small closed circles) resulting in a falsely low concentration result.

The magnitude of the Hook effect in such cases is proportional to the length of incubation until equilibrium is reached. Inadequate wash steps following incubation of the analyte with capture antibody may also lead to leftover free analyte in the assay wells; the free analyte can then bind detection antibody, and the complexes removed in

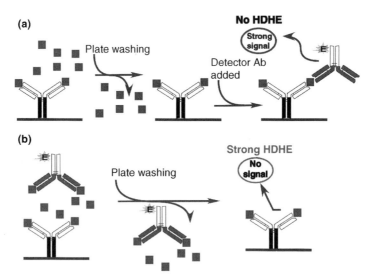

FIGURE 3.12 Schematic representation of HDHE. (a) A two-site ELISA with a wash step eliminates excess analyte resulting in a strong signal and no HDHE. (b) In a one-step ELISA, excess analyte binds to the detection Ab preventing completion of the sandwich complex and resulting in a loss of signal.

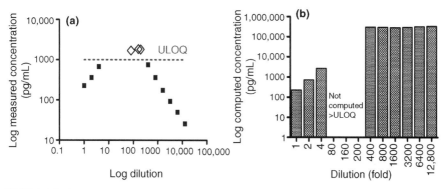

FIGURE 3.13   Hook effect revealed by dilutional linearity experiment. (a) The analyte when assayed neat resulted in a low measured concentration. When reassayed at multiple dilutions, the measured concentration for several dilutions was greater than the assay ULOQ. (b) The results, when corrected for the dilution factor, showed dilutional linearity at dilutions greater than 400-fold, indicating the presence of a HDHE.

subsequent wash steps. It has also been reported that antigens with multiple binding sites, such as ferritin, can cause desorption of antigen–antibody complexes after analyte has been captured [34]; experimental data suggests that the rate of desorption may be particularly rapid when the analyte concentration is very high, thus leading to a HDHE.

A representative example of the HDHE is shown in Fig. 3.13. Khan and Wang [35] reported that a sample from a dose-escalating study in which a high concentration of drug was expected when assayed "neat" (without dilution) in a one-step ELISA produced a low measured concentration. In troubleshooting experiments, the sample was reassayed at a wide range of dilutions. The graphs in Fig. 3.13 demonstrate that increasing dilutions (80 to 200-fold) resulted in measured concentrations greater than the ULOQ of the assay. Successive dilutions from 400 to 12,800-fold, when corrected for the dilution factor, showed dilutional linearity, suggesting that computed concentrations provided a realistic estimate of sample drug concentration at these dilutions. The example clearly illustrates the importance of evaluating HDHE and establishing dilutional linearity during immunoassay development.

3.4.9   Analyte Stability in Biological Matrix

Analyte stability is a great source of concern, and it often varies with matrix type as each matrix has a distinct combination of binding proteins, lipids, and proteolytic enzymes that may act on the drug. Analyte stability can be determined in experiments meant to mimic the conditions encountered by study samples such as room temperature or refrigerator incubations and multiple freeze–thaw cycles. Analyte stability determined for one matrix may not be extrapolated to another matrix as an analyte found to be stable in monkey or human serum could be highly unstable in rat or mouse serum. Where an analyte stability issue is anticipated, it is recommended that the study samples are collected in the presence of a protease inhibitor cocktail and kept on ice during analysis. In some cases, this may also require optimizing the assay at low temperature (as opposed to ambient temperature). It should also be noted that protease inhibitors may cause interference in the assay and should be evaluated before their addition on a routine basis.

3.5   OPTIMIZATION OF COMMERCIAL KIT-BASED ASSAYS

Commercial kits are available for the measurement of a wide range of analytes, including many biomarkers, in biological samples. Kits are designed for use in research laboratory environments and must be adapted to GLP-compliant bioanalytical work. The composition and format of QC samples in the kits should be restructured for monitoring the assay performance, making assay acceptance decisions, and most especially for assessing the kit lot-to-lot variability. Commercially available multiplexed assay kits present a unique challenge in adaptation and validation for analyte measurement. A detailed discussion of commercial kit use is presented in Chapter 7.

3.6   TROUBLESHOOTING IMMUNOASSAYS

Immunoassays developed along the recommendations provided above should perform consistently and generate reliable data over time. However, occasional failures happen; variations in laboratory environmental conditions, reagent quality, operator skill, and instrument performance, for example, make systematic troubleshooting skills invaluable in discerning the cause for assay failures.

Immunoassay troubleshooting is a sequential, cumulative process whereby one first looks at the calibration curve, then QCs, and finally the sample results. If the curve is not acceptable, the assay fails. If the curve is acceptable, then one reviews QC performance; if QC performance is unacceptable, the assay fails. If QCs are acceptable, then one examines individual sample results. If the assay fails as the result of an apparent technical error, the error is corrected and the assay is repeated. If the cause for the failure is not apparent or the assay has failed consistently, then a troubleshooting process should be initiated prior to further analysis (and depletion) of study samples. A summary of the calibrator/QC/sample result troubleshooting process is depicted in Fig. 3.14.

3.6.1   Calibration Curve Issues and Solutions

A visual examination of the calibration curve can reveal a variety of problems. One should first look at the abnormalities in curve shape or range of signal; a properly designed ELISA calibration curve has a low nonspecific background (ideally ≤ 0.1 OD), and the difference in OD response between the zero and highest calibrator should be greater than 1.0 OD. If the calibration curve OD response range has decreased, note whether the NSB (or blank calibrator) value is higher or the highest calibrator OD

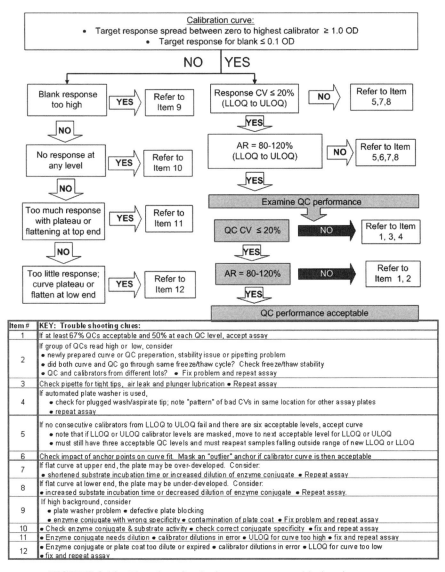

FIGURE 3.14 Flowchart for the immunoassay troubleshooting process.

values are lower than previously observed values. The points below further discuss possible causes and solutions.

- A high background impacts the entire calibration curve and can result from reagents used in the assay, matrix interference, improper blocking, or inadequate washing. Reagents must be carefully evaluated for potential interactions; a blocking reagent may generate a high background, or, in rare cases, a high background may result from cross-reactivity of detection components and blocking reagents. High background resulting from BSA can be reduced by substitution with HSA, casein, or fish gelatin. Alternatively, ready-to-use blocking buffers from which we have observed satisfactory performance in our laboratory are available commercially.

- A high background may also result from the matrix, requiring a sample dilution before use. The MRD for the matrix in a particular assay system should be evaluated during the method development stage. If matrix-related background problems persist, check that the appropriate population was used for the generation of the blank pool, and that the MRD chosen is correct.

- Inadequate washing can lead to a high background and washing at each step must be carefully controlled. Sometimes, it is more effective to briefly soak the assay plate between wash cycles than to increase the number of wash cycles.

- In addition to high background, underdevelopment of the plate can also impact the calibration curve. Underdevelopment may stem from inadequate or inconsistent plate mixing, incorrect substrate addition, not bringing all reagents to room temperature, matrix interference, omission of capture or detector antibody, overdilution of substrate or enzyme-conjugated antibody, or addition of stop solution before the assay was fully developed. If no color is present, the quality of detector reagents can be tested by mixing a solution of substrate with the enzyme-conjugated detection antibody in a separate tube or well. Color development in such test wells ensures that the detection components of the assay are functional.

- A plateau or flattening at the top of the curve may be the result of plate overdevelopment or erroneous calibrator dilutions. Overdevelopment can be rectified by further dilution of the enzyme conjugate; for a suspected error in dilution, one should check for consistency with previous assays. Also consider if the appropriate ULOQ level was selected during assay setup. Or, if the maximum signal has dropped, the coating antibody or detection conjugate may be rate limiting and the concentration of either coating antibody or detection conjugate or both should be increased.

- If weak color development causes flattening at the low end of the curve resulting in a loss of sensitivity or failure of the LLOQ calibrator level, the enzyme conjugate may be too dilute, expired, or calibrator dilutions are in error. If this is a bridging assay with an Ig analyte, the concentration of the capture antibody used in plate coating could be too high or too low and require reoptimization.

3.6.1.1 *Calibrator Precision*   A calibration curve containing a calibrator with unacceptable replicate precision (e.g., CV >20%) may still pass the overall assay acceptance criteria. If there is an insufficient number of acceptable calibrators from LLOQ to ULOQ, or if adjacent calibrators fail precision, consider whether the curve is too "flat" at the points of failure. If replicate %CV of the signal (OD, in the case of ELISA) is

less than 5% yet the calculated concentration backfit values have >15% replicate CV, chances are that the measurement is being made in a flat or plateau region at the top or bottom end of the calibration curve. A plateau at the upper end of the curve can result from insufficient plate coat or too little enzyme conjugate. A low-end plateau and loss of sensitivity shows underdevelopment of plate (low response signal), which can be caused by reagent deterioration, lower incubation temperatures, or shorter incubation times.

3.6.1.2 Calibrator Backfit Accuracy   As with calibrator precision, curves with consecutive calibrators not meeting %AR criteria (outside the suggested $100 \pm 20\%$ of the nominal concentration) or with less than six acceptable calibrators are usually failed. Before rejecting the calibration curve for unacceptable %AR near LLOQ or ULOQ, try masking selected anchor points outside the curve working range that may be impacting the curve-fit algorithm. Although it is not appropriate to mask calibrator levels solely to make a QC set pass acceptance criteria, it is generally acceptable to mask calibrator anchor points to improve %AR of apparently failing calibrators. Note that a typical 4PL curve fit may not fit an asymmetrical curve (e.g., with plateau at only one end), and an alternate curve-fit model may be required.

3.6.2 QC Issues and Solutions

It is an industry recommended practice to bracket study samples on an assay plate with two sets of duplicate QCs at three levels (low, mid, and high). Acceptable QC performance typically requires that at least 67% of all QC samples, with at least 50% at each level, must satisfy preestablished precision and accuracy criteria. Consistent QC failure warrants a serious look at the assay performance up to that point in time.

3.6.2.1 QC Precision Troubleshooting   If multiple QCs fail acceptance criteria, but the calibration curve is acceptable for precision over the working range, consider the following: (1) a systematic wash error (plugged tip on plate washer); (2) possible pipetting error (leaking tip or fibrin clot when plasma is used as the matrix); or (3) defective plate resulting in well-to-well variation (as described in Section 3.4.2). If the calibration curve is relatively flat at the end where the QCs are failing, consider the suggested solutions for calibration curve flattening to fix the problem.

3.6.2.2 QC Accuracy Troubleshooting   For poor analytical recovery of the QC samples, check for a possible edge effect. Are the failing QCs mostly around the edges of the assay plate? The difference in OD between wells on the edge and wells in the central region of the plate may be due to difference in temperature or due to a difference in the time to add the reagents across the plate. The polystyrene microtiter plate is a poor conductor of heat; temperature at the edges is potentially unlike the central region and the difference may be more acute when incubation time is short and incubation temperature is 37°C. To prevent edge effects, ensure the substrate and microtiter plate are at the same temperature prior to use and avoid stacking of plates.

Changing tips between pipetting of each QC set also improves overall QC accuracy. Also check that a new QC lot has been properly qualified. Other questions to consider include the following: Are the calibrators and the QCs prepared in the same lot of pooled matrix? If not, do the two matrix pools exhibit comparable spike recovery of the analyte? Are the calibrators and QCs prepared from different lots of source material? If yes, check respective certificates of analysis for purity. Is there a sensitivity to freeze/thaw? Check for validated stability of QC samples against storage conditions. Have the standard calibrators and QC samples experienced the same number of freeze/thaw cycles? Answers to these questions often lead to the determination of the causes of failures.

3.6.3 Sample Result Issues and Solutions

If the calibration curve and QCs meet the acceptance criteria, sample results falling on the curve working range (between LLOQ and ULOQ) are reportable if their replicates have acceptable precision (generally $\leq 20\%$ CV). Results falling below the LLOQ may be reported as <LLOQ if tested at the method MRD. Other samples falling below LLOQ or above ULOQ are repeated at an appropriate dilution within the validated range of dilutional linearity. Samples falling on the reportable range of the calibration curve, but with unacceptable precision ($>20\%$ CV), are to be repeated. Visible fibrin (if plasma is used as matrix) or other debris in the sample should be removed to improve precision.

3.6.4 Resolving Issues Due to Heterophilic Antibodies

3.6.4.1 Detection and Measurement of Interference Due to Heterophilic Antibodies   Often, a method is used to quantify an endogenous analyte associated with particular clinical signs. When the clinical signs and obtained result do not correlate, it may provide an early indication of interference due to heterophilic antibodies. However, information about the patient's clinical signs is not always readily available to the bioanalytical scientist, making it difficult to recognize this type of interference. The following indications and experiments may also suggest the presence of interfering antibodies:

- The sample fails to show parallelism between dilution and computed concentration.
- The analyte concentration differs significantly before and after the use of commercially available heterophilic antibody blocking reagents.
- Discrepancies between methods of measurement that use different antibodies or platforms, for example, ECL and ELISA.
- Perform a bridging assay in which the same antibody is used as both capture and detector antibody. If the assay signal in a predose sample is increased above the capture or detector antibody blank signal, interference should be suspected; an increase in signal indicates likely presence of heterophilic antibodies cross-linking

the capture and the detection reagents, resulting in positive interference [36]. Similarly, a decrease in signal in the presence of added analyte suggests inhibition, or negative interference, of the test analyte by heterophilic antibodies.

- Perform an analyte recovery test as follows: spike a known amount of analyte into both the suspect test sample and a normal sample from a healthy subject. Quantify the analyte over a series of dilutions and compare results from the test and normal samples; interference is likely if the amount of sample recovered is not what is expected.

3.6.4.2 *Elimination and Reduction of Interfering Antibodies*   Interfering antibodies or components can be eliminated or removed in several ways depending upon the nature of the analyte [36]. If the analyte of interest is a relatively small molecule (e.g., polypeptide hormone, cytokine, etc.), both heterophilic and auto-antibodies may be removed by PEG precipitation [37] or absorption with protein L [36,38] without precipitating the analyte of interest. These steps may improve the assay, but it is often not practical to treat the large number of samples from a clinical trial in this manner; thus, other measures must be considered.

Preincubation of the study samples with animal antibodies or serum has been reported to substantially decrease positive interference due to heterophilic antibodies by preventing, for example, heterophilic human antimouse antibodies present in the study samples from cross-linking the reagent antibodies [37,39]. These types of reagents are produced commercially for such purposes.

Replacement of the capture and/or the detection antibody is also an effective measure as substantial improvements can be achieved by altering the assay design. Larsson and Mellstedt [40] observed that the use of chicken antibodies as capture or detection reagents in immunoassays avoided heterophilic antibody interference since the human heterophilic antibodies did not react with the chicken IgY. Hennig et al. [41] used rabbit $F(ab')^2$ fragments as reagents to alleviate reported false-positive levels of interferon α and β in up to 27% of sera from otherwise healthy individuals. Use of Affibody® molecules by Andersson et al. [42] and single-chain antibodies by Warren et al. [43] has also resulted in avoidance of positive interference due to heterophilic antibodies. Affibodies are engineered binding proteins of approximately 6 kDa that mimic monoclonal antibodies in function. Although the generation of such reagents requires additional resources during early assay development, it may be worth the cost in large studies where testing of thousands of samples is anticipated.

The above troubleshooting guide does not cover every possible cause for an assay failure, but it discusses the most common problem origins. Other resources are available on company web sites and in assay design guidebooks.

3.7 CONCLUSIONS

In the arena of large molecule drug development, ligand-binding assays are the bioanalytical techniques of choice. Assays supporting preclinical and clinical studies undergo structured and rigorous prestudy validation prior to their use in study sample analysis. Generally, only a limited amount of time is allotted for method validation, which soon leads to commencement of sample analysis; thus, we strongly recommend that a robust method suitable for the intended use is skillfully developed before initiating the validation phase. Method specificity, selectivity, dilutional linearity, and reproducibility should be established during the method development phase along with procurement of high quality critical reagents in quantities sufficient to support method development, validation, and sample analysis. A method selectivity evaluation, if not given necessary attention, may lead to serious problems during validation and sample analysis. This chapter not only provides a comprehensive discussion on appropriate choice of reagents and a step-by-step guide for the development of a robust and reproducible method, but also includes an extensive troubleshooting section that any development scientist will find useful.

ACKNOWLEDGMENTS

We extend our sincere gratitude to Neel Neelkantan, Matthew Stinchcomb, Laura Kelly, Jim Weaver, Mitra Moussazadeh and Michele Rasamoelisolo for their timely assistance in reviewing this chapter and providing valuable recommendations.

REFERENCES

1. Findlay, J.W., Smith, W.C., Lee, J.W., Nordblom, G.D., Das, I., DeSilva, B.S., Khan, M.N., and Bowsher, R.R. (2000) Validation of immunoassay for bioanalysis: a pharmaceutical industry perspective. *Journal of Pharmaceutical and Biomedical Analysis*, **21**, 1249–1273.

2. DeSilva, B., Smith, W., Weiner, R., Kelley, M., Smolec, J., Lee, B., Khan, M., Tacey, R., Hill, H., and Celniker, A. (2003) Recommendations for the bioanalytical method validation of ligand-binding assay to support pharmacokinetics assessment of macromolecules. *Pharmaceutical Research*, **20**, 1885–1900.

3. Wadhwa, M., Bird, C., Dilger, P., Gaines-Das, R., and Thorpe, R. (2003) Strategies for detection, measurement and characterization of unwanted antibodies induced by therapeutic biologicals. *Journal of Immunological Methods*, **278**, 1–17.

4. Mire-Sluis, A.R., Barrett, Y.C., Devanarayan, V., Koren, E., Liu, H., Maia, M., Parish, T., Scott, G., Shankar, G., Shores, E., Swanson, S.J., Taniguchi, G., Wierda, D., and Zuckerman, L.A. (2004) Recommendations for the design and optimization of immunoassays used in the detection of host antibodies against biotechnology products. *Journal of Immunological Methods*, **289**, 1–16.

5. Shankar, G., Devnarayan, V., Amaravadi, L., Barrett, Y.C., Bowsher, R., Finco-Kent, D., Fiscella, M., Gorovits, B., Kirschner, S., Moxness, M., Parish, T., Quarmby, V., Smith, H., Smith, W., Zukerman, L.A., and Koren, E. (2008) Recommendations for the validation of immunoassays used for detection of host antibodies against biotechnology products. *Journal of Pharmaceutical and Biomedical Analysis*, doi: 10.1016/j.jpba.2008.09.020.

6. Lee, J.W., Devanarayan, V., Barrett, Y.C., Weiner, R., Allinson, J., Fountain, S., Keller, S., Weinryb, I., Green, M., Duan, L., Rogers, J.A., Millham, R., O'Brien, P.J., Sailstad, J., Khan,

M., Ray, C., and Wagner, J.A. (2006) Fit-for-purpose method development and validation for successful biomarker measurements. *Pharmaceutical Research*, **23**, 312–328.

7. Khan, M. (1999) Immunoassay in drug development arena: an old player with new status. *Journal of Clinical Ligand Assay*, **22**, 242–245.

8. Crowther, J.R. (2001) *The ELISA Guidebook, Methods in Molecular Biology*, Vol. **149**, Humana Press, Totowa, NJ.

9. Wild, D. (ed.) (2001) *The Immunoassay Handbook*, 2nd edition. Nature Publishing Group, New York, NY.

10. Wu, J.T. (2000) *Quantitative Immunoassay: A Practical Guide for Assay Establishment, Troubleshooting, and Clinical Applications*. AACC Press, Washington, DC.

11. Viswanathan, C.T., Bansal, S., Booth, B., DeStefano, A.J., Rose, M.J., Sailstad, J., Shah, V. P., Skelly, J.P., Swann, P.G., and Weiner, R. (2007) Workshop/Conference Report— Quantitative bioanalytical methods validation and implementation: best practices for chromatographic and ligand binding assays. *The AAPS Journal*, **9**, E30–E42.

12. Rup, B., and O'Hara, D. (2007) Critical ligand binding reagent preparation/selection: when specificity depends on reagents. *The AAPS Journal*, **9**, E148–155.

13. Hollemans, H.J., and Bertina, R.M. (1975) Scatchard plot and heterogeneity in binding affinity of labeled and unlabeled ligand. *Clinical Chemistry*, **21**, 1769–1773.

14. Lappalainen, M., and Hedman, K. (2004) Serodiagnosis of toxoplasmosis. The impact of measurement of IgG avidity. *Annals of 1st Super Sanita*, **40**, 81–88.

15. Perciani, C.T., Peixoto, P.S., Dias, W.O., Kubrusly, F.S., and Tanizaki, M.M. (2007) Improved method to calculate the antibody avidity index. *Journal of Clinical Laboratory Analysis*, **21**, 201–206.

16. Shekarchi, I.C., Sever, J.L., Lee, Y.J., Castellano, G., and Madden, D.L. (1984) Evaluation of various plastic microplates with measles, toxoplasma, and gamma globulin antigens in enzyme-linked immunosorbent assays. *Journal of Clinical Microbiology*, **19**, 89–96.

17. Cuvelier, A., Bourguignon, J., Muir, J.F., Martin, J.P., and Sesboüé, R. (1996) Substitution of carbonate by acetate buffer for IgG coating in sandwich ELISA. *Journal of Immunoassay and Immunochemistry*, **17**, 371–382.

18. Craig, J.C., Parkinson, D., Goatley, L., and Knowles, N. (1989) Assay sensitivity and differentiation of monoclonal antibody specificity in ELISA with different coating buffers. *Journal of Biological Standard*, **17**, 281–289.

19. Sadhu, C., Hendrickson, L., Dick, K.O., Potter, T.G., and Staunton, D.E. (2007) Novel tools for functional analysis of CD11c: activation-specific, activation-independent, and activating antibodies. *Journal of Immunoassay and Immunochemistry*, **29**, 42–57.

20. Gibbs, J. (2001) Effective Blocking Procedures. ELISA Technical Bulletin No. 3, Corning Life Sciences, Kennebunk, ME, pp. 1–6.

21. Plaksin, D. (2008) PolyHRP Detection Users Guide: Ultra-Sensitive Two-Site (Sandwich) ELISA Systems Utilizing Streptavidin-PolyHRP Conjugates. RDI Division of Fitzgerald Industries Intl, Concord, MA. Available at http://www.researchd.com/rdioem/polysdt.htm.

22. Gerlach, R.W., White, R.J., Deming, S.N., Palasota, J.A., and van Emon, J.M. (1993) An evaluation of five commercial immunoassay data analysis software systems. *Analytical Biochemistry*, **212**, 185–193.

23. Debad, J.D., Glezer, E.N., Wohlstadter, J., and Sigal, G.B., and Leland, J.K. (2004) Clinical and biological applications of ECL. In: Bard, A.J. (ed.), *Electrogenerated Chemiluminescence*. Marcel Dekker, New York, pp. 43–78.

24. Selby, C. (1999) Interference in immunoassay. *Annals of Clinical Biochemistry,* **36**, 704–721.

25. Marks, V. (2002) False-positive immunoassay results: a multicenter survey of erroneous immunoassay results from assays of 74 analytes in 10 donors from 66 laboratories in seven countries. *Clinical Chemistry,* **48**, 2008–2016.

26. Sponholtz, D.K. (1995) Immunoassays in Microplate Wells: Optimization of Binding by Passive Adsorption. Technical Bulletin, IVD Technology, pp. 12–15. Available at http://www.devicelink.com/ivdt/95/03.html.

27. Guidance for Industry: Bioanalytical Method Validation. U.S. Department of Health and Human Services FDA (CDER and CVM). 2001. Available at http://www.fda.gov/cder/guidance/4252fnl.pdf.

28. Miller, K.J., Bowsher, R.R., Celniker, A., Gibbons, J., Gupta, S., Lee, J.W., Swanson, S.J., Smith, W.C., and Weiner, R.S. (2001) Workshop on bioanalytical method validation for macromolecules: summary report. *Pharmaceutical Research,* **18**, 1373–1383.

29. Findlay, J.W., and Dillard, R.F. (2007) Appropriate calibration curve fitting in ligand binding assays. *The AAPS Journal,* **9**, E260–E267.

30. Maciel, R.J. (1985) A standard curve fitting in immunodiagnostics: a primer. *Journal of Clinical Immunoassay,* **8**, 98–106.

31. Gottschalk, P.G., and Dunn, J.R. (2005) The five-parameter logistic: a characterization and comparison with the four-parameter logistic. *Analytical Biochemistry,* **343**, 54–65.

32. Plikaytis, B.D., Holder, P.F., Pais, L.B., Maslanka, S.E., Gheesling, L.L., and Carlone, G. M. (1994) Determination of parallelism and nonparallelism in bioassay dilution curves. *Journal of Clinical Microbiology,* **32**, 2441–2447.

33. Rodbard, D., Feldman, Y., Jaffe, M.L., and Miles, L.E. (1978) Kinetics of two-site immunoradiometric ('sandwich') assays. II. Studies on the nature of the 'high-dose hook effect'. *Immunochemistry,* **15**, 77–82.

34. Fernando, S.A., and Wilson, G.S. (1992) Studies of the 'hook' effect in the one-step sandwich immunoassay. *Journal of Immunological Methods,* **151**, 47–66.

35. Khan, M., and Wang, N. (2008) Method development for preclinical bioanalytical support. In: Gad, S.C. (ed.), *Preclinical Development Handbook.* John Wiley & Sons, Inc., Hoboken, NJ, pp. 117–150.

36. Ismail, A.A. (2005) A radical approach is needed to eliminate interference from endogenous antibodies in immunoassays. *Clinical Chemistry,* **51**, 25–26.

37. Boscato, L.M., and Stuart, M.C. (1986) Incidence and specificity of interference in two-site immunoassays. *Clinical Chemistry,* **32**, 1491–1495.

38. de Jager, W., Prakken, B.J., Bijlsma, J.W., Kuis, W., and Rijkers, G.T. (2005) Improved multiplex immunoassay performance in human plasma and synovial fluid following removal of interfering heterophilic antibodies. *Journal of Immunological Methods,* **300**, 124–135.

39. Ismail, A.A., Walker, P.L., Barth, J.H., Lewandowski, K.C., Jones, R., and Burr, W.A. (2002) Wrong biochemistry results: two case reports and observational study in 5310 patients on potentially misleading thyroid-stimulating hormone and gonadotropin immunoassay results. *Clinical Chemistry,* **48**, 2023–2029.

40. Larsson, A., and Mellstedt, H. (1992) Chicken antibodies: a tool to avoid interference by human anti-mouse antibodies in ELISA after *in vivo* treatment with murine monoclonal antibodies. *Hybridoma,* **11**, 33–39.

41. Hennig, C., Rink, L., Fagin, U., Jabs, W.J., and Kirchner, H. (2000) The influence of naturally occurring heterophilic anti-immunoglobulin antibodies on direct measurement of serum proteins using sandwich ELISAs. *Journal of Immunological Methods*, **235**, 71–80.

42. Andersson, M., Rönnmark, J., Areström, I., Nygren, P.A., and Ahlborg, N. (2003) Inclusion of a non-immunoglobulin binding protein in two-site ELISA for quantification of human serum proteins without interference by heterophilic serum antibodies. *Journal of Immunological Methods*, **283**, 225–234.

43. Warren, D.J., Bjerner, J., Paus, E., Børmer, O.P., and Nustad, K. (2005) Use of an *in vivo* biotinylated single-chain antibody as capture reagent in an immunometric assay to decrease the incidence of interference from heterophilic antibodies. *Clinical Chemistry*, **51**, 830–838.

CHAPTER 4

Validation of Ligand-Binding Assays to Support Pharmacokinetic Assessments of Biotherapeutics

BINODH S. DESILVA

Amgen Inc., Thousand Oaks, CA, USA

RONALD R. BOWSHER

Millipore, St. Charles, MO, USA

4.1 INTRODUCTION

Biological macromolecules represent many structural and chemical classes, including proteins, such as hormones and antibodies, as well as nucleic acid derivatives, such as oligonucleotides, including antisense molecules, aptamers, and spiegelmers. These molecules have been described by a variety of terms by different organizations and individuals. Thus, macromolecules derived through the use of DNA technology involving genetic manipulation of cells have been described as "biotherapeutics" or "biopharmaceuticals." However, biological macromolecules produced by extraction and purification from a biological source, such as blood products, vaccines, enzymes, and some hormones, have been described by some by the broad term, "biologicals." These two descriptors do not encompass macromolecules, such as oligonucleotides, which are often prepared by chemical synthesis. In this chapter, the term "biotherapeutics" will be used broadly to include all biological macromolecules, regardless of the methods used to produce them.

Over the past several years, there has been a marked increase in the number of biological macromolecules undergoing development as potential therapeutics by pharmaceutical and biotechnology companies [1]. Biotherapeutics now account for 4 out of 10 preclinical candidates and 1 in 4 submissions for marketing approval in the United States [2]. As shown in Table 4.1, in 2007, the top-10 selling

Ligand-Binding Assays: Development, Validation, and Implementation in the Drug Development Arena. Edited by Masood N. Khan and John W.A. Findlay
Copyright © 2010 John Wiley & Sons, Inc.

TABLE 4.1 Top-Selling Biopharmaceuticals in 2007

Product	Companies	Projected 2007 Sales ($ Billion)
Enbrel	Amgen/Wyeth/Takeda	5.12
Remicade	J&J/S-P/Tanabe	4.92
Rituzan/MabThera	Biogen/Genentech/Roche	4.40
Aranesp	Amgen	3.94
Herceptin	Genentech/Roche	3.88
Procrit/Epres	J&J	3.16
Avastin	Genentech/Roche	3.12
Neulasta	Amgen	3.08
Epogen	Amgen/Kirin	2.80
Lantus	Sanofi-Aventis	2.56

Source: Adapted from *Nature Biotechnology* (2007), **25** (12), 1342.

biotherapeutics were projected to generate approximately $37 billion in sales [2]. The preferred bioanalytical method for determination of these macromolecules in biological matrices for the support of pharmacokinetic (PK), toxicokinetic (TK), or bioequivalence studies is ligand-binding assay (LBA), with immunoassay typically being the most common analytical format. Given the importance of biotherapeutics, appropriate validation of LBAs for their bioanalysis is most important. The Good Laboratory Practices (GLP)-compliant bioanalysis of biotherapeutics presents bioanalytical scientists with a different set of challenges for bioanalytical method validation (BMV) from those for bioanalysis of conventional small-molecule xeno-biotic drugs (Table 4.2). These challenges arise, in part, from the use of LBA methodology (e.g., immunoassay) as the principal analytical technology and issues inherent in measuring macromolecules in biological matrices. Table 4.3 summarizes some of the key technological differences between LC–MS, the principal technology for small-molecule bioanalysis, and LBA technology. These combined factors

TABLE 4.2 Differences in Bioanalytical Characteristics between Small-Molecule Drug and Biotherapeutics

Characteristic	Small Molecules	Macromolecules
Size	Small (<1000 Da)	Large (>1000 Da)
Structure	Relatively simple organic molecules	Biopolymers. Complex structures with multiple subunits
Purity	Homogenous	Mostly heterogeneous
Solubility	Often hydrophobic	Often hydrophilic
Stability	Chemical	Chemical, physical, and biological
Presence in matrix	Xenobiotics (foreign)	Could be endogenous
Synthesis	Organic synthesis	Produced biologically or synthetically
Catabolism	Defined	Not well defined
Serum binding	Albumin	Specific carrier proteins

TABLE 4.3   LC–MS and LBA Technological Differences

Characteristic	LC–MS Assays	Ligand-Binding Assays
Basis of Measure	Analyte properties	Analyte binding to macromolecule
Detection method	Direct	Indirect
Analytical reagents	Widely available	Unique, often with limited availability and lot-to-lot variability
Analytes	Small molecules and peptides	Generally macromolecules (e.g., molecular weight ≥ 1 kDa)
Sample clean up	Yes	Usually no (may include sample dilution)
Calibration model	Linear	Nonlinear (usually 4/5-PL model)
Assay range	Usually broad	Limited (e.g., 2 log range)
Assay environment	Usually contains an organic modifier	Aqueous (often physiological conditions, e.g., pH 6–8)
Assay development time	Weeks	Months (antibody preparation is usually rate limiting)
Imprecision (interassay)	Low (<10%CV)	Moderate (<15%CV)
Imprecision source	Intrabatch	Interbatch
Analysis mode	Series, batch	Batch

often make application of traditional GLP BMV approaches more challenging for biotherapeutics. Moreover, the evolving diversity of biotherapeutics undergoing development further complicates efforts at LBA BMV standardization. Some common issues that impact bioanalysis of biotherapeutics include the use of unique reagents (e.g., antibodies), low circulating concentrations (high potency), reference standard heterogeneity, specificity/selectivity, absence of sample cleanup, presence of endogenous equivalents/homologues, existence of high-affinity binding proteins (especially antidrug antibodies), nonlinear calibration curves, and limited calibration range, need for dilutional linearity and parallelism, analyte instability (chemical, physical, and biological), and the tendency for greater analytical imprecision than LC–MS. This last point was the genesis for a proposal within the LBA community to adopt "total error" (TE) as an additional criterion for GLP LBA method acceptance [3–5,9]. However, this concept has led to some misunderstanding and confusion about how to use and apply this additional prestudy validation criterion. The topic of total error will be discussed in more detail in Section 4.3.

4.2   ASSAY DEVELOPMENT AND VALIDATION PARADIGM

Because LBAs are conceptually simple and operationally easy to perform, there is often a perception among scientists that LBA method development and validation should be fairly straightforward and simple to conduct. In reality, establishment of LBAs for GLP-compliant bioanalysis to support PK/TK assessments of biotherapeutics is often a challenging task. Successful LBA establishment involves a systematic

Development
(Early-phase development)
⬇
Prevalidation
(Late-phase development ⇨ optimization)
⬇
Prestudy validation
(Validation phase ⇨ method acceptance)
⬇
In-study validation
(Implementation phase ⇨ batch acceptance)

FIGURE 4.1 Method development and validation paradigm for establishment of a LBA.

and stepwise process (Fig. 4.1). Aspects of this process are highlighted in other chapters in this book. As Dr. Shah stated in the original Crystal City meeting, the ultimate goal of BMV is "to demonstrate a method is suitable for its intended purpose" [6,7]. Finally, we adhere to the philosophy that the goal of BMV is to develop a valid assay, as opposed to validating a developed method [9]. The key point here is that the analytical capabilities needed to support the pharmacokinetic assessment of a biotherapeutic should dictate the design, development, and optimization of a GLP-compliant LBA.

The developmental phase begins with early-phase activities, such as method conceptualization, generation and testing of unique reagents, and selection of method format, and strategy for detection. Following creation of a "prototypic" LBA, the assay is optimized in the prevalidation phase specifically to meet the intended purpose and analytical objectives (e.g., sensitivity/LLOQ and range of quantification). Some key considerations here include investigation of the impact of matrix, definition of calibrator range and calibration model, and optimization of sensitivity [4,9]. Upon completion of the optimization phase, the assay is evaluated systematically during the prestudy method validation phase to ensure that it meets *a priori* defined criteria for method acceptance. For LBAs to support pharmacokinetic assessments of bio-pharmaceuticals, recommendations for validation design and acceptance criteria are described in guidance documents and published "white" papers [3–7,9,11]. After successful completion of prestudy validation, the LBA is deemed suitable for use to quantify the "analyte of interest" in support of PK, TK, or bioequivalence/comparability studies. In-study validation refers to use of specific criteria for acceptance of assay batches (i.e., assay runs) of study samples. As described in numerous publications, in-study validation often involves application of a 4-6-X rule, where $X = \pm 20$–30% of the nominal concentration in quality control samples [4,9,10]. This topic will be discussed in more detail in later sections.

4.3 PRESTUDY VALIDATION PHASE

At this stage, it is assumed that the analytical method that is being validated has been developed and optimized, as described in the previous section. Accordingly, the main objective of prestudy validation is to evaluate and confirm that the method possesses acceptable accuracy, precision, selectivity, and specificity. Prior to initiating validation experiments, it is necessary to document the intent of the validation and the experimental plan for assessing the parameters that are being validated for the method. Most organizations have an appropriate standard operating procedure (SOP) that outlines these requirements for a validation. In the absence of a formal SOP, we recommend development of a validation plan that outlines the experimental design to evaluate each performance characteristic, including target acceptance criteria. Upon completion of the validation experiments, a report that comprehensively describes the experiments, the results obtained and the conclusions should be written. It is also important to finalize the analytical method that was validated with updated information and the final acceptance criteria.

4.4   ANALYTICAL PERFORMANCE CHARACTERISTICS

Table 4.4 lists the analytical performance characteristics that need to be confirmed during the prestudy validation phase [4–5,9]. In addition, this table highlights the activities that are needed to progress from method development to help ensure the method will meet the prestudy *a priori* criteria for method acceptance and for successful acceptance of batch runs (in-study validation).

4.4.1   Reference Material

Even though Chapter 9 provides details and recommendations for macromolecular reference materials, a discussion concerning GLP BMV of biotherapeutics is not complete without at least a brief discussion of the reference material. Often a "gold standard" reference standard, as understood for a conventional small-molecule drug, is not available for a biotherapeutic. This is particularly true in nonclinical and early clinical studies prior to Phase II and III studies. Consequently, use of a well-characterized material may be the only option during the prestudy BMV and in-study analyses of the test samples. Some of the issues inherent for reference standards of biotherapeutics are described in Table 4.5. Stability is more complicated for biotherapeutics than conventional small molecules, as they are susceptible to chemical (e.g., deamidation, disulfide bond cleavage, etc.), physical (e.g., aggregation, adsorption, precipitation), and biological instability (e.g., matrix-based proteases). Therefore, documentation (e.g., certificate of analysis) on the origin and characteristics of a reference material is pivotal for BMV of biotherapeutics. Moreover, it is important to clearly state the source of the material and refer to any documentation describing characteristics of that material. Ideally, the reference standard is formulated in a buffer-based medium that provides maximum long-term storage stability. Usually, frozen storage conditions (e.g., -70°C) are preferable for macromolecules. When feasible, the standards, the validation samples, and QC samples should be prepared from separate aliquots of the same source material. In circumstances of limited availability of reference standard material, standards

TABLE 4.4 Summary of Analytical Performance Characteristics [4,5]

Performance Characteristic	Method Development	Prestudy Validation (Validation Phase)	In-Study Validation (Implementation Phase, Sample Analysis Phase)
Assay reagent selection/stability/ assay format/batch size	Identify; establish	Confirm	Monitor, lot changes require confirmation of performance
Specificity and Selectivity	Establish	Confirm	Confirm in diseased states as available
Matrix selection/sample preparation/minimum required dilution	Establish	Confirm, for modified matrices, QCs must be prepared in relevant neat matrix	Monitor; with changes to lot of matrix, comparability must be demonstrated
Standard calibrators and standard curves	Select model	Confirm	Monitor
Precision and accuracy	Evaluate imprecision and bias	Establish imprecision and bias	Total error or 4-6-30
Range of quantification	Evaluate	Establish	Apply
Sample stability	Initiate	Establish	Ongoing assessment and extension
Dilutional linearity	Evaluate	Establish	Monitor and establish dilutions not covered in prestudy validation
Parallelism	N/A	Investigate where possible	Establish with incurred samples
Robustness/ruggedness	Evaluate	Establish	Monitor
Partial validation/method transfer/cross-validation	N/A	N/A	Apply as appropriate
Run acceptance criteria	N/A	Runs accepted based on standard curve acceptance criteria	Standard curve and QC acceptance criteria. Apply 4-6-30 rule or other appropriate statistical criteria that align with the prestudy acceptance criteria

TABLE 4.5   Issues for Reference Standards of Biotherapeutics

Often heterogeneous (e.g., product differs in posttranslational modification or degree
   of substitution with polyethylene glycol)
Variability within and between lots
Less well characterized than small-molecule drugs
Absence of "gold standard" method for characterization
Impurities are "biological" for protein therapeutics
Susceptibility to change with process modifications and scale-up
Physical characterization may not predict "bioactivity"
Official reference may not be available until registration studies

and QC samples can be prepared from single aliquots after checking the
comparability between lots or other commercial sources. Lot numbers, batch numbers, and supporting documentation should be monitored and documented carefully.

    Because biotherapeutics have a greater potential for lot-to-lot variability in terms of
their purity and potency, it is usually advisable to develop and validate bioanalytical
methods using a reference material that is equivalent to the relevant study drug.
The reference material used in the nonclinical/clinical study may have different
properties (e.g., posttranslational modifications), which could theoretically result in
the alteration of binding and analytical performance, rendering the method unsuitable
for its intended purpose. This situation is depicted in Fig. 4.2. This issue is also relevant
to immunoassays of biotherapeutic drugs that are analogues or truncated forms of
endogenous proteins/peptides. We recommend that new lots of reference standards
undergo a systematic evaluation to qualify them prior to utilization in supporting
PK and TK assessments.

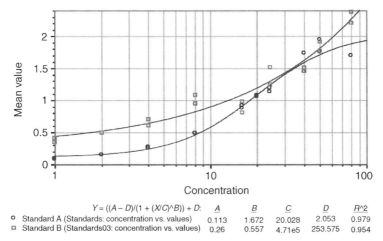

FIGURE 4.2   Graphical representation of a standard curve performance after a change in
reference material. Standard A (open circles) was used during prestudy validation, while
Standard B (open squares) was the reference material used during the clinical study.

An additional aspect of having the appropriate reference material is critical in the quantification of therapeutics when an endogenous counterpart is in the matrix. The assay specificity and the accuracy of the measurements must be evaluated carefully under these conditions to account for the endogenous counterpart, as the exogenously administered drug may or may not be immunoanalytically equivalent. Accordingly, depending on the binding properties of the ligands used in the assay, there could be either an underestimation or an overestimation of the measured concentrations when an endogenous protein is present in the biological matrix.

4.4.2 Specificity and Selectivity

As defined in ICH Q2(R1), specificity is the concept that expresses the ability of an analytical method to assess unequivocally an analyte of interest (i.e., macromolecular therapeutic) in the presence of other components that are expected to be present in the test sample [11]. For LBAs, the degree of specificity of the macromolecular binder (i.e., antibodies, receptors, etc.) for the ligand of interest (i.e., biotherapeutic) is the principal factor that governs a method's specificity and, therefore, the suitability of a LBA for its intended purpose. The macromolecular binder needs to be highly specific for the biotherapeutic, as LBAs are used typically without sample pretreatment procedures, such as extraction. Ideally, the antibody (i.e., macromolecular binder) is specific for the biotherapeutic of interest and lacks cross-reactivity with variant forms (i.e., metabolites and degraded forms) and other structurally related materials (i.e., endogenous equivalents) that may be present in the test sample. Following administration of a biotherapeutic, it is not uncommon for different cleaved forms to be found in the circulation. Sometimes it may be impossible to discern the effect of truncated forms and their immunoreactivity completely. However, attempts should be made to understand how these different variant forms affect the measured concentration. Moreover, these results should be communicated to the pharmacokineticist for the proper interpretation of the pharmacokinetic parameters. For example, if the assay is a bridging assay for a fusion protein and it is necessary for the fusion protein to be intact for the detection by the antibody reagents used, one can be reasonably assured that the assay determines the intact molecule and does not detect those metabolites that have lost this key molecular feature. Although specificity of a method for a particular macromolecule can neither be measured directly nor demonstrated absolutely, it can be evaluated empirically by assessing systematically the cross-reactivity of any available structurally related materials that might be expected to be present in the test sample.

Selectivity, a concept related to specificity, is a measure of the extent to which the method can determine the analyte of interest in a biological matrix without interference from other constituents in the test sample (i.e., matrix components). Again, because LBAs determine analytes in the biological matrix without sample pretreatment, this methodology is prone to interference from components present in the sample matrix. Specificity and selectivity evaluations are conducted in prevalidation and confirmed early in prestudy validation.

For LBA methodology, it is helpful to categorize nonspecificity into two types, specific nonspecificity and nonspecific nonspecificity [9,13,14]. *Specific nonspecificity* results from the assay interference from compounds that have similar physicochemical properties to that of the analyte (i.e., endogenous compounds, isoforms, metabolites, degraded forms, and variants with different posttranslational modifications but similar binding epitopes). *Specific nonspecificity* is evaluated usually by performing experiments to evaluate the extent of cross-reactivity from potential interfering substances. Accordingly, cross-reactivity experiments require insight into the structure of potentially cross-reactive substances and their availability in purified form to permit testing in the LBA.

Nonspecific nonspecificity results from interference of matrix components that are structurally unrelated to the analyte of interest. Examples of such interfering matrix components would include serum proteins, lipids, heterophilic antibodies, rheumatoid factor, proteases, and so on. *Nonspecific nonspecificity* is often referred to as "matrix effect." Figure 4.3 depicts the impact of matrix on the assay performance. Matrix interference is one of the chief reasons that LBAs often require more method development and validation prior to switching from one species matrix to another or even within the same species. In addition, we recommend during clinical study support that matrix from the relevant disease populations be tested for matrix effects as soon as that matrix becomes available. Matrix effects should be evaluated by comparing the concentration–response relationship of both spiked and unspiked samples of the biological matrix (recommendation is 10 or more lots of individual sources) to a comparable buffer solution. It is recommended that the spiked sample

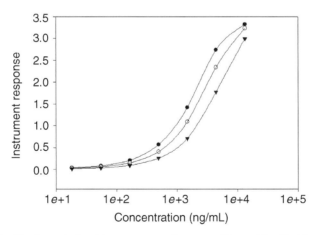

FIGURE 4.3   The impact of matrix on assay performance. The matrix effect (nonspecificity) could be additive or inhibitory. The open circles represent the standard curve when the macromolecular therapeutic was spiked into a buffer matrix. The solid circles represent an additive effect when the standard curve was prepared in 100% matrix, and the closed triangles represent an example where there was an inhibitory effect when the standards were prepared in 100% matrix.

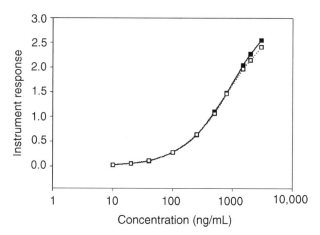

FIGURE 4.4 Elimination of matrix effect with minimum required dilution. The open squares are for the standard curve in buffer and the closed squares represent a standard curve prepared in pooled serum, pretreated 1:30 with I-block buffer.

concentrations be at the low and high ends of the dynamic range. Often *nonspecific nonspecificity* can be reduced or eliminated by dilution of the matrix with a buffer. The least dilution of matrix required to eliminate or reduce matrix interference to acceptable levels is referred to as the minimal required dilution (MRD). Figure 4.4 depicts an example where the matrix effect was eliminated by using a MRD of 1:30 in a buffer. In the cases where sample dilution is not an option, other sample cleanup procedures may be employed. Some examples include selective precipitation, liquid–liquid, solid-phase, and immunoaffinity extractions, where interferences are more pronounced. It is important to remember that sensitivity, or lower limit of quantification (LLOQ), needs to be reported in terms of the concentration of the therapeutic in the original undiluted test sample.

During prestudy validation, the performance of the assay with respect to specificity and selectivity is confirmed with the most relevant compounds and matrices. Selectivity is expressed as acceptable recovery, using the same criteria that are applied during the assessment of accuracy. The recommended target acceptance criterion for selectivity is that acceptable recovery (e.g., 80–120% relative to buffer control) is obtained in at least 80% of the matrices evaluated.

4.4.3 Calibration Model Assessment

The topic of nonlinear calibration for LBAs, such as immunoassays, has been reviewed in detail in a number of publications [4,8,9,15–17]. Typically, immunoassay calibration curves are inherently nonlinear [9]. Because the response–error relationship is a nonconstant function of the mean response, weighting is needed to account for the heterogeneity in response variances. The four- or five-parameter logistic models are accepted widely as the standard models for fitting nonlinear sigmoidal calibration data [3–5,8,9,16,17]. This model can be described arithmetically by the following equation:

$$Y = D + \left(\frac{A-D}{[1+(X/C)^{\wedge}B]} \right)$$

where Y is the expected response, A is the response at zero concentration, D is the response at infinite concentration, C is the concentration at the halfway point between A and D responses, and B is the slope factor (typically near 1.0). The four-parameter logistic model is a specific case of the more generalized five-parameter logistic model in which the dose–response relationship is assumed to be symmetric around the inflection point (ED_{50}) [15,16]. This is usually a valid assumption for competitive assays, such as RIAs. However for noncompetitive assays (i.e., sandwich ELISAs) in which the upper asymptote is not well defined, a better overall fit is often obtained with the five-parameter logistic model that does not assume symmetry in the dose–response relationship. Examples of four- and five-parameter logistic model curve fits are depicted in Fig. 4.5, which illustrate the symmetrical and asymmetrical nature of these models, respectively.

Statistical approaches for selection of the calibration models are described elsewhere in this book. The best practices with respect to selecting the calibration model and assessing the placement of calibration points will be discussed below. During the method development phase, it is recommended that standard curve concentration–response data from a minimum of three independent batch runs be analyzed when establishing a calibration model. A greater number of standard points and replicates should be included during method development to facilitate a detailed investigation of the concentration–response relationship. The number of standard points and replicates should be large enough to provide a reliable assessment of all competing regression models. Standard calibrators should span the anticipated concentration range for diluted study samples with concentrations approximately evenly spaced on a logarithmic scale. A minimum of 10 nonzero standard points in duplicate are recommended for the early characterization of a concentration–response relationship fit using the four- or five-parameter logistic (4/5PL) functions [4,5]. Standard points outside of the range of quantification (anchor calibrators) are often useful for assisting in fitting these nonlinear regression models [8–10,12,14–16]. Even though the utility of anchor calibrators has been a topic of discussion and debate, a sound mathematical argument can be made for including them to optimize curve fitting for sigmoidal dose–response relationships. As the intricacies of nonlinear calibration become more understood, it is likely the use of anchor calibrators will become less of a topic of discussion within the bioanalytical community and regulatory bodies. Inclusion of duplicate curves in each of the assays is highly desirable to permit an evaluation of the intrabatch standard curve repeatability.

The appropriateness of a model is judged by analysis of the relative error (RE) for back-calculated standard points. In general, the absolute RE for each back-calculated standard point should be $\leq 20\%$ for most points within a curve. For a calibration model to be considered acceptable, the accumulated back-calculated values from all the

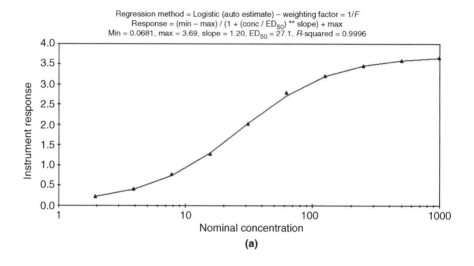

Regression method = Logistic (auto estimate) – weighting factor = $1/F$
Response = (min – max) / (1 + (conc / ED_{50}) ** slope) + max
Min = 0.0681, max = 3.69, slope = 1.20, ED_{50} = 27.1, R-squared = 0.9996

(a)

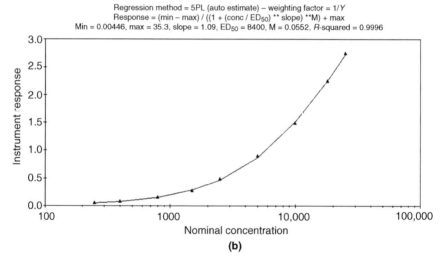

Regression method = 5PL (auto estimate) – weighting factor = $1/Y$
Response = (min – max) / ((1 + (conc / ED_{50}) ** slope) **M) + max
Min = 0.00446, max = 35.3, slope = 1.09, ED_{50} = 8400, M = 0.0552, R-squared = 0.9996

(b)

FIGURE 4.5 (a) Typical four-parameter regression model. (b) Typical five-parameter regression model.

curves should have an absolute *mean* RE of $\leq 10\%$ and a coefficient of variation (CV) of $\leq 15\%$ for all concentrations within the anticipated validated range. A systematic deviation (trend) in the mean RE versus calibrator concentrations (i.e., calculated concentrations consistently above or consistently below the nominal concentrations) is evidence for a "lack of fit" that can invalidate a model (i.e., result in unacceptable accuracy and precision for validation samples). A lack of fit can result from use of either an inappropriate mean function (e.g., using the 4PL function when the response curve is asymmetric) or a weighting procedure. Once a few standard curves have been established, it is advisable to fit the data to a few different models and calculate the RE for each of the models to select the appropriate regression model and

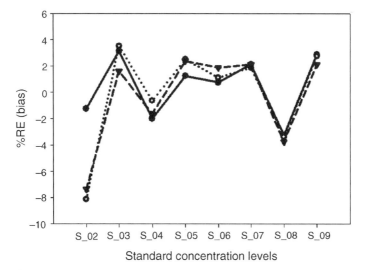

FIGURE 4.6   An example showing the use of weighting factors and regression models to a validation data set. Solid circle represents a 5PL curve fitting with weighting, open circle represents a 5PL curve without weighting, and the inverted triangle represents a 4PL curve without weighting. It is apparent that the use of weighting reduces the %bias at the lower end of the curve. Use of the 4 or 5-parameter regression models without weighting does ot reduce the %bias at the lower end of the curve.

the weighting factor. If use of weighting results in better curve fits, particularly near the extremes of the standard curve, this is evidenced by a reduction in the mean RE (Fig. 4.6) at lower concentrations.

Once the method has been optimized during prevalidation (i.e., calibration model and weighting are selected but not confirmed), it is necessary to finalize the concentrations of the calibration standards that will be used in the prestudy validation. Usually, a minimum of six nonzero calibrators in duplicate should be included within the anticipated validated range for a concentration–response relationship fit using the 4/5PL function, excluding anchor points. The regression model established during method development should be confirmed in a minimum of six independent prestudy validation runs. These are typically the same runs in which the method precision and accuracy are assessed. The target acceptance criteria established during the method development phase need to be clearly stated prior to execution of the prestudy validation runs. The standard concentrations should not be changed once assay validation has begun. During prestudy validation, the general recommendation for the curve within a run to be acceptable is that the %RE of the back-calculated values for at least 75% of the standard points, not including anchor points, should be within 20% of the nominal concentration, except at the LLOQ where the value should be within 25%. At the end of validation, the cumulative mean %RE and percent CV from all runs should be calculated for each calibrator. Accordingly, the regression model is judged to acceptable if the cumulative mean RE and CV are ≤15% for each standard calibrator, not including anchor points, except at the LLOQ where both should be $\leq 20\%$. The use of the correlation coefficient is strongly discouraged for making conclusions regarding a model's "goodness of fit" [4,9,17,19,20].

In some instances, these recommended *a priori* acceptance criteria for model acceptance may be too restrictive and more lenient criteria may be appropriate with suitable justification and documentation. Model confirmation should precede the reporting of analytical results for validation samples. The standard curve for each in-study run (study sample analysis) should be monitored using the same criteria used during prestudy validation.

Criteria and procedures for editing of standard points during the prestudy validation, as well as during the sample analysis phase, should clearly be documented and comply with internal SOPs. Generally, standard points are run in duplicate and the mean of the response should be fitted instead of the individual responses. In situations where the RE or the %CV between the replicates is outside of the acceptance criteria (e.g., >20%), the standard point can be edited. Unless prior data, or other rationales, exist to support the elimination of a specific replicate, our recommended practice is to eliminate both replicates and fit the standard curve through the remaining calibrators. If a standard point is edited, the curve must be refitted before assessing the validity of the validation samples or the QC samples. The final number of standard calibrators remaining after editing must be either $\geq 75\%$ of the total or a minimum of six, not including anchor calibrators. The details of standard curve calibration point selection to be used during method validation are described in detail in DeSilva et al. [4] and Findlay et al. [9].

4.4.4 Precision/Accuracy and Role of QCs

For this discussion, the definitions of accuracy and precision are those that have been reported in recent publications concerning BMV of LBAs [3–5,9,10,18,20]. It is worth pointing out that mean bias is used to approximate method accuracy. Even though accuracy is usually considered to be the same as "trueness" (difference between the *mean* measured amount and the accepted true concentration, ICH Q2(R1) [9,11,21]), acceptable spike recovery data during BMV do not guarantee good accuracy for analyses of test samples. This is because quantification is based on immunoreactivity (i.e., antigen recognition). As such, a validated immunoassay may not be able to detect the structural differences among macromolecules that are closely related, such as metabolites, degraded forms, endogenous homologues, and products of posttranslational modifications.

Method precision (random error, variation) and accuracy (systematic error, mean bias) for LBAs should be evaluated by analyzing validation samples (QC samples) that are prepared in a biological matrix that is judged scientifically to be representative of the anticipated study samples [18]. This topic has been reviewed in other publications [3–6,9,10,20]. These performance characteristics should be evaluated during the method development phase, taking into consideration the factors known to vary in the method (e.g., analysts, instruments, reagents, different days, etc.). Several concentrations are required during the method development phase and are assayed in replicates. Factors known to vary between runs (e.g., analyst, instrument, and day) that may affect the variation in analytical results should be identified and documented (see later section on robustness and ruggedness evaluation for more details). Method accuracy, intrabatch (within-run) precision, and interbatch (between-run) precision should be established preliminarily during method development and confirmed in prestudy validation. QC samples are used during in-study sample analysis to monitor assay performance characteristics. Design and analysis recommendations for precision and accuracy assessments of LBAs for biotherapeutics are summarized in Table 4.6 [4].

Prestudy precision and accuracy assessments require the comparison of calculated performance measures with *a priori* target limits that specify the amount of (analytical) error allowable without compromising the intended use and interpretation of test results [22]. Limits for the minimum acceptable precision and accuracy should be established before or during method development and used throughout the assay life cycle. At least five or more concentration levels (anticipated LLOQ, less than three times LLOQ, mid, high, and anticipated upper limit of quantification (ULOQ)), with at least two independent determinations per assay should be run during the prestudy validation phase. Because the interbatch variance component is usually higher in LBAs than the intrabatch variance component, it is recommended that at least six independent (for each run dilutions prepared for each calibrator) batch runs be conducted during prestudy validation to provide more reliable estimates of the method's accuracy, precision, and the total error. For each validation sample, the repeated measurements from all runs should be analyzed together using an appropriate statistical method [4,9,10].

4.4.5 Range of Quantification (LLOQ/ULOQ)

The range of quantification, commonly referred to as the "validated range," is the concentration range between the established lowest (LLOQ) and highest (ULOQ) validation samples that meet the targeted precision and accuracy criteria. Due to the inherently nonlinear sigmoidal nature of LBA standard curves, it is necessary to define both the lower and upper ends of the quantification range. Although the FDA guidance [18] states that the lower limit of quantification should be the lowest standard on the standard curve, this may not be feasible in fitting nonlinear regression models.

The preliminary estimates of the range of quantification can be established during the method development phase using multiple standard curves. The % bias (RE) can be calculated from each of the regression models in a similar manner that was used to establish the model as described above. The LLOQ and the ULOQ can be estimated by examining the precision profile (Fig. 4.7). The variability in LBAs arises mainly from the interassay component and it is essential to include data from multiple runs over a period of time in the compilation of the precision profile. Data generated during the method development phase will enable setting of the targets for the LLOQ and the ULOQ, and must be confirmed using the data from the prestudy validation experiments.

During the prestudy validation phase, samples should be spiked at the anticipated LLOQ and the ULOQ of the assay. These validation samples should be assayed as part

TABLE 4.6 Precision and Accuracy Assessment Criteria

Assessment Topic	Method Development	Prestudy Validation	In-Study Validation
Design:			
1. Number of batch runs	≥ 3	≥ 6	1
2. Number of VS or QC sample concentrations	≥ 8	≥ 5	≥ 3
3. Concentration levels	Span calibrator range	LLOQ, LQC, MQC, HQC, ULOQ	LQC, MQC, HQC
4. Number of replicate results/batch	≥ 2	≥ 2	≥ 2
Analysis:			
5. Compute performance statistics	Use appropriate statistical methods to compute these values. For example, EXCEL program for computation of accuracy/precision summary statistics for prestudy methods validation (http://www.aapspharmaceutica.com/inside/sections/biotec/applications/lba.asp)	%RE of QC result	

TABLE 4.6 (Continued)

Assessment Topic	Method Development	Prestudy Validation	In-Study Validation
6. Compare statistics to target limits			
a. Bias (%RE)	±20 (25 at LLOQ and ULOQ)	±20 (25 at LLOQ and ULOQ)	—
b. Intrabatch precision (%CV)	≤20 (25 at LLOQ and ULOQ)	≤20 (25 at LLOQ and ULOQ)	—
c. Interbatch precision (%CV)	≤20 (25 at LLOQ and ULOQ)	≤20 (25 at LLOQ and ULOQ)	—
d. Total error (%RE)	—	—	±30 (±40% at the LLOQ and ULOQ)
Acceptance criteria:			
Part 1: Apply limits separately	Calculated bias and precision satisfy 6a, 6b, 6c	"4-6-30 rule"	
Part 2: Combined limit	|Bias %RE| + interbatch precision %CV ≤30		

Recommended analysis and acceptance criteria apply to each sample concentration. HQC = high-quality control sample; LQC = low-quality control sample; MQC = middle quality control sample; ULOQ = upper limit of quantification sample; %CV = percent coefficient of variation; %RE = percent relative error [4].

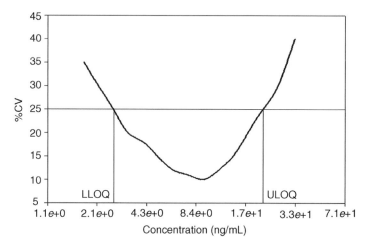

FIGURE 4.7 A typical precision profile.

of the accuracy and precision assessment. The validation samples should be prepared in the undiluted matrix of the anticipated samples. In circumstances where there is a minimum required dilution prior to the analysis, the range of quantification should be reported as the concentration in 100% matrix. As an example, a standard curve of 100–1000 ng/mL in neat matrix is equivalent to an in-assay/on-plate standard curve range of 10–100 ng/mL with an MRD of 10 (i.e., 10% matrix). However, the assay LLOQ remains at 100 ng/mL due to the MRD of 1:10 for all samples being assayed. The recommended acceptance criteria for establishing the range of quantification are determined by the lowest and highest validation samples for which the precision (interbatch %CV) and accuracy (absolute %RE) are both ≤20% (25% at the LLOQ and ULOQ) and the sum of the two is ≤30% [4,10,23].

Once the range of quantification is confirmed during the prestudy validation phase, this should be the calibrator range used during in-study sample analysis for reporting test sample results. The LLOQ and the ULOQ of the assay can be monitored by inclusion of standard curve points at these levels during in-study sample analysis. Any study samples that fall above the ULOQ need to be reanalyzed after appropriate dilution so that the results will fall within the standard curve's range of quantification. Any study samples that are below the LLOQ and are at the lowest dilution would be reported as below the quantifiable limit (BQL), taking into account any required MRD.

There may be situations during sample analysis in which the LLOQ or the ULOQ standard point is removed due to a technical error or other *a priori* determined acceptance criterion. The practical outcome is a truncated standard curve, that is, in the case where the LLOQ standard is revised, then the next highest level standard becomes the LLOQ for this run. This revised standard curve should then be used in the evaluation of the study samples from that particular run, rejecting (for repeat analysis) any study samples read below the new LLOQ. In general, the study samples that fall between the revised LLOQ and the original assay LLOQ are repeated in a separate run to avoid having samples reported against two LLOQ values in the pharmacokinetic data. Appropriate SOPs or documentation that clearly describe the reporting of the data in these situations must be in place prior to sample analysis phase. Alternatively, this issue can be mitigated by inclusion of anchor calibrators below and above the limits of quantification.

A common phenomenon that occurs during the sample analysis phase is a change in the matrix for studies in different patient populations. Even though the prestudy validation should be reflective of the in-study sample analysis, during the clinical development of a therapeutic candidate, multiple indications can be recommended. In situations such as these, if the patient matrix has interferences that were not anticipated during the prestudy validation phase, these need to be evaluated as described in the selectivity section. However, the range of quantification may be affected based on this evaluation and must be re-evaluated if needed (e.g., if a rheumatoid arthritis population is being tested, then the interference from rheumatoid factor or autoantibodies may necessitate the use of a higher MRD). If this occurs, then the range of quantification may need to be revised for analysis of samples from these clinical trials.

4.4.6 Dilutional Linearity and Parallelism

Dilutional linearity and parallelism are important analytical performance characteristics due to the indirect and limited range nature of LBAs [4,9]. As noted in previous sections, the quantification range (i.e., validated range from LLOQ to ULOQ) is more limited for LBAs due to their nonlinear calibration curves. LBAs are typically designed to provide maximal sensitivity to allow definition of the terminal elimination phase of a biotherapeutic. As a consequence, peak drug concentrations (i.e., near C_{max}) are often above the ULOQ due to the limited quantification range (usually about 2 logs). Therefore, in prestudy validation, it is necessary to document analyte recovery after dilution (i.e., dilutional linearity), as a means of achieving analyte concentrations within the standard curve's validated range. Dilutional linearity experiments are performed by "spiking" a pool of matrix deemed to be equivalent to the test sample matrix with the analyte of interest at a concentration that exceeds the anticipated highest matrix concentration for a nonclinical/clinical study [4,9]. Thus, for designing dilutional linearity experiments in prestudy validation, it is helpful to have input on anticipated matrix concentrations of the macromolecule and planned routes of administration. For dilutional linearity experiments, it is not uncommon to utilize matrix samples that have the biotherapeutic spiked at 100–1000 times higher than the anticipated ULOQ [4]. As reported previously, dilutional linearity experiments can be utilized to help detect the presence of a "high-dose Hook effect" in noncompetitive immunoassays [4]. We recommend that a minimum of three dilutions of the spiked sample into the standard curve range should be utilized to evaluate dilutional linearity. The resultant concentrations, after dilution, should "target" different ranges of the standard curve (e.g., lower third, mid-range near EC_{50}, upper third) to enable detection of nonlinearity. Prestudy acceptance criteria for dilutional linearity require that the *mean* cumulative back-calculated concentration, after correction for dilution, needs to be within $\pm 20\%$ of the nominal concentration at each dilution evaluated [4].

If repeated measures are performed, a predefined percentage of the diluted samples also needs to meet the specified ±20% criterion (e.g., at least two-thirds). The precision (CV) of the cumulative back-calculated concentrations should also be within ±20%. If a systematic deviation is found after dilution, additional investigation may be warranted to explain the observed bias. Dilutional QC samples are utilized sometimes during in-study analyses. In these situations, it is important to have *a priori* criteria for run acceptance.

Procedurally, dilutional linearity should not be confused with the MRD of an assay. The MRD is a designed integral part of an analytical method and involves a predefined dilution of test samples, QC samples and, often, calibrators usually with a buffer-based matrix. In contrast, dilution linearity is used only to support analysis of study samples that exceed the assay's ULOQ and involves dilution(s) intended to result in an analyte concentration within the standard curve's validated range. Another notable difference is that, while MRD is usually performed in buffer, dilutional linearity is performed in matrix, often the same one used to prepare the standard curve.

Parallelism for an analyte in a test sample is a necessary condition for method validity when the analytical response is displayed as a function of the log of the analyte concentration [10]. Parallelism is assessed by analyzing a high-concentration study sample (e.g., around the maximum plasma concentration) at multiple dilutions and then examining for a constant recovery of the measured analyte. Because parallelism involves analysis of test samples after *in vivo* drug administration, it provides insight into whether biotransformation or serum–protein binding produces potential interference by detection of nonlinearity after dilution. As a target, it is recommended that the CV between samples in a dilution series be ±30% [4,9]. Demonstration of nonparallelism indicates a problem that requires some follow-up action. Conversely, demonstration of parallelism is not an indication of accuracy, as there could still be interfering compounds that may have parallel curves to that of the analyte of interest. It should be pointed out that parallelism can only be assessed once *in vivo* studies have been conducted and samples are available. For this reason, parallelism is usually not included during prestudy validation but is conducted later on and reported as an addendum to the validation report. Finally, even though parallelism is a useful diagnostic for method validity, acceptance criteria for suitable parallelism should be defined *a priori*. We do not recommend that investigators test statistically for a lack of parallelism (i.e., no change in recovery as a function of dilution), as an acceptable method could have a small but acceptable degree of nonparallelism.

4.4.7 Sample Stability (In-Process, Frozen, and Freeze–Thaw)

The concentration data that are being derived from any bioanalytical method, irrespective of the technology used, are determined from analysis of the therapeutic candidate in biological matrix. In most cases, study samples are frozen and shipped to the laboratories for analysis. It is crucial that the stability of the therapeutic in the biological matrix be evaluated under the conditions of storage and processing [10]. The stability of the therapeutic in the desired matrix plays an important part in the selection of the matrix. For example, a labile therapeutic that may not withstand the process of clotting and the time required to prepare serum may have to be assayed in plasma. Another aspect to consider is the effect of freezing and thawing of the therapeutic in the chosen matrix. Although most bioanalytical assays are performed on samples that have been stored frozen for logistical reasons, the effects of storage conditions must be monitored and evaluated as a component of assay validation.

During the method development phase, preliminary stability experiments must be evaluated, for example, stability in blood, suitable matrix (plasma or serum), and length of time the drug can be exposed to ambient room temperature conditions, and so on. Processing and storage conditions assessed usually include benchtop stability, short-term and long-term storage, and stability to multiple freeze–thaw cycles. If the intended application of the LBA method requires the preparation and storage of "intermediate" concentrated stocks of standard solutions, the stability of these solutions under the conditions of storage should be investigated. The formal stability evaluations must be conducted during the prestudy validation phase with the assay that will support the planned studies.

Stability experiments should mimic, as best possible, the conditions under which study samples will be collected, stored, and processed. It is necessary to evaluate the stability conditions with at least two concentrations that represent the lower and the higher concentration ranges. Evaluation of the stability samples should be conducted with a freshly prepared standard curve. On the contrary, the assay QCs (in-study batch QCs) may be from the batches stored frozen within the established stability, or prepared fresh. There is still ongoing discussion regarding this topic. In either situation, what is necessary is a sound scientific justification for evaluation of the stability samples. Another facet to this is the situation where altered matrices are used for standard curve and QC preparations; in this case, stability samples must be prepared in the unaltered matrix.

An important issue that pertains specifically to LBAs is the availability of reference material and matrix during the long-term stability evaluations. The stability QCs may be prepared with a reference material that was from an initial manufacturing lot (e.g., during the first-in-human study support) and may not have been placed on an extended stability program for the reference material itself. Subsequent preparations of the standards and assay QCs for the evaluation of long-term stability samples may be affected in these scenarios; for example, the immunoreactivity may be different. A similar situation may occur for the matrix, where the matrix lot used for the preparation of stability QCs may not match the matrix in which the later standards and assay QCs are prepared. These scenarios or case studies are important for LBAs since specificity and selectivity parameters are critical in LBA validations. In both of these situations, it is recommended that aliquots of the reference material and adequate quantities of matrix be secured to perform the long-term stability evaluations. As discussed briefly above, if the matrix in the diseased patient population is different, then long-term stability evaluations should be considered in the relevant patient-derived matrix.

Stability assessments are often conducted by spiking the macromolecular therapeutic into whole blood, as well as into the resultant matrices after whole blood processing (plasma and/or serum). The stability evaluations should be conducted with spiked samples in the matrix deemed to be equivalent to that of anticipated study samples. For clinical studies, it is common practice to use matrix from normal healthy adults to evaluate stability. However, we recommend evaluating stability in the matrix from patients with disease or the matrix of the study samples, even when the matrix is rare and difficult to obtain (e.g., fetal serum, CSF, different oncology populations, etc.). Because differences in the matrix components (e.g., enhanced protease activity) can affect the stability of the therapeutic, it is valuable to understand the physiochemical properties of the macromolecule during the evaluation of the stability (e.g., whether there is a need for adding a protease inhibitor cocktail during collection, or whether the molecule is relatively hydrophobic, which may warrant the use of highly proteinaceous buffers for storage, etc.).

The details of the assessment of stability data are under intense discussion within the scientific community. A majority of laboratories evaluate data with acceptance criteria relative to the nominal concentration of the spiked sample. The rationale for this is that it is not feasible to introduce more stringent criteria for stability evaluations than that of the assay acceptance criterion. Another common approach is to compare data against a "baseline concentration" (or day zero concentration) of a bulk preparation of "stability samples" established by repeated analysis, either during the accuracy and precision evaluations, or by other means. This evaluation then eliminates any systematic errors that may have occurred in the preparation of the stability samples. A more statistically acceptable method of stability data evaluations would be to use confidence intervals or perform trend analysis on the data [24]. In this case, when the observed concentration or response of the stability sample is beyond the lower confidence interval (as set *a priori*), the data indicate a lack of analyte stability under the conditions evaluated.

For most antibody therapeutics, the stability in blood is not evaluated. However, the stability in blood should be evaluated for other proteins; for example, if the protein has a heparin-binding domain, collection of plasma using heparin as the anticoagulant needs to be evaluated. This evaluation should be done on a case-by-case basis based on the properties of the therapeutic.

A common approach to performing the above evaluation is to draw blood from subjects, add the appropriate concentrations of the therapeutic into the blood, then process the blood, either to plasma or to serum, under common clinical laboratory conditions. Examples of such conditions may include processing immediately following collection, leaving the blood sample for at least 2 h at room temperature prior to processing or storing in the refrigerator, and so on. Depending on the drug development phase, it may be necessary to evaluate storage for longer periods of time in blood. This may be useful when large clinical studies are conducted at multiple sites to generate a set of sample-specific processing requirements, with limits, that the clinical sites must follow. Once the plasma or serum is obtained, the most common stability conditions that are evaluated pertain to the container used for storage of the sample. Typically, polypropylene containers are used to store the samples; however, the use of caps with and without silicone O-rings may become an important parameter to evaluate. Other conditions include the size of the vials, especially during the preclinical phases, where the sample volume is smaller and the container size should be appropriate for the size of the sample.

The freeze–thaw stability evaluation should take into account the anticipated freeze–thaw cycles during routine sample analysis. A standard approach is four freeze–thaw cycles with no less than 12 h frozen storage between unassisted thaws. The rate of freezing and thawing should take into account the known properties of the therapeutic as well as the manner in which samples will be handled as they are being thawed before assaying. For example, labile molecules may require a slow thawing process on ice.

Benchtop stability (sometimes also referred to as short-term stability) involves evaluation of the stability of the therapeutic during the execution of the assay, for example, testing the limits of time the samples can be on the bench during processing, testing whether the samples can be pretreated (MRD performed) and stored overnight under refrigerated conditions, and so on [25].

The determination of long-term storage stability must take into account the storage at both the sample collection site and at the testing facility. It is essential to show that the samples are stable throughout the lifetime of a study, including the time required to complete all required reanalyses. The intervals for stability testing depend on the needs of the study. For clinical studies that span a very long period, stability analysis may need to be conducted at more frequent intervals, and for a longer period, to ensure that samples can be stored until the end of a study before sample analysis is conducted, if need be. The need to conduct studies on samples stored at both $-20°C$ and -70 to $-80°C$ may depend on the duration of storage at $-20°C$. If samples are to be frozen at $-20°C$, followed by storage at $-80°C$, the stability samples should be prepared in the same manner, with the time at $-20°C$ modeled as well as can be predicted. In many cases, long-term stability assessments often continue during the sample analysis.

The most recent white paper on the best practices for chromatographic and LBAs highly recommends the formal testing of stability of the reagents used in LBAs [10], for example, antibodies, antibody conjugates (e.g., horse radish peroxidase, biotin, and avidin conjugates). Therefore, during method development and validation, proper storage of these reagents should be clearly documented and maintained during the in-study support. Suitable stability data should be generated to demonstrate acceptable performance of the critical reagents over longer periods of time under the specified storage conditions. In most situations, the data are generated at the same time that the sample analysis is being performed. The recommendations in this white paper also allow the use of manufacturer's data if the reagents are commercially available and stored as per the manufacturer's recommendations.

4.4.8 Robustness and Ruggedness

Robustness and ruggedness are two analytical performance characteristics that are related closely, and often not easy to distinguish. The main focus of any robustness/ruggedness investigation is to address the question of whether the assay will be able to withstand changes in the standard laboratory conditions. The robustness of an analytical procedure is a measure of its capacity to remain unaffected by small, but deliberate variations in method parameters and provides an indication of its reliability during normal usage [11]. The ruggedness of an assay is determined by its consistency when routine changes are implemented resulting in different operational conditions [28].

Elements in an immunoassay that could impact its robustness include incubation temperatures, light exposure (enzyme-linked immunosorbent assay, ELISA), and different lots of matrix (plasma, serum CSF). The ruggedness of the analytical method can be tested by implementing changes to the analysts, different instruments, batch size, and the day, time, or other environment factors otherwise should not greatly impact the consistency of the assay.

During the prestudy evaluation phase, an attempt should be made to evaluate the variety of conditions that may reflect the execution and performance of the method during the in-study phase. The final conditions should be clearly documented in the analytical procedures prior to in-study sample analysis. As an example, robustness assessment could include incubation time tolerances, while ruggedness assessment could include changes in analysts and batch size (Table 4.7). Most robustness and ruggedness evaluations are empirical in nature; however, more formal evaluations can also be used [29].

4.4.9 Prestudy Method Acceptance

Since the publication of the white paper by DeSilva et al. [4], broader discussions have taken place regarding BMV method acceptance for support of PK/TK studies of both small and large molecules [10,23]. As a result, BMV recommendations have undergone refinement for LBAs. Based on the recent information from the literature, conferences, and workshops (3rd AAPS/FDA Bioanalytical Workshop, Round Table discussion at the AAPS Annual Meeting and Exposition, AAPS Bioanalytical Method Validation of Ligand-Binding Assays to Support Pharmacokinetic Assessments of Macromolecules: A Post-Crystal City III Perspective 2006 [10,23]), a LBA method can be regarded as acceptable for generating pharmacokinetic and toxicokinetic data if the prestudy interbatch precision (%CV) and the absolute mean bias (%RE) are both $\leq$20% (25% at LLOQ and ULOQ) and the method total error (sum of the %CV and absolute %RE) is $\leq$30% (40% at the LLOQ, ULOQ).

TABLE 4.7   An Example of Assay Parameters Tested for Robustness

Assay Step	Ambient Temperature (22–28°C)	Refrigerated Temperature (2–8°C)
Plate coating incubation time	NA	12–72 h
Plate blocking incubation time	1–2 h	NA
Sample incubation time	1 h 50 min–2 h 10 min	NA
Secondary antibody incubation time	50–70 min	NA
Reporter incubation time	25–35 min	NA

However, in situations where more stringent criteria are needed to support a clinical (e.g., bioequivalence study, or pivotal preclinical study), additional efforts may be warranted to develop and validate a LBA that exhibits more stringent performance criteria. Conversely, more lenient criteria may be proposed if a sound scientific rationale is provided.

The use of total error has been advocated for prestudy BMV of LBAs in publications and at meetings [3–5,9]. Even though this criterion was proposed to aid interpretation of BMV data for judging the suitability of a method for in-study sample analyses, this proposal has led to some confusion. The goal of introducing this criterion was to bring more consistency between prestudy method acceptance and the 4-6-X criteria used in-study for batch/run acceptance. It is worth pointing out that the proposed calculation TE = interassay CV (intermediate precision, random error) + |%RE| (absolute value of %RE, systematic error) is an approximation (surrogate) of total error. A more detailed description for the computation of TE can be found at http://www.westgard.com/essay111.htm. For a given validation sample concentration, an immunoassay that shows high TE (e.g., >30%) will have a greater probability of failing to meet the in-study 4-6-20/30 run acceptance criteria. Thus, rather than viewing TE as a strict rule for method acceptance, one should consider this additional prestudy validation criterion (TE < 30%) as a useful diagnostic to aid in judging the suitability of an analytical method for application in in-study sample analysis. In the end, formal method acceptance of prestudy BMV data is based on whether the assay in question met its stated *a priori* criteria for accuracy and precision.

4.5 IN-STUDY VALIDATION PHASE

4.5.1 Batch/Run Acceptance Criteria

The acceptability of in-study batches/runs is based on the performance of standard calibrators and quality control samples run in an assay. As mentioned previously, it is desirable to have prestudy method acceptance criteria consistent with the in-study batch acceptance criteria. If not, a higher percentage of assay failures can be expected. This rationale was the genesis for the 4-6-30 rule as recommended by DeSilva et al. [3–5]. The standard curve acceptance criteria for macromolecule LBAs are that at least 75% of the standard points should be within 20% of the nominal concentration (%RE of the back-calculated values), except at the LLOQ and ULOQ where the value should be within 25%. This requirement does not apply to "anchor concentrations," which are typically outside the validation range of the assay and are used to facilitate and improve the nonlinear curve fitting.

Run acceptance criteria that have been embraced for both chromatographic and LBAs require at least two-thirds of all QC results for a run to be within a specific percentage (e.g., 15%, 20%, 25%, or 30%) of the corresponding nominal reference values, with at least 50% of the results within the specified limit for each QC concentration. Assays of conventional small-molecule drugs have adopted a 4-6-15 rule [7,10,18]. In contrast, a 4-6-30 rule was proposed for LBAs of macromolecules at the March 2000 AAPS workshop [3]. As noted above, this recommendation was discussed in detail at the 3rd AAPS/FDA Bioanalytical Workshop in 2006, and results of a survey indicated that most responders did not use the total error criterion during the assessment of validation data and that the commonly used run acceptance criterion for LBAs was 20/25%. Although there was much discussion at this workshop on the use of point estimates for run acceptance criteria, the use of relevant statistical approaches (e.g., total error, confidence intervals, tolerance intervals) that describe the data from the prestudy validation was supported in assigning the run acceptance criteria during in-study validation, primarily based on the intended use of the study data [8,20,26,27]. At this time, the 4-6-20 rule represents the default criteria for run acceptance in support of regulatory-compliant LBAs [10]. The committee did recognize that in certain situations, those wider acceptance criteria (e.g., 4-6-30) are appropriate upon documented justification [10,23].

4.5.2 Incurred Sample Reanalysis

The topic of incurred sample reanalysis (ISR) was introduced at the Crystal City III Conference in May 2006 to help understand the poor reproducibility of results found by FDA in some cases when samples from studies were reanalyzed. The recommendation from the workshop report [10] on this topic is that an adequate evaluation of incurred sample reproducibility should be conducted for each species used for GLP toxicology experiments and in selected clinical studies. It is also recognized that the degree of reproducibility could be different in human samples in comparison to the animal samples. Selection of the studies to be evaluated for ISR was left up to the sponsor.

Subsequent to this meeting, a workshop held on this topic in February 2008 provided more clarity to the initial recommendations [31]. The FDA recommendation was that ISR was a requirement to demonstrate reproducibility of the analytical methods that support regulated studies, and that the sponsor should have an SOP describing their ISR procedure. The following general recommendations were provided: (a) ISR must be considered if pharmacokinetics is the primary end point of the study, (b) ISR must be performed with individual samples and not with pooled study samples, (c) the analysis of samples from more subjects with fewer samples per subject should give a better chance of finding anomalous samples or subjects, (d) the recommended sampling points were one sample near C_{max} and one near end of elimination phase. There was also a request from the FDA to report the data in the relevant study reports rather than in validation reports.

For nonclinical studies, ISR should be conducted at least once in each species, preferably in the first toxicology study. This could be a validation activity. Guidance was to follow the recommendations from the 2007 white paper [10]. Evaluation of ISR in clinical studies was recommended for all bioequivalence/comparability studies and, where applicable, for the first-in-human study and diseased patient population studies.

The guidance from the workshop on when to conduct the ISR was flexible, taking into account the efficiency of the laboratory processes. It was strongly recommended to do this evaluation earlier in the animal study rather than later (with the exception of small toxicology studies). For studies in which samples were received intermittently, ISR should be done as soon as reasonably possible.

The acceptance criterion recommendation for large molecules was that two-thirds of the values derived from the ISR should be within 30% of the original value. This was discussed extensively, and other appropriate statistical approaches such as Bland–Altman analysis were also presented [30]. An important issue that was highlighted in this discussion was that unacceptable ISR data would not result in acceptance or rejection of a study, but would lead to an investigation of the causes of the failed ISR and agreement on follow-up actions.

4.6 PARTIAL VALIDATIONS/METHOD TRANSFER/CROSS-VALIDATION

A full validation assessing all of the performance characteristics discussed above should be performed for a new method. Unlike for small molecules, for biotherapeutics it is recommended that a full validation be conducted when there is a change in species (e.g., rat to mouse) and a change in matrix within a species (e.g., rat serum to rat urine). In all the situations discussed in detail below, it is necessary to have a validation plan with *a priori* established acceptance criteria.

4.6.1 Partial Validation

Partial validations can range from one intra-assay accuracy and precision run to several runs, depending on the complexity of the change. Some examples for conducting partial validations include qualification of analysts, change in an anticoagulant, and a change in lots of a key reagent (e.g., matrix, antibody, or detection conjugate). Most often in this situation, it is expected that the partial validation would meet the acceptance criteria of the original validation. We recommend that investigators develop internal SOPs to govern partial validation.

4.6.2 Method Transfer

Method transfers are typically done between laboratories, where a method has been validated at one laboratory and is being transferred to another laboratory. This requires at least a partial validation that is documented and agreed upon by both parties. It is highly recommended that blinded spiked samples as well as incurred samples be tested during a method transfer to compare the performance of both laboratories. Method transfer studies should employ appropriate statistical design and data analysis.

4.6.3 Cross-Validation

Cross-validation is conducted when two bioanalytical methods are being used in a single study or a submission, for example, ELISA and a LC/MS method. It is recommended that both spiked samples and incurred samples be used to cross-validate the two methods. Appropriate statistical criteria should be used to compare the data.

4.7   DOCUMENTATION

The conference report from the Crystal City III Workshop outlines the documentation requirements in detail [10]. The degree of documentation should be sufficient to recreate the validation. Prior to initiating a prestudy validation, an appropriate standard operating procedure or a detailed validation plan should be written. This plan can be a stand-alone document or can be contained in a laboratory notebook or some comparable format. The documentation should clearly state the intended use of the method and a summary of the performance parameters to be validated. The plan should include a summary of the proposed experiments and the target acceptance criteria for each performance parameter evaluated.

4.7.1   Prestudy Validation

After completion of the validation experiments, a comprehensive report that details the results, performance of the assay, observations, any deviations, and the conclusions should be written.

4.7.2   In-Study Validation

Cumulative standard curve and quality control (QC) data tables containing appropriate statistical parameters should be generated and included with the study sample values in the final study report. Additional documentation with respect to the failed runs, dates of these runs, and the reason for failure should be documented. All deviations, impact to the study results, and supporting data should also be included in the final report.

4.8   CONCLUSIONS

Currently, LBAs are essentially the only bioanalytical option with sufficient performance capabilities (e.g., sensitivity) to support the PK/TK of macromolecular biotherapeutics. For this reason and others, considerable energy has gone into defining appropriate methods for BMV of LBAs. Prior to 2000, LBA BMV approaches varied considerably across the pharmaceutical and biotechnology industries and were dictated largely by intracompany policies. Following the initial Crystal City macromolecule meeting in March 2000, LBA BMV has been a topic of frequent discussion at meetings and in publications. These efforts have resulted in increased standardization in procedures and harmonization of LBA BMV methods. In spite of this progress, an ongoing effort is needed for harmonization of LBA BMV due, in part, to the evolving diversity and complexity of biotherapeutics. In conclusion, in this chapter, we have attempted to capture the intent of regulatory guidance and report the latest trends in describing the BMV of LBAs in support of PK/TK assessments of biopharmaceuticals.

REFERENCES

1. 2008 PhRMA Report, Medicines in Development Biotechnology, Available at http://www. phrma.org/files/Biotech%202008.pdf. Accessed December 24, 2008.

2. Lawrence, S. (2007) Pipelines turn to biotech. *Nature Biotechnology*, **25**, 1342.

3. Miller, K.J., Bowsher, R.R., Celniker, A., Gibbons, J., Gupta, S., Lee, J.W., Swanson, J.S. J., Smith, W.C., and Weiner, R.S. (2001) Workshop on bioanalytical methods validation for macromolecules: summary report. *Pharmaceutical Research*, **18**, 1373–1383.

4. DeSilva, B., Smith, W., Weiner, R., Kelley, M., Smolec, J.-M., Lee, B., Khan, M., Tacey, R., Hill, H., and Celniker, A. (2003) Recommendations for the bioanalytical method valid-ation of ligand-binding assays to support pharmacokinetic assessments of macromole-cules. *Pharmaceutical Research*, **20**, 1885–1900.

5. Smolec, J.-M., DeSilva, B., Smith, W.C., Weiner, R., Kelley, M., Lee, B., Khan, M., Tacey, R., Hill, H., and Celniker, A. (2005) Workshop Report—Bioanalytical method validation for macromolecules in support of pharmacokinetic studies. *Pharmaceutical Research*, **22**, 1425–1431.

6. Shah, V.P., Midha, K.K., Dighe, S.V., McGilveray, I.J., Skelly, J.P., Yacobi, A., Layloff, T., Viswanathan, C.T., Cook, C.E., McDowall, R.D., Pittman, K.A., and Spector, S. (1992) Conference Report—Analytical methods validation: bioavailability, bioequivalence and pharmacokinetic studies. *Pharmaceutical Research*, **9**, 588–592.

7. Shah, V.P. (2007) The history of bioanalytical method validation and regulation: evolution of a guidance document on bioanalytical methods validation. *The AAPS Journal*, **9**, E43–E47.

8. Smith, W.C., and Sittampalam, G.S. (1998) Conceptual and statistical issues in the valid-ation of analytic dilution assays for pharmaceutical applications. *Journal of Biopharma-ceutical Statistics*, **8**, 509–532.

9. Findlay, J.W.A., Smith, W.C., Lee, J.W., Nordblom, G.D., Das, I., DeSilva, B.S., Khan, M. N., and Bowsher, R.R. (2000) Validation of immunoassays for bioanalysis: a pharmaceutical industry perspective. *Journal of Pharmaceutical and Biomedical Analysis*, **21**, 1249–1273.

10. Viswanathan, C.T., Bansal, S., Booth, B., DeStefano, A.J., Rose, M.J., Sailstad, J., Shah, V.P., Skelly, J.P., Swann, P.G., and Weiner, R. (2007) Quantitative bioanalytical methods validation and implementation: best practices for chromatographic and ligand binding assays. *The AAPS Journal*, **9**, E30–E42.

11. ICH Harmonised Tripartite Guideline (2005) Validation of Analytical Procedure: Text and Methodology, Q2(R1). Available at http://www.ich.org/LOB/media/MEDIA417.pdf.

12. Findlay, J.W.A. (1995) Validation in practice: experience with immunoassay. In: Blume, H. H., and Midha, K.K. (eds), *Bio-International 2: Bioavailability, Bioequivalence and Pharmacokinetic Studies*. Medpharm Scientific Publishers, Stuttgart, pp. 361–370.

13. Chard, T. (1987) An introduction to radioimmunoassay and related techniques. In: Burdon, R.H., and van Knippenberg P.H. (eds), *Laboratory Techniques in Biochemistry and Mole-cular Biology*, 3rd edition, Vol. 6, Part 2. Elsevier Press, New York, NY, pp. 175–193.

14. Lee, J., and Ma, H. (2007) Specificity and selectivity evaluations of ligand binding assay of proteins therapeutics against concomitant drugs and related endogenous proteins. *The AAPS Journal*, **9**, E164–E170.

15. Dudley, R.A., Edwards, P., Ekins, R.P., Finney, D.J., McKenzie, I.G.M., Raab, G.M., Rodbard, D., and Rodgers, R.P.C. (1985) Guidelines for immunoassay data processing. *Clinical Chemistry*, **31**, 1264–1271.

16. Rodbard, D., and Frazier, G.R. (1975) Statistical analysis of radioligand assay data. *Methods in Enzymology*, **37**, 3–22.

17. Findlay, J.W.A. and Dillard, R.F. (2007) Appropriate calibration curve fitting in ligand-binding assays. *The AAPS Journal*, **9**, E260–E267.

18. Guidance for the Industry: Bioanalytical Method Validation. U.S. Department of Health and Human Services FDA (CDER and CVM). May 2001. Available at http://www.fda.gov/cder/guidance/4252fnl.pdf.

19. Hartmann, C., Smeyers-Verbeke, J., Massart, D.L., and McDowall, R.D. (1998) Validation of bioanalytical chromatographic methods. *Journal of Pharmaceutical and Biomedical Analysis*, **17**, 193–218.

20. Kelley, M., and DeSilva, B. (2007) Key elements of bioanalytical method validation for macromolecules. *The AAPS Journal*, **9**, E156–E163.

21. Boulanger, B., Dewe, W., Hubert, P., Govaerts, B., Hammer, C., and Moonen, F. (2006) Objectives of analytical methods, objective of validation and decision rules. *AAPS Workshop*, Crystal City, VA, May 1–3, 2006.

22. Westgard, J.O. (1998) Points of care in using statistics in method comparison studies. *Clinical Chemistry*, **44**, 2240–2242.

23. Nowatzke, W., and Bowsher, R. (2007) A macromolecule perspective on the 3rd AAPS/FDA workshop/conference report—quantitative bioanalytical methods validation and implementation: best practices for chromatographic and ligand binding assays. *AAPS Newsmagazine*, **10**, 21–23.

24. Timm, U., Wall, M., and Dell, D. (1985) A new approach for dealing with the stability of drugs in biological fluids. *Journal of Pharmaceutical Sciences*, **74**, 972–977.

25. Kringle, R., and Hoffman, D. (2001) Stability methods for assessing stability of compounds in whole blood for clinical bioanalysis. *Drug Information Journal*, **35**, 1261–1270.

26. Hartmann, C., Smeyers-Verbeke, J., Penninckx, W., Vander Heyden, Y., Venkeerberghen, P., and Massart, D.L. (1995) Reappraisal of hypothesis testing for method validation; detection of systematic error by comparing the means of two methods or two laboratories. *Analytical Chemistry*, **67**, 4491–4499.

27. Hartmann, C., Massart, D.L., and McDowall, R.D. (1994) An analysis of the Washington Conference Report on bioanalytical method validation. *Journal of Pharmaceutical and Biomedical Analysis*, **12**, 1337–43.

28. Riley, C.M., and Rosanke, T.W. (1996) *Development of Validation of Analytical Methods: Progress in Pharmaceutical and Biomedical Analysis*, Vol. 3. Elsevier, Pergamon, NY.

29. Plackett, R.L., and Burman, J.P. (1946) The design of optimum multifactorial experiments. *Biometrica*, **33**, 305–325.

30. Rocci, M.L., Jr., Devanarayan, V., Haughey, D.B., and Jardieu, P. (2007) Confirmatory reanalysis of incurred bioanalytical samples. *The AAPS Journal*, **9**, E336–E343.

31. Fast, D.M., Kelley, M., Vishwanathan, CT., O'Shaughnessy, J., King, S.P., Chaudhary, A., Weiner, R., DeStefano, A. J., and Tang, D. (2009) Workshop report and follow-up—AAPS workshop on current topics in GLP bioanalysis: assay reproducibility for incurred samples—implications of crystal city recommendations. *The AAPS Journal*, **11**, 238–241.

CHAPTER 5

Statistical Considerations in the Validation of Ligand-Binding Assays

BRUNO BOULANGER

UCB Pharma SA, Braine-L'alleud, Belgium

VISWANATH DEVANARAYAN

Abbott Laboratories, Souderton, PA, USA

WALTHÈRE DEWÉ

GSK Biologicals, Rixensart, Belgium

5.1 INTRODUCTION

In the pharmaceutical industry, analytical procedures are the necessary eyes and ears of all experiments performed and data produced. If the quality of an analytical procedure is inadequate, the resulting measurements may be questionable and the scientific validity of the study conclusions may be compromised. Therefore, appropriate evaluation of the data from an analytical procedure is critical from both the statistical and scientific perspectives.

Regulatory documents [1–3] related to analytical and bioanalytical method validations suggest that all analytical methods should comply with specific acceptance criteria to be recognized as validated procedures. The primary aim of these documents is to provide guidelines on the type of evidence needed from the analytical methods to demonstrate that they are suitable for their intended use. There are, nevertheless, some inconsistencies between these documents with respect to the definition of the performance characteristics and their acceptance criteria. In addition, appropriate ways for analyzing the data and estimating the performance characteristics are not provided.

Ligand-Binding Assays: Development, Validation, and Implementation in the Drug Development Arena. Edited by Masood N. Khan and John W.A. Findlay
Copyright © 2010 John Wiley & Sons, Inc.

In this chapter, we will provide a statistical overview of some important concepts, performance characteristics, and acceptance criteria related to analytical validation. We will also attempt to resolve the inconsistencies noted above and clarify the link between the performance criteria established during analytical validation and the required performance of the measurements during the routine use of the analytical method during the in-study phase.

5.1.1 Method Classification Based on Data Types

The ultimate goal of an assay or an analytical procedure is to measure accurately a quantity or a concentration of an analyte, or to measure a specific activity, as in some assays for biomarkers. However, many activity assays, such as cell-based and enzyme activity assays, may not be very sensitive, may lack precision, and/or do not include the use of definitive reference standards. Assays based on measurements of physicochemical (such as chromatographic methods) or biochemical (such as ligand-binding assays) attributes of the analyte assume that these quantifiable characteristics are reflective of the quantities, concentration, or biological activity of the analyte. For the purpose of bioanalytical method validation, we will follow the recently proposed classifications for assay data by Lee et al. [4,5]. These classifications, as summarized below, provide a clear distinction with respect to analytical validation practices and requirements.

- *Qualitative methods* generate data that do not have a continuous proportionality relationship with the amount of analyte in a sample; the data are categorical in nature. Data may be nominal positive/negative data such as a present/absent call for a gene or gene product. Alternatively, data may be ordinal in nature, with discrete scoring scales (1–5, −, +, +++, etc.) such as for immunohistochemistry assays.

- *Quantitative methods* are assays where the response signal has a continuous relationship with the quantity or activity of the analyte. These responses can therefore be described by a mathematical function. Inclusion of reference standards at discrete concentrations allows the quantification of sample responses by interpolation. A well-defined reference standard may or may not be available, or may not be representative of its content or activity, so quantification may not be absolute. To that end, three types of quantitative methods have been defined.

  - *Definitive quantitative assay* uses calibrators fitted to a known model to provide absolute quantitative values for unknown samples. Typically, such assays are only possible where the analyte is not endogenous, for example, a small-molecule xenobiotic drug.

  - *Relative quantitative assay* is similar in approach, but generally involves the measurement of endogenously occurring analytes. Since in this case even a "zero" or blank calibrator will contain some amount of analyte, quantification can only be done relative to this "zero" level. Examples of this include immunoassays for cytokines such as interlueken-6 or certain gene expression assays (e.g., RT-PCR).

- *Quasi-quantitative assay* does not involve the use of calibrators mostly due to the lack of suitable reference material, so the analytical result of a test sample is reported only in terms of the assay signal (e.g., optical density in ELISA).

This chapter deals with the assessment of definitive and relative quantitative assays. A good reference on the analytical validation of a quasi-quantitative assay is a white paper on immunogenicity by Mire-Sluis et al. [6] and the guidance on assay development and validation for high-throughput screening developed by scientists from NIH and Eli Lilly & Company [7].

5.2 OBJECTIVES OF ASSAY VALIDATION

5.2.1 Objective of an Assay

The objective of a definitive or a relative quantitative analytical procedure is to quantify as accurately as possible *each* of the unknown quantities that the laboratory intends to measure. In other words, a laboratory should expect the difference between the observed/measured value (X) and the unknown "true value" (μ_T) of the test sample to be small or within an acceptance limit λ:

$$-\lambda < X - \mu_T < \lambda \Leftrightarrow |X - \mu_T| < \lambda \qquad (5.1)$$

The acceptance limit λ varies depending on the requirements of the laboratory and the intended use of the measured results. The objective is to link this acceptance limit to the requirements usually employed in specific applications. For example, this might be 1% or 2% on bulk drug, 5% on pharmaceutical specialties such as tablets, 15% for biological samples in a bioequivalence study, λ% for clinical applications where λ depends on factors such as the physiological variability and the intent of use.

5.2.2 Objective of the Prestudy Validation Phase

As already pointed by other authors [8,9], the life cycle of an assay includes three major phases: development, prestudy validation, and in-study validation. Since this life cycle is a continuum, what matters is to "develop a valid (acceptable) method" rather than to simply "validate (accept) a developed method." The aim of the prestudy validation phase is to generate enough information to guarantee that during the in-study phase, the analytical procedure will provide measurements close to the true value [10–13] without being affected by other components present in the sample. In other words, the prestudy validation phase should demonstrate that a large proportion of the future results will fulfill the condition described in Equation 5.1. The difference between the measurement X and its true value μ_T is composed of a systematic error δ_M (bias or trueness) and a random error σ_M of the method (variance or imprecision). The true values of these parameters δ_M and σ_M, also called performance characteristics (parameters) of the procedure, are unknown and therefore estimated based on the validation experiments. The reliability of these estimates depends on the adequacy of the design of the experiments. Consequently, given the estimates of bias δ_M and variance σ_M of the procedure, the objective of the validation phase [14–16] is to evaluate whether the expected proportion π of future results that will fall within the acceptance limits is greater than a predefined minimal proportion, say π_{min}. This can be expressed mathematically as follows:

$$\pi = E_{\hat{\delta}_M, \hat{\sigma}_M}\{P[|X - \mu_T| < \lambda]|\hat{\delta}_M, \hat{\sigma}_M\} \geq \pi_{min} \qquad (5.2)$$

If the expected proportion π of results that will fall within the acceptance limits $[-\lambda, \lambda]$ is greater than the minimum acceptance level π_{min} (e.g., 80%), then the analytical procedure will be declared "valid" and expected to produce reliable results in the future, assuming that there are no significant deviations in the operational protocol and the specific conditions in the assay. It is important at this stage to notice that an assay should be declared valid or invalid based on the quality of the results it is expected to produce in the future. Such a decision should not be based only on its past performances as estimated by its bias δ_M and its precision σ_M. It is often assumed in practice that if the analytical procedure has apparently "good" performance today, then it will produce "good" results tomorrow. There is no guarantee that this will be the case. The validation criteria required by regulatory documents do not provide an adequate link between the prestudy validation and in-study validation. The "missing" link between the performance (δ_M and σ_M) of an assay estimated during prestudy validation experiments and the accuracy ($X - \mu_T$) of its future results during the in-study phase is shown in Equation 5.2. Therefore, the objective of the prestudy validation is to first provide estimates of the performance of the analytical procedure and use that information to predict the expected proportion of accurate results it will provide for future samples (during the in-study phase). If these results are satisfactory, the procedure will then be used in study for routine determination of unknown samples.

5.2.3 Objective of the In-Study Validation Phase

Once a decision has been made to use an assay for testing study samples (in-study phase), it is necessary to routinely assess whether it continues to produce accurate results, because some aspects of the operational or environmental conditions of the method may have changed significantly enough to affect its performance characteristics. This is usually achieved by including some quality control (QC) samples in each assay run (batch). Stated in a more statistical way, if used routinely, it is assumed that the true $\pi > \pi_{min}$, as long as correct decisions were made at the prestudy validation phase, that is, those decisions comply with Equation 5.2, and as long as the method is operated under normal conditions. The objective of the in-study validation process can then be described in Equation 5.3:

$$P(\text{Accept run}|\pi \geq \pi_{min}) > \gamma_{min} \qquad (5.3)$$

where γ_{min} is the minimum proportion of runs that the laboratory would like to accept. Once a run is accepted based on the QC samples, it is assumed that most of the measurements obtained over that run are likely to fall within the acceptance limits.

5.3 VALIDATION CRITERIA

The main validation parameters widely recommended by various regulatory documents (ICH and FDA) and commonly used in analytical laboratories [17] are as follows:

- Specificity/selectivity
- Calibration curve
- Linearity (of the result)
- Precision (repeatability and intermediate precision)
- Accuracy (trueness)
- Measurement error (total error)
- Limit of detection (LOD)
- Lower limit of quantification (LLOQ)
- Assay range: LLOQ to upper limit of quantification (ULOQ)
- Sensitivity

In addition, according to the domains concerned, other specific criteria can be required such as follows:

- Analyte stability
- Recovery
- Effect of dilution

The validation parameters mentioned above must be established, as much as possible, in the same matrix as that of the samples intended to be analyzed. Every new analytical procedure will have to be validated for each type of matrix (e.g., for each type of biological fluid and for each animal species). In addition, expectations on characteristics such as precision, sensitivity, assay range, should be stated *a priori* depending on the intended use of the assay (target population, matrix, study objectives, etc.).

The primary focus of this section will be on the criteria that apply to most analytical methods and that must be adequately estimated and documented for ensuring compliance with regulations. Criteria that entail significant statistical considerations will be discussed in this chapter.

5.3.1 Calibration Curve

The calibration curve of an analytical procedure is the relationship between the assay response (signal, e.g., area under the curve, peak height, and absorption) and the concentration (quantity) of the analyte in the sample. The calibration curve should preferably be a simple, monotonic response function that gives accurate measurements.

The requirements on the calibration curve are frequently confused with the dilutional linearity criteria. Dilutional linearity is the relationship between the dilutions of the sample and corresponding back-calculated results. This is typically misunderstood to imply that the calibration curve should also be linear. Not only is this not required, as for ligand-binding methods, but this is also irrelevant and often paradoxically leads to large errors in the measurements [17].

Statistical models for calibration curves are usually either linear or nonlinear in their parameter(s). The choice between these two families of models can depend on the type of method or the range of concentration of interest. If the calibration range is very narrow, then a linear model may suffice, while a wider range typically requires more advanced nonlinear models. In addition, an inherent feature of most analytical methods is that the variability of the assay signal is a function of the analyte level or quantity to be measured. This has to be taken into consideration by weighting the curve proportionally to the changing variability across the analyte range; this is usually referred to as weighting. Calibration curves for HPLC methods are mostly linear, especially in the log scale, while for ligand-binding assays they are typically nonlinear, often requiring weighting.

The methodologies used for fitting calibration curves depend on whether they are linear or nonlinear. Model fitting basically consists of finding values of the model parameters that minimize the deviation between the fitted curve and the observed data (i.e., to get the curve to fit the data as perfectly as possible). For linear models, estimates of the parameters such as the intercept and slope can be derived analytically. However, this is not possible for most nonlinear models. Estimation of the parameters in most nonlinear models requires computer-intensive numerical optimization techniques that require the input of starting values by the user (or by an automated program), and the final estimates of the model parameters are determined based on numerically optimizing the closeness of the fitted calibration curve to the observed measurements. Fortunately, this is now automated and available in most user-friendly software.

As mentioned above, if the variability of signal across the analyte range is heterogeneous, it is recommended to weight the observations proportionately when fitting the curve. This usually results in significant improvement in the accuracy of measurements at lower concentrations, and thus has a tremendous impact on the sensitivity of assay. Based on our experience with ligand-binding assays, the use of appropriate weighting methods when fitting nonlinear calibration curves typically results in at least five-fold improvement in assay sensitivity, thus saving months of additional assay development work that may otherwise be necessary to improve the assay sensitivity.

When replicate measurements are available at each calibrator concentration, the calibration curve can be fitted to either all the replicate data or just the average (means or medians) of the replicates. However, if the replicates are not independent, as is often the case (for example, if replicates are obtained by analyzing the same preparation or some steps of the preparation were common), calibration curves should be fitted on the average of the replicates instead of the individual measurements. This is because most statistical models that are available in user-friendly software assume that the replicate observations are independent.

The statistical models for calibration curves are typically fitted on either the linear or log scale of assay signal and the calibrator concentrations. Use of the log scale for assay signal may help account for the proportionately increasing variability across the analyte concentration range; however caution should be exercised when using this as an alternative to the weighting approach described above. If the samples are serially diluted, as is the case in most ligand-binding assays, then the use of log scale for the calibrator concentrations is recommended for plotting and fitting the calibration curves. A significant source of variability and bias in an analytical method can come from the choice of the statistical model used for the calibration curve.

The most frequently used nonlinear calibration curve models [18] are the four- and five-parameter logistic models (4PL and 5PL). For example, the four-parameter logistic model is expressed mathematically as follows:

$$y = f(x) = \beta_1 + \frac{\beta_2 - \beta_1}{1 + \left(\frac{x}{\beta_3}\right)^{\beta_4}} \tag{5.4}$$

where β_1, β_2, β_3, and β_4 are the top asymptote, the bottom asymptote, the concentration corresponding to half distance between β_1 and β_2, and the slope, respectively.

5.3.2 Linearity

As defined in ICH-Q2A [1], linearity of an analytical procedure is its ability, within a defined range, to obtain results directly proportional to the concentrations of the analyte in the sample. This is sometimes misinterpreted to imply that the assay response should be a linear function of the analyte concentration. The linearity criteria should be applied only to the back-calculated (calibrated) results, that is, the back-calculated results should be directly proportional to the analyte concentrations of the sample within the range in which the study samples are expected to fall.

5.3.3 Accuracy and Precision

5.3.3.1 Accuracy (Trueness)   The accuracy of an analytical procedure, according to ICH and related documents, expresses the closeness of agreement between the *mean* value obtained from a series of measurements and the value that is accepted either as a conventional true value or an accepted reference value (international standard, standard from a pharmacopoeia). This is also referred to as trueness [19].

Trueness is a measure of the systematic error (δ_M) of the calculated result introduced by the analytical method from its theoretical true/reference value. This is usually expressed as percent recovery or relative bias/error. The term "accuracy" is used to refer to bias or trueness in the pharmaceutical regulations as covered by ICH (and related national regulatory documents implementing ICH Q2A and Q2B). Outside the pharmaceutical industry, such as in those covered by the ISO [20,21] or NCCLS (food industry, chemical industry, etc.), the term "accuracy" is used to refer to total error, which is the aggregate of both the systematic error (trueness) and random error (precision). In addition, within the ICH Q2R (formerly, Q2A and Q2B) documents, two contradictory definitions of "accuracy" are given: one refers to the difference between the calculated value (of an individual sample) and its true value (total error), while the other refers to the difference between the *mean* of results and its true value (systematic error, i.e., trueness) [19].

5.3.3.2 Precision

The precision of an analytical procedure expresses the closeness of agreement (usually expressed as coefficient of variation) between a series of measurements obtained from multiple sampling of the same homogeneous sample (independent assays) under prescribed conditions. It quantifies the random errors produced by the procedure and is evaluated with respect to three levels: repeatability, intermediate precision (within laboratory), and reproducibility (between laboratories).

Repeatability   Repeatability expresses the precision under conditions where the results of independent sample results are obtained from the same assay run and same analytical procedure on identical samples in the same laboratory, with the same operator and using the same equipment, and during a short interval of time.

Intermediate Precision   Intermediate precision expresses the precision under conditions where the results of independent assays are obtained by the same analytical procedure on identical samples in the same laboratory, possibly with different operators and using different instruments, and during a given time interval. This represents the total random error from individual sample results, taking into consideration all the assay variables.

Reproducibility   Reproducibility expresses the precision under conditions where the results are obtained by the same analytical procedure on identical samples in different laboratories, and possibly with different operators and different equipment. This is rarely used when the tendency is to use central laboratories.

5.3.3.3 Total Error or Measurement Error

The measurement error of an analytical procedure expresses the closeness of agreement between the value measured and the value that is accepted either as a conventional true value or an accepted reference value. This is also the definition of "accuracy" in ICH Q2R. This closeness of agreement represents the sum of the systematic and random errors, that is, the total error associated with the observed result. Consequently, the measurement error is the expression of the sum of the trueness and precision, that is, the total error [19,22].

$$X = \mu_T + \text{bias} + \text{precision}$$
$$\Leftrightarrow X - \mu_T = \text{bias} + \text{precision}$$
$$\Leftrightarrow X - \mu_T = \text{total error}$$
$$\Leftrightarrow X - \mu_T = \text{measurement error} \tag{5.5}$$

As shown in Equation 5.5, the observed sample result, X, is an aggregate of the true value, μ_T, of the sample, the bias of the method, and the precision, which is equivalent to say that the difference between a measure and the true value is the result of both systematic and random errors, that is, the total error or the measurement error.

5.3.4   Limits of Quantification and Dynamic Range

The limits of quantification of an analytical procedure are the lowest and largest amounts of the targeted substance in the sample that can be quantitatively determined under the prescribed experimental conditions with well-established measurement error (analytical bias and precision). Consequently, the dynamic range of an analytical procedure is the range between the lower and the upper limits of quantification within which a measured result is expected to have acceptable levels of bias and precision.

5.3.5   Limit of Detection

The limit of detection of an assay is the lowest amount of the targeted substance in the sample that can be detected almost surely, but not necessarily quantified with acceptable level of bias and precision using the experimental conditions prescribed. A popular method for estimating the LOD that has been widely used in the literature is to interpolate the concentration corresponding to mean plus 3SD of the assay signal of a background sample. From experience, LOD tends to be three times less than LLOQ.

5.4   ESTIMATING ASSAY PERFORMANCE CHARACTERISTICS

Performance characteristics of ligand-binding assays are estimated using calculated concentrations from the spiked validation samples during prestudy validation and/or from the quality control samples during in-study validation.

5.4.1   Prestudy Validation

The primary performance measures of a ligand-binding assay are bias/trueness and precision. These measures along with the total error are then used to derive and evaluate several other performance characteristics such as sensitivity (LLOQ), dynamic range, and dilutional linearity. Estimation of the primary performance measures (bias, precision, and total error) requires relevant data to be generated from a number of independent runs (also termed as experiments or assays). Within each run, a number of concentration levels of the analyte of interest are tested with two or more replicates at each level. The primary performance measures are estimated independently at each level of the analyte concentration. This is carried out within the framework of the analysis of variance (ANOVA) model with the experimental runs included as a random effect [23]. Additional terms such as analyst, instrument, etc., may be included in this model depending on the design of the experiment. This ANOVA model allows us to estimate the overall mean of the calculated concentrations and the relevant variance components such as the within-run variance and the between-run variance.

The model is written as follows:

$$X_{ijk} = \mu_j + \alpha_{ij} + \varepsilon_{ijk} \tag{5.5}$$

where X_{ijk} is the measured value of the kth sample at the jth concentration level from the ith run, μ_j is the overall mean concentration at the jth concentration level, α_{ij} is the difference between the mean concentration of the ith run and μ_j at the jth concentration level, and ε_{ijk} is the experimental error associated with this measurement. The differences α_{ij} (run effect) are assumed to be normally distributed with a mean equal to 0 and variance $\sigma_{B,j}^2$, representing the between-run variability. In addition, the error term ε_{ijk} is assumed to be normally distributed with a mean equal to 0 and variance $\sigma_{W,j}^2$, representing the within-run variability. The overall mean $\hat{\mu}_j$ gives an estimate of $\mu_{T,j}$, the true value of the samples at concentration level j.

The trueness of the method can be represented by the percent relative error (bias). At concentration level j, it is given by

$$\mathrm{bias}_j(\%) = 100\frac{\hat{\mu}_j - \mu_{T,j}}{\mu_{T,j}}$$

Repeatability and intermediate precision are derived from the variance components of the above ANOVA model. Repeatability (R) is estimated by the within-run variance and the intermediate precision (IP) is the sum of both components. The coefficients of variation are

$$\mathrm{CV}_{R,j}(\%) = 100\frac{\sqrt{\hat{\sigma}_{W,j}^2}}{\mu_{T,j}}$$

$$\mathrm{CV}_{IP,j}(\%) = 100\frac{\sqrt{\hat{\sigma}_{W,j}^2 + \hat{\sigma}_{B,j}^2}}{\mu_{T,j}}$$

The measurement error criterion is defined by the so-called tolerance interval within which we would expect a certain proportion of all the possible measurements to fall. Suppose that the objective of an analytical method is to produce at least 90% of the results within 15% of the true value. In that case, we would calculate a 90% tolerance interval [16,24,25] on the relative scale and we would consider the method valid if this interval is between -15% and 15%. Indeed, we would have some guarantees that at least 90% of the results generated in the future by the method will actually be within 15% of the true value.

A $\beta\%$ tolerance interval is obtained as follows:

$$\mathrm{Bias}_j(\%) \pm Q_t\left(v_j; \frac{1+\beta}{2}\right)\sqrt{1 + \frac{1}{pn_jB_j^2}}\,\mathrm{CV}_{IP,j}(\%)$$

where

$$R_j = \frac{\hat{\sigma}_{B,j}^2}{\hat{\sigma}_{W,j}^2}$$

$$B_j = \sqrt{\frac{R_j+1}{n_jR_j+1}}$$

$$v_j = \frac{(R_j+1)^2}{\left(\left(R_j+\frac{1}{n_j}\right)^2 \Big/ (p-1)\right)+\left(\left(1-\frac{1}{n_j}\right)\Big/ (pn_j)\right)}$$

and Q_t is the quantile of a t distribution, p is the number of runs, and n_j is the number of replicates within each run at the jth concentration level.

When the experimental design consists of more than one level of concentration, the lower and upper limits of the tolerance intervals are connected, respectively, across the concentration levels resulting in two curves that represent the so-called measurement-error profile, as illustrated in Fig. 5.1.

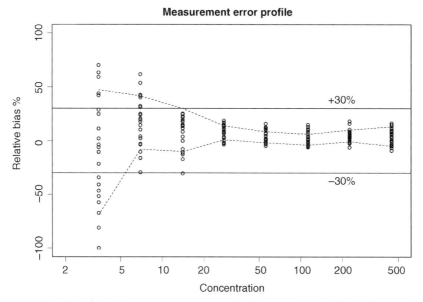

FIGURE 5.1 Example of measurement-error profile. The central dotted line is the mean bias (trueness). The outer lines are obtained by connecting the upper and lower limits of the tolerance intervals. Open circles represent the values obtained from individual validation samples from multiple experimental runs.

5.4.2   In-Study Validation

In-study validation entails the routine monitoring of the quality control samples to determine whether the analytical method is performing consistently over time and whether data from a particular plate or run are acceptable. In addition, especially for biomarker assays, evaluation of parallelism using incurred samples is carried out to confirm the validity and suitability of the reference standard.

A common criterion for accepting a run/plate is based on the proportion of QC sample results that fall within pre-specified limits. Adequate numbers of QC samples are prepared at different concentration levels, typically at the low, middle, and high levels of the assay dynamic range. These samples are analyzed in each run/plate and the concentration values are estimated. The proportion of results falling within the pre-specified acceptance limits is then calculated at each concentration level and also across the entire concentration range.

5.5   DECISION RULES AND RISK ASSESSMENT IN PRESTUDY VALIDATION

A decision about the validity/suitability of an analytical method for routine testing of study samples is taken, based on the estimated measurement error profile. Such a decision is possible only when no more than one section of the concentration range has its measurement error profile within the acceptance limits. For example, it is not reasonable to consider a method to be valid in a certain section of low concentrations and a different section of higher concentrations. In such cases, the measurement error profile is probably not precise enough to define a unique section of the range where the method is valid. In such cases, it is recommended to add a few more runs in the experimental design to obtain a more reliable estimate of the measurement error profile.

The different cases where a decision can be taken are as follows:

- The measurement error profile is within the acceptance limits across the entire concentration range tested during prestudy validation. In other words, the tolerance intervals calculated at different concentration levels are all within the acceptance limits. In such a case, the method is declared valid across the entire range. The lower and upper limits of quantification are defined, respectively, by the lowest and highest concentrations of this tested range (see Fig. 5.1).
- None of the calculated tolerance intervals are within the acceptance limits. In such a case, the method is declared invalid for the entire range and the lower limit of quantification is not estimable.
- The tolerance intervals of a single section of the concentration range are within the acceptance limits. The analytical method is considered valid within this concentration range. The lower and upper limits of quantification are the lowest and highest concentrations, respectively, for which the measurement error profile is within the acceptance limit.

There are two types of risks when making this decision: the consumer perspective [26], that is, the risk of validating/accepting an invalid method, and the producer perspective, that is, the risk of invalidating/failing a valid method. The consumer risk is typically more important to control as this can impact the selection of an appropriate dose for the patients or disease diagnoses based on a biomarker depending on the context. The producer risk results in extra cost to the sponsor due to the additional development and optimization that may be necessary if the method is declared invalid.

Taking a decision based on the measurement error profile with the tolerance intervals as described above provides better control over the consumer risk [27]. If the method is truly incapable of providing a desired proportion of the results that are close enough to their true value, it will most likely be declared invalid based on this measurement error profile.

However, the producer risk is controlled by the number of runs and replicates used in the prestudy validation experiment. This is partially due to the fact that there are two penalties in the tolerance intervals calculated at each concentration level. The first penalty depends on the precision of the mean result: the lower the precision of the mean, the broader the tolerance interval. Increasing the sample size improves the precision resulting in narrower interval. The second penalty depends on the degrees of freedom available to estimate the variance components: the smaller the degrees of freedom, the broader the tolerance interval. Increasing the sample size increases the degrees of freedom. Ensuring smaller between-run variability relative to the within-run variability also contributes to the increase in the degrees of freedom.

However, if the analytical bias is relatively high, but the method is truly valid (borderline situation), the producer risk can be quite high. Use of a larger sample size will not reduce this risk.

5.6 DECISION RULES DURING IN-STUDY PHASE AND ASSOCIATED RISKS

Unlike the prestudy validation phase, where the experiments are relatively time consuming and need to be rigorous, validation rules during the in-study phase should be simple and inexpensive. An in-study rule that is largely accepted in the bioanalytical community is the "4–6–15" rule and is defined in the FDA guidance [3] as "... At least four of every six QC samples should be within 15% of their respective nominal values ..." to accept a run. This rule provides a simple and practical guide for routine follow-up.

The properties of such a decision rule need to be examined carefully from the perspective of both the sponsor/laboratory and client [28]. Indeed, the probability of accepting a run with respect to the quality level π of the assay depends on its performance criteria, bias and precision (δ_M) and (σ_M), as seen in Equation 5.2. As performance of the assay deteriorates, a smaller proportion of results is expected to fall within the pre-specified acceptance limits. Then, from both the sponsor and regulatory perspectives, it would be better to have an acceptance criterion that is more likely to reject the runs when the expected proportion π of results within the acceptance limits

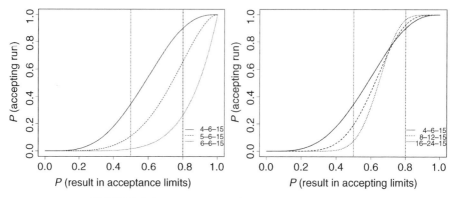

FIGURE 5.2   Power of s–n–λ as a function of s and n.

is low, say 50%, to reduce customer's risk [29]. Symmetrically, everyone will prefer the same rule to have a high chance to accept the runs when the expected proportion π of results within the acceptance limits is high, say 80%, to reduce producer's risks. Figure 5.2 shows the probabilities of accepting a run as a function of the expected proportion π of results that fall within the acceptance limits for various values of s and n in the s–n–15 rule, namely, 6–6–15, 5–6–15, and 4–6–15 on the left panel and 4–6–15, 8–12–15, and 16–24–15 on the right panel. As evident from the left panel of Fig. 5.2, when the proportion π is about 50–60%, that is, not acceptable for the customer, then there is still a 40–50% chance of accepting the run when it should be rejected. This is too much risk for the customer, say a patient. On the other side, as evident from the left panel of Fig. 5.2, when proportion π is greater than 80%, that is, acceptable for the customer and the laboratory, then there is over 90% chance of accepting the run. In summary, the 4–6–15 rule suffers from a lack of power to reject unacceptable runs, but is appropriately powered to accept good runs. A simple way to improve this asymmetrical behavior and to guarantee the protection of the customer is to increase the number of QC samples in the run. The right panel of Fig. 5.2 shows that with a 8–12–15 rule (i.e., doubling the size of the original rule of 4–6–15), the probability of accepting runs that should be rejected is reduced to about 25%.

5.7   RECONCILING VALIDATION AND ROUTINE DECISION RULES

The basic aim when applying prestudy and in-study validation procedures to a measurement method is to reconcile the objectives of the two validation phases. When the tolerance interval approach is used for prestudy validation and the 4–6–λ rule is used during in-study validation, the common objective is to control the proportion π of measurement results $(X - \mu_T)$ that fall within the acceptance limits $[-\lambda, +\lambda]$.

The ability to reconcile the prestudy and in-study rules and risks depends then on the adequacy of the parameters chosen. These parameters should ensure that a laboratory that has proved an assay to be valid based on prestudy validation will see most of the runs getting accepted during the in-study phase, as long as the performance of the method remains stable over time. Indeed, it would be counterproductive to maintain an analytical method that frequently leads to runs getting rejected when the method is still valid.

The alignment of risk between the prestudy and in-study validation phases can be envisaged in two ways, as shown by Boulanger et al. [29]. On the one hand, if the number of QC samples, n, to be used and the minimum, s, of QC samples within the acceptance limits in the s–n–λ rule are fixed (e.g., 4–6–15), the value of π_{min} should be chosen so as to ensure that if the method remains valid, the s–n–λ rule is accepted in most cases (e.g., with a minimum probability γ_{min}). On the other hand, for a given prestudy validation scheme (π_{min} and λ fixed), the value of s QC samples within the acceptance limits (for a given n) should guarantee that most of the runs will be accepted if the method remains valid.

Let us now consider the particular case of the 4–6–λ rule. As stated above, a good prestudy validation rule should be based on a value of π_{min} that ensures acceptance of a routine test in most cases (say $\gamma_{min} = 90\%$) if the method is valid, that is,

$$P(Y \geq s | \pi > \pi_{min}) > \gamma_{min}$$

For a given s and n, this π_{min} is obtained by inverting the binomial (n, π) distribution function, as shown in Fig. 5.3.

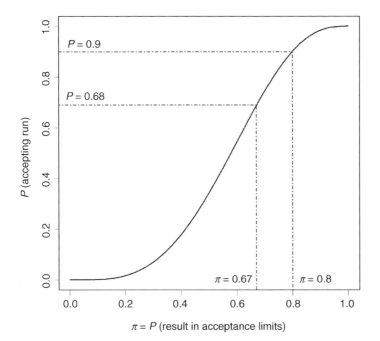

FIGURE 5.3   Reconciling prestudy validation value of π_{min} with the 4–6–λ rule.

For the 4–6–λ rule, we have $\pi_{min} = 0.8$. This means that in the prestudy validation experiment, the laboratory should demonstrate that at least 80% of the measurements fall within the acceptance limits $[-\lambda + \lambda]$. This will ensure that the 4–6–λ rule will accept 90% of the runs in routine use if the process remains valid $(\pi > \pi_{min})$. This contrasts with the (intuitive) proposal frequently encountered in the literature [3,28] that 4/6 or 66.7% of the results should fall within the acceptance limits. Adopting 66.7% as the value for π_{min} in prestudy validation can lead to up to 32% of the "valid" runs being rejected, as can be seen in Fig. 5.3.

5.8 CONCLUSIONS

In this chapter, we have covered the ways to understand, estimate, and interpret various criteria required for assessing the validity of an analytical method. Whatever the complexity or simplicity of computations and models needed, the primary objective of an analytical method should never be forgotten: Can each measurement be trusted or, equivalently, is the measurement error acceptable? All the information needed to make a decision is contained in the measurement error profile. The key performance characteristics such as the linearity, accuracy, precision, limits of quantification, and sensitivity are readily obtained from this profile and can easily be understood and interpreted by an analyst.

The acceptance criteria used during prestudy validation and in-study validation should be consistent with each other. Lack of consistency can result in a validated method failing more often than expected during the in-study phase or vice versa. To ensure this consistency, either the commonly used in-study acceptance criteria such as the 4–6–15 rule can be modified by increasing the number of QC samples (e.g., 8–12–15 rule) or the prestudy validation criteria based on tolerance intervals can be altered to ensure that a higher proportion of the measured results fall within the acceptance limits.

REFERENCES

1. International Conference on Harmonization (ICH) of Technical Requirements for the Registration of Pharmaceuticals for Human Use, Validation of Analytical Procedures. ICH–Q2A, Geneva, 1995.

2. International Conference on Harmonization (ICH) of Technical Requirements for the Registration of Pharmaceuticals for Human Use, Validation of Analytical Procedures: Methodology. ICH–Q2B, Geneva, 1996.

3. FDA Guidance for Industry, Bioanalytical Methods Validation. U.S. Department of Health and Human Services, Food and Drug Administration, Center for Drug Evaluation and Research (CDER), May 2001.

4. Lee, J.W., Nordblom, G.D., Smith, W.C., and Bowsher, R.R. (2003) Validation of bioanalytical assays for novel biomarkers: practical recommendations for clinical investigation of new drug entities. In: Bloom J., and Dean R.A. (eds), *Biomarkers in Clinical Drug Development*. Marcel Dekker, New York, pp. 119–148.

5. Lee, J.W., Devanarayan, V., Barrett, Y.C., Weiner, R., Allinson, J., Fountain, S., Keller, S., Weinry, I., Green, M., Duan, L., Rogers, J.A., Millham, R., O'Brien, P.J., Sailstad, J., Khan, M., Ray, C., and Wagner, J.A. (2006) Fit-for-purpose method development and validation for successful biomarker measurement. *Pharmaceutical Research*, **23**, 312–328.

6. Mire-Sluis, A.R., Barrett, Y.C., Devanarayan, V., Koren, E., Liu, H., Maia, M., Parish, T., Scott, G., Shankar, G., Shores, E., Swanson, S.J., Taniguchi, G., Wierda, D., and Zuckerman, L.A. (2004) Recommendations for the design and optimization of immunoassays used in the detection of host antibodies against biotechnology products. *Journal of Immunological Methods*, **289**, 1–16.

7. Assay Guidance Manual Version 5.0 (2008). Eli Lilly and Company and NIH Chemical Genomics Center. Available at http://www.ncgc.nih.gov/guidance/manual_toc.html. Last accessed 2008 June 21.

8. Finney, D. (1978) *Statistical Methods in Biological Assays*. Charles Griffin, UK.

9. Smith, W.C., and Sittampalam, G.S. (1998) Conceptual and statistical issues in the validation of analytical dilution assays for pharmaceutical applications. *Journal of Biopharmaceutical Statistics*, **8**, 509–532.

10. Hubert, P., Nguyen, J.J., Boulanger, B., Chapuzet, E., Chiap, P., Cohen, N., Compagnon, P.A., Dewe, W., Feinberg, M., Lallier, M., Laurentie, M., Mercier, N., Muzard, G., Nivet, C., and Valat, L. (2004) Harmonization of approaches for validation of quantitative analytical procedures: a SFSTP proposal. *Journal of Pharmaceutical and Biomedical Analysis*, **36**, 579–586.

11. Miller, K.J., Bowsher, R.R., Celniker, A., Gibbons, J., Gupta, S., Lee, J.W., Swanson, S. J., Smith, W.C., and Weiner, R. (2001) Workshop on bioanalytical methods validation for macromolecules: summary report. *Pharmaceutical Research*, **18**, 1373–1383.

12. Desilva, B., Smith, W., Weiner, R., Kelley, M., Smolec, J., Lee, B., Khan, M., Tacey, R., Hill, H., and Celniker, A. (2003) Recommendations for bioanalytical method validation of ligand-binding assays to support pharmacokinetic assessments of macromolecules. *Pharmaceutical Research*, **20**, 1885–1900.

13. Findlay, J.W.A., Smith, W.C., Lee, J.W., Nordblom, G.D., Das, I., Desilva, B.S., Khan, M.N., and Bowsher, R.R. (2000) Validation of immunoassays for bioanalysis: a pharmaceutical industry perspective. *Journal of Pharmaceutical and Biomedical Analysis*, **21**, 1249–1273.

14. Boulanger, B., Hubert, P., Chiap, P., Dewe, W., and Crommen, J. Analyse statistique des résultats de validation de méthodes chromatographiques. Journées GMP. Bordeaux, 2000.

15. Boulanger, B., Hubert, P., Chiap, P., and Dewe, W. (2000) *Objectives of Pre-Study Validation and Decision Rules*. AAPS APQ Open Forum, Washington.

16. Boulanger, B., Chiap, P., Dewe, W., Crommen, J., and Hubert, P. (2003) An analysis of the SFSTP guide on validation of chromatographic bioanalytical methods: progresses and limitations. *Journal of Pharmaceutical and Biomedical Analysis*, **32**, 753–765.

17. Hubert, Ph., Nguyen-Huu, J.-J., Boulanger, B., Chapuzet, E., Chiap, P., Cohen, N., Compagnon, P.-A., Dewe, W., Feiinberg, M., Lallier, M., Laurentie, M., Mercier, N., Muzard, G., Nivert, C., and Valat, L. (2004) Harmonization of strategies for the validation of quantitative analytical procedures: a SFSTP proposal. Part I. *Journal of Pharmaceutical and Biomedical Analysis*, **36**, 579–586.

18. O'Connell, M.A., Belanger, B.A., and Haaland, P.D. (1993) Calibration and assay development using the four-parameter logistic model. *Chemometrics and Intelligent Laboratory Systems*, **20**, 97–114.

19. Rozet, E., Ceccato, A., Hubert, C., Ziemons, E., Oprean, R., Rudaz, S., Boulanger, B., and Hubert, P. (2007) An analysis of recent pharmaceutical regulatory documents on analytical method validation. *Journal of Chromatography A*, **1158**, 111–125.

20. International Organization for Standardization, Sampling Procedures for Inspection by Attributes. ISO/DIS (1995) 2859 (Part 0).

21. International Organization for Standardization, Sampling Procedures for Inspection by Variables. ISO/DIS (2005) 3951 (Part 0).

22. Hubert, P., Nguyen-Huu, J.J., Boulanger, B., Chapuzet, E., Cohen, N., Compagnon, P.A., Dewé, W., Feinberg, M., Laurentie, M., Mercier, N., Muzard, G., and Valat, L. (2006) Quantitative analytical procedures: harmonization of the approaches. Part III. *STP Pharma Pratique*, **16**, 1–35.

23. Boulanger, B., Devanaryan, V., Dewé, W., and Smith, W. (2007) Statistical considerations in the validation of analytical methods. In: Dimitrienko, A., Chuang-Stein, C., and D'Agostino, R. (eds.) *Statistical Considerations in the Validation of Analytical Methods.* SAS Institute Inc., pp. 69–94.

24. Mee, R.W. (1984) β-expectation and β-content tolerance limits for balanced one-way ANOVA random model. *Technometrics*, **26**, 251–254.

25. Mee, R.W. (1988) Estimation of the percentage of a normal distribution lying outside a specified interval. *Communication in Statistics: Theory and Methods*, **17**, 1465–1479.

26. Hoffman, D., and Kringle, R. (2005) Two-sided tolerance intervals for balanced and unbalanced random effects models. *Journal of Biopharmaceutical Statistics*, **15**, 283–293.

27. Boulanger, B., Dewe, W., Hubert, P., Rozet, E., Moonen, F., Govaerts, B., and Maumy, M. Conciliating Objectives of Analytical Methods and Objectives of Validation: A Statistical Perspective. Institute of Validation Technology, Philadelphia, December 7, 2005.

28. Kringle, R.O. (1994) An assessment of the 4–6–20 rule for acceptance of analytical runs in bioavailability, bioequivalence, and pharmacokinetic studies. *Pharmaceutical Research*, **11**, 556–560.

29. Boulanger, B., Dewé, W., Gilbert, A., Govaerts, B., and Maumy, M. (2007) Risk management for analytical methods based on the total error concept: conciliating the objectives of the pre-study and in-study validation phases. *Chemometrics and Intelligent Laboratory Systems*, **86**, 198–207.

CHAPTER 6

Development and Validation of Ligand-Binding Assays for Biomarkers

JEAN W. LEE

PKDM, Amgen Inc., Thousand Oaks, CA, USA

YANG PAN

Amgen Inc., Seattle, WA, USA

PETER J. O'BRIEN

Pfizer Inc., San Diego, CA, USA

REN XU

Amgen Inc., Seattle, WA, USA

6.1 INTRODUCTION

Biomarkers have been used for many years in the diagnosis of disease and in monitoring its progression and response to treatment. Prominent examples of this dual utility are seen in the diagnosis and treatment of diabetes, cancer, and cardiovascular disease and areas where the utility of biomarkers has been extended to clinical trials of new drugs. Familiar biomarkers from diabetes, oncology, and cardiovascular disease therapy are now used routinely in drug trials to monitor progress ahead of clinical outcomes. Diabetes trials commonly employ measurement of blood glucose, hemoglobin A1c, and circulating insulin; oncologists may use circulating prostate-specific antigen (PSA), carcinoembryonic antigen (CEA), and other tumor markers to monitor drug responses, while blood pressure and C-reactive protein are used in cardiovascular disease trials. More recently, the use of novel biomarkers has become a prominent component of decision-making processes in drug development, where

Ligand-Binding Assays: Development, Validation, and Implementation in the Drug Development Arena. Edited by Masood N. Khan and John W.A. Findlay
Copyright © 2010 John Wiley & Sons, Inc.

these newly described and/or validated clinical measurements aid in "quick hit, quick kill" decisions often adopted in early-phase clinical trials.

This new application requires new operating principles, including quickly evolving concepts surrounding the circumstantial "validity" of a given measurement. The central premise of this "fit-for-purpose" validation strategy is that the level of technical rigor and documentation applied to a given biomarker measurement should reflect the intended use and implementation of the resultant data. This chapter focuses on the application of this principle to biomarker assay validation, specifically in the realm of ligand-binding assays.

6.1.1   New Approaches to Drug Discovery and Development Necessitate New Bioanalytical Approaches

Novel approaches to biomedical research, particularly in the past decade, have caused a massive shift in our understanding of the underlying mechanisms of disease and therapy. New and exciting technologies have facilitated new insights into underlying disease genetics and signaling events that drive normal and disease biology. The introduction of immunoassay into standard clinical practice necessitated a new vocabulary, as well as new methods of data analysis and interpretation. New and often radically different data, such as multiplex assays covering target and related pathway biomarkers, are now commonplace in early-phase drug development, demanding still more tools.

Pharmaceutical companies use a more mechanistic approach to drug targeting than in the past, but still face the same biological hurdles to effectively "hitting" drug targets. Mechanism and proximal biomarkers offer evidence that a target is hit, information that increasingly influences "go, no-go" decision making on costly clinical trials. The number of new data types and potential interpretations has grown proportionally, as new drug targeting strategies necessitate new methods of measuring whether a drug target has been modulated by a given therapy. This trend is only likely to increase, since the U.S. Food and Drug Administration (FDA) has endorsed the use of biomarkers to aid in drug development in its Critical Path Initiative Report in March 2004 [1], and many pharmaceutical companies have adopted this strategy [2].

Many of the bioanalytical principles applied to drug development in the past arose from the diagnostics industry and clinical laboratory sciences. The application of biomarker assays and data in drug development often differs markedly from those approaches, particularly in the case of "novel" biomarker assays. It is important, therefore, to clarify definitions and use of terms.

A *biomarker* is defined as a characteristic that is objectively measured and evaluated as an indicator of normal biological or pathological processes, or pharmacological response to a therapeutic intervention [3]. A *clinical end point* quantifies a characteristic of a patient's condition (e.g., how they feel or function, or the survival rate of a population) and is used to determine the outcome of a clinical trial. A *surrogate end point* predicts the safety and efficacy of a drug based on subjective and quantitative data and can be used as a substitute for the clinical end point.

Owing to the clinical and analytical rigor required to achieve surrogacy, there are only few surrogate end points approved for drug development, such as blood glucose and glycosylated hemoglobin (Hb$_{A1c}$) for type 2 diabetes, and LDL cholesterol for atherosclerosis. Biomarkers are nonetheless used to support interim decisions regarding the design and progress of clinical trials, including reporting to regulatory agencies on the apparent efficacy and safety of new drug candidates. This is especially relevant in those cases where changes in a biomarker reflect alterations in underlying pathology or otherwise reflect a clinically relevant alteration of disease progression. This can occur under several different circumstances, even when the mechanism by which a biomarker reflects pathology is unknown, where mechanism is understood but biomarker changes are not reflective of therapeutic dose, and in cases where dose–response relationships have established ties to mechanism [4].

The variety and number of novel biomarkers emerging from contemporary genomics and proteomics studies are too great to enumerate here. Changes in gene expression and protein abundance or modification are the most common novel biomarkers today. By their very nature, protein biomarkers are typically more closely linked to disease-specific pathways and are more typically reflective of whether a drug has "hit" its target to alter its function. Such target and proximal biomarkers are contrasted with distal biomarkers, where a given protein is involved in disease progression and indirectly reflects the action of a drug at its target. Distal markers are often "downstream" from the pathogenic driver, where signal magnification affords increased sensitivity to changes at a drug target [5]. Biomarker measurement in disease or other relevant target tissue is preferred, but often measurement in surrogate biological fluids (e.g., peripheral blood) is necessary to make correlations between treatments and clinical end points. A common example of the use of biomarkers in clinical trials is the establishment of pharmacodynamic (PD)–pharmacokinetic (PK) relationships, that is, the relationship between the PK of a drug and relative changes in a PD biomarker (i.e., the PK/PD relationship). Comparison of these dose–exposure effects can be considered in light of toxicity–dose relationships in the selection of lead candidates and appropriate dose ranges for clinical trials [6].

6.1.2 Data Type and Technologies for Biomarker Analysis

Biomarker assays differ considerably in the type of data generated using the wide spectrum of available bioanalytical technologies, and the intended use of the data. As with biomarker types, the range and nature of data are rapidly changing, and a flexible nomenclature has been developed to address most eventualities as described by Lee and colleagues [7,8]. A *definitive quantitative assay* uses a well-characterized reference standard that is fully representative of the endogenous biomarker. Absolute quantitative values for unknown samples are calculated from a regression function. Such assays are common for drug analysis for PK studies, but only applicable to a small fraction of biomarkers such as small molecule analytes (e.g., steroids). Instead, most biomarker assays are *relative quantitative assays* where the reference standard is not well characterized, not available in a purified form, or not fully representative of the endogenous form (e.g., cytokine immunoassays). Results from these assays are expressed in continuous numeric units of the relative reference standard. When no reference standard is available for use as a calibrator, an alternative *quasi-quantitative assay* can be used if the analytical response is continuous (numeric), with the analytical results expressed in terms of a characteristic of the test sample. Examples are anti-drug antibody assays (where the readout is a titer or % bound), enzymatic assays (where activity might be expressed per unit volume), and flow cytometric assays [9]. In contrast to the "quantitative" categories, *qualitative assays* of biomarkers generate discrete (discontinuous) data, which are reported in either ordinal (e.g., low, medium, and high, or scores ranging from 1 to 5) or nominal (yes/no, positive/negative) formats. In general, qualitative methods are suitable for differentiating marked effects such as an all or none effect on gene expression, activation or inhibition in relatively homogenous cell populations in discrete scoring scales such as immunohistochemical assays. The techniques used in molecular biology and proteomics to quantify biomarkers are usually qualitative or quasi-quantitative methods that detect changes of several folds in concentration. These include gene expression analysis using hybridization arrays or quantitative amplification, Western blot, mass spectrometry coupled to capillary gel electrophoresis, and multidimensional HPLC [10,11].

Consistent with a recurring theme in biomarker implementation, the choice of assay format and measurement type are often dependent upon the intended use of the data that the assay will generate. The ultimate goal of a biomarker assay is typically to evaluate the drug effect on the biomarker activity *in vivo*, and a method that measures this accurately is most desirable. Direct measurement of changes to a drug target in cells, tissues, or organs in response to a drug is rarely feasible, and given current drug potencies, activity assays rarely have adequate sensitivity and precision. Moreover, cell-based and activity assays are usually laborious, low throughput, and often lack definitive reference standards.

In contrast, ligand-binding assays (LBAs) provide higher sensitivity and more precise, quantitative data. If biomarker reference material is available as a standardized calibrator, a quantitative method can be developed. Since many biomarkers are proteins that can be cloned and purified, molecular techniques are also useful in generating reference materials and calibrators appropriate for LBA. Thus, these methods are often chosen for biomarker analysis over activity measurements. So far, LBAs are the most common choices for protein quantification because of their sensitivity, versatility in application, relatively high throughput, and low cost. The focus of this chapter is on the method development and validation of protein biomarkers using LBA in support of drug development.

6.1.3 Fit-for-Purpose Method Development and Validation

A range of biomarker implementations has been demonstrated across all phases of drug development, from biomarker discovery and target validation in preclinical models and early-phase clinical trials, through preclinical and early-phase clinical trial PK/PD modeling for dose selection in later stages of development, and into post-marketing patient monitoring [12–14]. In general, the intended application dictates the required rigor of biomarker method validation and the nature of its documentation. In exploratory and proof-of-concept studies, PD correlations are typically unknown, data are used mainly for internal decision making, and the output will generally not be subjected to regulatory review. The extent of method validation can thus be limited to a

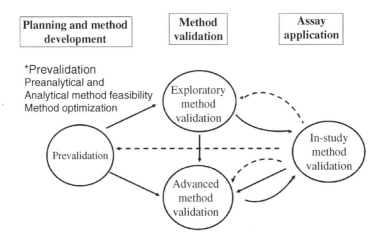

FIGURE 6.1 Conceptual diagram of "fit-for-purpose" biomarkers method validation. The method validation processes include four activity circles: prevalidation (preanalytical consideration and method development), exploratory method validation, in-study method validation and advanced method validation. The processes are continuous and iterative, dictated by the purpose of the biomarker application. The solid arrows depict the normal flow of biomarker development (prevalidation), method validation (exploratory or advanced), and application (in-study method validation). The process could include moving the chosen biomarkers from exploratory mechanistic pilot studies to advanced validation and confirmatory studies, or from exploratory validation to advanced validation after changes in critical business decision. The broken arrows represent scenarios where validation data do not satisfy study requirements, necessitating assay refinement or modification.

few basic components to expedite the process and preserve resources without unduly slowing drug development [15]. In contrast, advanced applications that provide pivotal data for regulatory review or otherwise influence critical decisions are best performed using a GLP-like approach to method validation.

This philosophy, where a fit-for-purpose biomarker assay validation approach is used, was described by Lee and colleagues [15] and is conceptualized in Fig. 6.1. In general, the method validation process includes four activities: prevalidation (preanalytical consideration and method feasibility), method validation for exploratory applications, in-study method validation (during the exploratory application), and a more complete method validation for advanced applications in more mature or higher stakes biomarker programs. The solid arrows depict the normal flow of biomarker development (prevalidation), method validation (exploratory or advanced), and application (in-study method validation). The process might thus involve moving selected biomarkers from the mechanistic exploration to a pilot, in-study validation, then to an advanced validation for confirmatory studies. Another common path might see transition from the exploratory validation directly to the advanced validation due to an accelerated need for data for a critical business decision. The arrows with dotted lines represent scenarios where validation criteria are not satisfied and additional refinement or method modifications are necessary.

Different data types require differential consideration during method validation but, as is the case with assay monitoring in clinical diagnostics, methods are consistently better understood and validated through the appropriate use of reference samples. Biomarker assays thus monitored can be improved as validation proceeds. To ensure data quality, assay performance is evaluated during method validation with validation samples (VS) and monitored during sample analysis with quality control (QC) samples. VS are used in method qualification or validation to define intra- and interrun accuracy, precision, and sample stability, providing data to demonstrate the robustness and suitability of the assay for its intended application. On the other hand, QC samples are essential in determining run-acceptability during specimen analysis. It is acceptable to retain VS for use as QC after the prestudy validation, adding further economy to the process. The following section details the use of commercially and internally obtained reagents in generating assay performance data using VS during prestudy method validation. The subsequent section describes in-study validation and the implementation of the validated method for sample analysis.

6.2 PREANALYTICAL CONSIDERATIONS AND METHOD FEASIBILITY

Given the variety and depths of efforts necessary to validate a biomarker method, a work plan is extremely useful for the bioanalytical laboratory. Communicating the work plan to the project team brings clarity on the scope of work and intended application of the data. By laying out the intended purpose and required performance characteristics of a biomarker assay, focus can be facilitated, and the entire team becomes a source of insights and improvements. An example biomarker work plan is shown in Table 6.1 with a list of content and brief description. The preanalytical consideration and method feasibility workflow are depicted in Fig. 6.2. The intended purpose of the study is the key variable at this stage. Determining the level of necessary rigor allows the "right sizing" of the validation process, depicted in examples of exploratory and advanced validations in the workflow diagrams of Figs 6.3 and 6.4, respectively.

In reviewing the literature and other information sources, it is worthwhile to keep in mind that a useful biomarker has the following attributes: (1) measurable levels in blood (or other readily accessible biological matrix, such as saliva or urine), (2) exhibits measurable differences between normal populations and the intended target patient population, and (3) exhibits consistent or predictable levels within an individual over time (i.e., diurnal, seasonal, and food effects). A review of the scientific and commercial literature is often the first and best step toward an understanding of achievable assay ranges and sensitivities relative to expected conditions in relevant samples. Data on the relative stability of analytes and other reagents in the expected sample matrices and under expected storage and transportation conditions should be obtained to aid in the design of sample collection, handling, and storage protocols.

TABLE 6.1   Example of a Biomarker Work Plan

Content	Description
Summary of intended application, SOP	The intended application of the ELISA for BMK-X in <species> <matrix> is <exploratory, advanced>. The process will be carried out according to <SOP (if applicable)>
Material sources	Reference material from <vendor or in-house>. Kit components (coating plates and detector antibody) from <vendor or in-house>
Standard curve range	<More than six concentrations> pg/mL in protein/buffer matrix
VS/QC	<LLOQ, LQC, MQC, HQC, ULOQ concentrations> pg/mL in <protein buffer, biological matrix>
Accuracy and precision runs	$\geq N$ runs
Regression model selection	<4-PL> with <X> weighting factor
Sensitivity	LLOQ and LOD determination by $\geq N$ runs
Confirm selectivity	$\geq X$ individual lots
Specificity	<BMK-Y> at levels of <n> to <m>; test compounds <JJJ> at levels of <n> to <m>, and <KKK> at levels of <n> to <m> will be tested
Endogenous sample controls (SC)	<NA or start data collection>
Stability	
Freeze/thaw stability	N cycles will be tested.
Benchtop stability	N h at ambient temperature
Long-term storage	<NA or start data collection>
Report	<Report, memo> will be issued

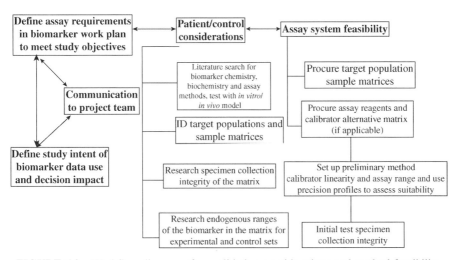

FIGURE 6.2   Workflow diagram of prevalidation considerations and method feasibility.

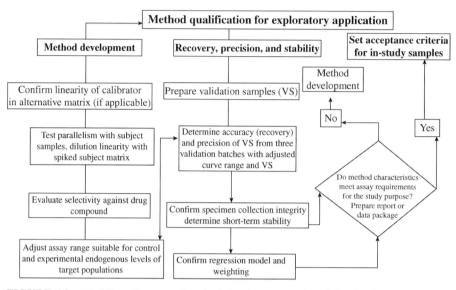

FIGURE 6.3   Workflow diagram of method development and qualification for exploratory application.

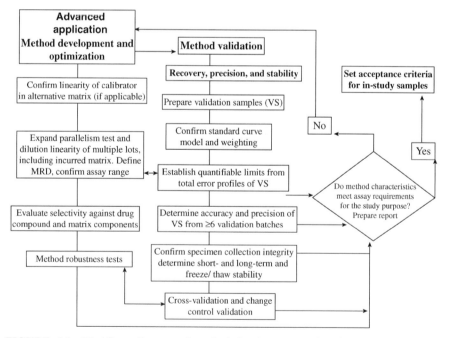

FIGURE 6.4   Workflow diagram of method development and validation for advanced application.

6.2.1 Procurement and Characterization of Critical Reagents

In general, LBA quantification of biomarkers depends upon custom-generated (in-house) or commercial (kit) reagents. Critical reagents should be procured and characterized during method feasibility assessment. Similar to LBA in PK studies, critical reagents include the reference standard material and the ligand-binding reagents. For example, in an enzyme-linked immunosorbent assay (ELISA), the ligand-binding reagents consist of capture and detection binding reagents (frequently antibodies), the latter being typically conjugated to a reporter enzyme, or to biotin or other detection amplifiers. In addition, a blank control (or alternative matrix) and sample matrices from target patient population(s) are essential. It is desirable to find a control matrix devoid of the endogenous biomarkers for standards and VS/QC preparations, but the nature of biomarker studies typically means that certain amounts will likely be present in the matrix of interest from target populations. In this case, an alternative matrix should be used. Target population sample matrices are used for method feasibility range finding, selectivity and parallelism experiments, and for the preparation of endogenous sample controls (SC).

6.2.1.1 *Reference Standard Material*   Key information that can aid in understanding the strengths and limitations of a given reference standard can often be found in the scientific literature, and it is time well spent to thoroughly understand the analyte in question early in the method validation process. The reference standard material is used for the preparation of standards, VS and QC. It is important to note that the reference material may not be fully representative of the endogenous analyte because of the heterogeneity of the biomarker of interest. However, a well-defined reference standard may serve the purpose as a scalar for the relative measurement of the endogenous species. Therefore, comprehensive documentation of the reference material is necessary to establish the basis of a reference range for a given assay.

At a minimum, documentation of the characterization and stability of a standard, such as a certificate of analysis (CoA) and/or a certificate of stability (CoS), is typically available from the suppliers. The certificate should be obtained and recorded. The quantity of reference standard is typically limited in commercial kits designed for research use, and it is not uncommon that the reference material values may differ substantially between lots and manufacturers [16]. Novel biomarkers rarely have established "gold standards" against which their potency and abundance can be calibrated. A comparison of available sources can be useful, and when validating an assay for advanced applications it is desirable to plan ahead to obtain and reserve a sufficient supply of the same reference material. The example in Fig. 6.5 compares three reference standard curves, each prepared from a concentrated stock solution from a commercial supplier, an in-house reference standard, and a commercial kit, respectively. The instrument responses (optical density, OD) were highest with the standard from the commercial stock, the lowest with the kit, while the in-house reference standard response was intermediate. In this case, either the same commercial stock or the in-house reference standard can be used throughout the clinical study.

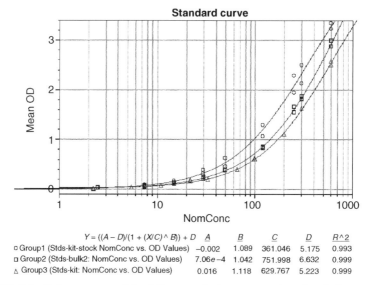

$Y = ((A − D)/(1 + (X/C)^B)) + D$	A	B	C	D	R^2
○ Group1 (Stds-kit-stock NomConc vs. OD Values)	−0.002	1.089	361.046	5.175	0.993
▫ Group2 (Stds-bulk2: NomConc vs. OD Values)	7.06e−4	1.042	751.998	6.632	0.999
△ Group3 (Stds-kit: NomConc vs. OD Values)	0.016	1.118	629.767	5.223	0.999

FIGURE 6.5 Reference materials differences in immunoreactive signal observed in an ELISA. Circles: standard prepared from a concentrated stock from the commercial supplier. Squares: standards prepared from a concentrated stock from in-house reference material. Triangles: standards prepared from a kit.

6.2.1.2 *Biomarker Concentration Range Finding*   As mentioned above, many biomarkers are found at detectable concentrations in a variety of biological matrices. In addition, endogenous protein biomarkers can be physicochemically heterogeneous, with multiple forms present simultaneously. The concentration and biological activity of each component are often unknown and may vary with health status, over time, and between individuals. Biological variability should be surveyed in samples from normal and diseased donors, especially in samples from the anticipated patient population. An initial survey should be performed against standard calibrators prepared in a defined solution of defined protein content in a relevant buffer system.

These range-finding results and data from the literature can be used to provide the initial target assay range. For example, erythropoietin concentrations in nonsmokers, smokers, and cancer patients are shown in Table 6.2. The concentrations, 9.2, 15.2, and 21.9 mU/mL for nonsmokers ($N = 25$), smokers ($N = 14$), and cancer patients ($N = 10$), respectively, illustrate the need for establishing normal ranges in a target population.

In addition, the effect of drug administration on the biomarker concentration should be factored in for the standard curve dynamic range. This is often a challenge during the exploratory phase with a novel biomarker because the modulation by a drug candidate may not be known and postdose incurred samples would not be available for the initial tests.

6.2.1.3 *Ligand-Binding Reagents and Assay Formats*   Antibody (ligand) pairs are typically chosen as capture and detection reagents. In general, the more

TABLE 6.2   Selectivity Test of Erythropoietin Using Spike Recovery

Spiked Concentration (mU/mL)		Nonsmokers (N = 25)	Smokers (N = 14)	Cancer Patients (N = 10)	Mean
0	Basal concentration	9.2	15.2	21.9	
6	Observed concentration	13.4	19.6	26.6	
	Corrected concentration	4.2	4.4	4.7	4.4
	% Recovery	70.2	72.7	77.9	73.6
60	Observed concentration	48.8	55.6	69.2	
	Corrected concentration	39.6	40.4	47.2	42.4
	% Recovery	66.0	67.3	78.7	70.7

Serum samples from nonsmokers, smokers, and cancer patients (breast, colon, prostate, head, and neck) on cytotoxic and protein therapies. Aliquots of the serum samples were spiked with 6 or 60 mU/mL erythropoietin. The unspiked and spiked samples were analyzed using an in-house ELISA method. The basal concentration (unspiked) was subtracted from the observed concentration of each individual to obtain the corrected concentration. The % recovery was calculated against the nominal spike concentration of 6 or 60 mU/mL.

selective antibody would be chosen as the capturing agent, especially if it is more readily available than the other of the pair. A tertiary, detector antibody can be used that is conjugated to a reporter enzyme, such as horseradish peroxidase (HRP). Alternately, a biotinylated detector antibody can be used together with a biotin-binding protein (e.g., anti-biotin antibody or an avidin-type protein) conjugated to a reporter enzyme. The sensitivity of an assay can be increased by varying the number of reporter enzyme molecules on the detection reagents, or by using multivalent strategies to increase the effective signal from each analyte captured.

Some assays use receptors or their fragments as binding partners, most often in concert with a specific second antibody. This arrangement can improve selectivity for specific ligands (e.g., a cytokine activated from a latent precursor, or a particular subtype of ligand with distinct binding characteristics from its homologs). The binding selectivity of such reagents can offer added biological relevance to quantitation and can suggest results that might be otherwise obtained only via functional assays. Special care should be taken to assess interference from other endogenous binding proteins and drugs that alter ligand interactions with the capture reagent, and to assure that the stability of the reagent is well characterized. In general, the stability of antibodies is unparalleled for use in LBA; so, in cases where advanced validation and application of an assay are expected, it may be worthwhile to develop antibody-based reagents.

6.2.1.4 *Preparation of Standards and Curves*   In the absence of a true blank control matrix, standards can be prepared in a protein buffer at multiple (generally 9–11) concentrations for the initial test of assay range. For method validation and sample assay, 6–8 nonzero concentrations of standards plus anchor points should be used to define a curvilinear standard curve. If a commercial kit is to be used, it is preferred that the standards be prepared from a bulk reference material to assure the consistencies of the standard as well as adding enough standard points to properly define the regression model. Before replacing the kit standards with those prepared

from the bulk reference material, an initial comparison should be performed between the prepared standards and those of the kit. Standards prepared from the bulk material should be run as unknowns against the kit standards, using the kit protocol to assure that calculated results are within the described performance parameters of the kit. If a bulk reference material is not available and the kit standards were to be used, additional standards should be added to the few kit standards, including upper (if possible) and lower anchor points.

Pooling of multiple lots of blank control matrix identified in initial screens can aid in the preparation of standard calibrators. Alternatively, a synthetic matrix can be prepared by depleting the endogenous analyte by using one of the several different processing methods. Matrix cleanup by charcoal stripping, high-temperature incubation, acid or alkaline hydrolysis, or affinity chromatography is often a suitable alternative, as is the use of protein-containing buffers or the matrix from another species with a non-cross-reactive homologue. These alternatives to native matrices require studies of matrix effects and parallelism during method development and validation to better understand how the potential differences between these matrices and patient samples will affect assay results.

Regression models are essential for interpreting data extrapolated from sigmoid curves like those used in LBA. The most commonly used four- or five-parameter logistic regression should be evaluated with weighting factors in the feasibility experiments. Final decisions on which curve-fitting model to use should rest on which offers the best fit for all the standards in the precision profile. In some cases, a less than optimal fit will suffice to allow for greater assay sensitivity. For example, for very low abundance biomarkers and for the assay of free, unbound target biomarkers that bind to the therapeutic agent, the concentrations of most samples would be in the low region of the curve. The strategy in curve fitting in such cases would be to minimize the %CV of the precision profile at the low end instead of trying to get the best fit over the entire range.

6.2.1.5 Initial Test of Matrix Effects

Assay matrices are typically the most troublesome component in LBA. There should be careful consideration of this variable during method validation. Two types of tests are used to address the two major concerns surrounding matrix effects. These are performed in consideration of (1) whether there is a matrix difference between the standards and anticipated study samples that impacts the relative accuracy of an assay and (2) whether there are inter-individual or disease-specific differences in matrix in the target patient population. Two types of tests are used to evaluate such matrix effects: spike recovery, where known amounts of analyte are mixed ("spiked") into characterized matrix, and parallelism in patient samples. However, limited availability of patient samples may prevent the latter testing during the method feasibility phase.

In spike-recovery tests, samples from individual lots of matrix (≥ 3 lots for exploratory and ≥ 10 for advanced studies) are spiked with concentrations of the reference standard from the lower and middle (upper) portions of the curve, assayed, and compared to the corresponding neat (unmodified or unspiked) samples. Spike recovery is calculated by subtracting calculated concentration in the unspiked samples (reflecting assay background or endogenous levels) from the spiked sample value and comparing the difference to the nominal (known) concentration spiked into the matrix (or the mean of the individual lots). The amount spiked should be high enough to show distinctive difference from the endogenous basal concentration. This process should be performed in matrix derived from both normal and disease populations, when possible.

For example, spike-recovery assays on the bone turnover marker N-telopeptides of type I collagen (NTx) were performed in urine from normal individuals and patients with osteoporosis, rheumatoid arthritis, or breast cancer. For an assay with a lower limit of quantification (LLOQ) of 62.5 nM bone collagen equivalent (BCE), the range was 27–2792 and 33–2245 nM BCE in healthy and patient populations, respectively. A concentration of 150 nM BCE was spiked into the test samples. To minimize the contribution from the basal values, only data from samples with $\leq$300 nM BCE were evaluated. The results in Fig. 6.6 illustrate that higher recovery bias occurred in samples where the basal values were greater than the spiked concentration. A target acceptance criterion of spike recovery was set at $\leq$30% difference from the nominal concentration. Samples falling within acceptance limits included 17 of 27 from patients and 24 of 30 from healthy subjects. Among samples with basal values below

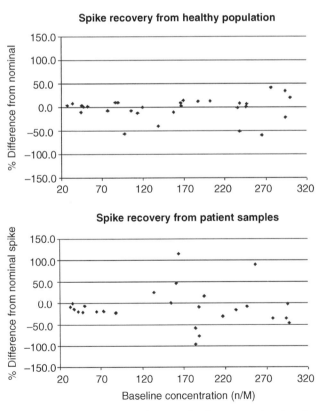

FIGURE 6.6   Spike recovery test of urine samples from normal and patients for NTx.

150 nM BCE, all 11 from patients and 12 of 14 from healthy subjects met the acceptance criterion, reinforcing the concept that a thorough understanding of matrix effects can significantly affect assay validation.

6.2.1.6 Initial Test of Specimen Collection Integrity As mentioned above, information on the properties of an analyte and its behavior under different handling and storage conditions is best obtained from literature, reagent vendors, and colleagues and then documented. Information is often lacking, particularly regarding stability in different matrices, after different isolation techniques, and under different handling conditions. In these cases, experiments should be conducted to assess the impact of anticipated clinical trial sample handling conditions, matrix types, and the impact of a range of likely handling and storage scenarios. It is best to perform comparisons of any preanalytical variable that might impact the design and execution of the biomarker study. These might include analyte stability and assay compatibility in serum and differently anticoagulated plasma types, in the presence of different sample additives and stabilizers, and a range of sample handling scenarios. The important consideration here is that the assay validation be performed under as similar a set of conditions as can reasonably be expected in a clinical trial. This can help eliminate uncontrollable variables, increasing the value and reliability of the biomarker data.

6.3 METHOD DEVELOPMENT AND METHOD QUALIFICATION FOR EXPLORATORY APPLICATIONS

Unlike analytes measured using clinical diagnostics assays, a novel biomarker typically requires extensive characterization before it is considered "qualified" for a variety of uses. This principle applies to methods validated for other matrices and uses, but used in a new way for biomarker measurements. As described above, the intended use of the biomarker data drives the level of rigor and documentation surrounding assay validation. Exploratory, proof-of-concept studies are among the least rigorous in biomarker research, typically occur earlier in drug development, and are almost exclusively used to drive internal decisions on the validity of a biomarker or the feasibility of its measurement. A typical workflow for this type of exercise is depicted in Fig. 6.3 and examples are given in this section for illustrations.

6.3.1 Assay Dynamic Range

In consideration of preclinical and published data, the work plan should set an initial target assay range. At this stage, if matrix effects are not an issue, standards can be prepared in a buffered protein solution. At least three qualification runs each consisting of one set of standards and at least two sets of VS are used to define assay dynamic range. For an ELISA method, each data point is usually calculated from the average of two readouts (e.g., OD from two wells). The standards include the ULOQ, LLOQ, and ~4–6 intermediate points evenly distributed across a log scale. In addition, because LBA standard curves are typically sigmoidal, curve fitting is improved using anchor points to better define the upper and lower asymptotes. Curve-fitting models, often four- or five-parameter logistic regression analyses, are evaluated with weighting factors. The variance is reduced and a lower LLOQ can be achieved with the appropriate regression model and proper weighting factor [15].

6.3.2 Preparation of Validation Samples, Quality Control and Sample Controls

Ideally, blank controls are found when screening samples for matrix assessment and can be used to prepare standards and VS/QC samples. Typically, however, true blank controls are rare, so the reference material is not a perfect representation of the endogenous biomarker that will be encountered in study samples. Under such circumstances, VS and QC are often prepared in the same buffer solution as the standards. Sample controls (SC) should therefore be prepared by pooling neat samples at high and low endogenous levels to reflect the real samples. The SC will be assayed during the qualification runs to determine their concentrations. True SC concentrations are then defined after sufficient data collection from pre- and in-study validation studies. For example, the mean of 30 runs and two standard deviations can be used to define the target concentration and acceptable range of the SC. Because the reference material may not fully represent the endogenous biomarkers, the SC should be used for stability tests (such as minimum test of exposure to ambient temperature and freeze/thaw cycle). In addition, the SC can be used for in-study, long-term storage stability analysis and to assess lot-to-lot variability of key assay reagents.

To evaluate assay performance, a set of VS prepared independently of the standards is used. At least five concentrations VS should be prepared, including the target LLOQ and ULOQ, low QC (~3 times of the LLOQ), mid-QC, and high QC (~75% of the ULOQ). Accuracy and precision can be evaluated from the total error (the sum of bias and precision) of VS data from the qualification runs in a similar way as for macromolecular protein drugs [17]. Given biological variability and other factors in biomarker research, more lenient acceptance criteria may be used for biomarker PD than for PK studies. Still, it should be recognized that accuracy and precision data of VS in buffer provide only a relative quantification, which may be quite different from measurements in the authentic matrix.

Figure 6.7 shows an example of the VS inter-day accuracy and precision of NTx assay in urine as a bone resorption biomarker. The standards were prepared in buffer, along with two sets of VS, one prepared in buffer and the other in blank urine (i.e., with undetectable NTx). The imprecision (%CV) was slightly higher for VS in urine than those in buffer, and total error was much higher at the two lowest concentrations. VS showed a higher degree of bias in urine, and results were more variable than in buffer, especially at the low concentrations. Although the VS were prepared in "blank" urine, the high positive bias at low concentrations most likely results from matrix component interference in the assay.

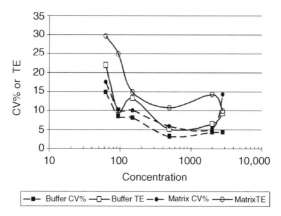

FIGURE 6.7 Total error (TE) and precision of validation samples. Data from inter-day method validation accuracy and precision runs. The standards were in buffer. Five levels of VS were prepared in buffer and in sample matrix. Open squares: TE% in buffer; solid squares: CV% in buffer; open circles: TE% in matrix; solid circles: CV% in matrix.

6.3.3 Confirmation of Sample Integrity

Biomarker measurements can be affected by numerous factors beyond one's control, increasing the importance of controlling as many variables as possible to understand the impact of uncontrollable events on assay performance. One of the more understandable and controllable factors in biomarker research is sample integrity. As implied by the term integrity, measurement of a biomarker after collection, transport, and storage should yield a result as close to that, which could be measured in as fresh a sample as possible. Variables that impact this potential difference are readily found during sample collection, shipping, and storage through sample analysis and the stability of the analyte in the matrix of choice. Biomarker selection should include consideration of analyte stability in available matrices, with robust biomarkers having greater stability across a range of handling conditions. Each stage of sample manipulation comes with potential pitfalls, so staff training and oversight procedures are essential for the monitoring and maintenance of sample integrity. Sample characteristics can vary over time, with feeding, or by age- and gender-specific factors, and by the methods used to prepare the sample. Sample handling can alter the sample irrevocably, so care must be used in collection, separation, addition of anticoagulants and other additives, and myriad other preanalytical circumstances. A careful review of potential confounding variables is essential prior to advanced validation. In some biomarker studies, it is possible to use normalization to correct for some of this preanalytical variability. Urine samples, for example, can be normalized to control for hydration status using urine creatinine concentration.

The study protocol should include procedures for sample collection, shipping, and analysis, as well as sample storage and disposal. If the procedures involve complex processing, on-site training of the clinical staff may be warranted. Control and standardization of sample collection are especially necessary to minimize variability from multiple clinical sites. For example, a common mistake is improper centrifugation at clinical sites, which can introduce significant variation in some biomarker quantification. Standardization of centrifuge speeds for different model centrifuges can minimize this problem.

Sample stability assessment includes the likely range of conditions to which a sample might reasonably be exposed. This includes process stability, assessing the impact of short-term storage under less than optimal conditions (as can occur on the laboratory benchtop during processing) and at least one cycle of freeze–thaw.

6.3.4 Assay Sensitivity

For PK/PD support, assay sensitivity is defined by the assay LLOQ, which is the lowest concentration that has been demonstrated to be measurable with acceptable levels of bias and precision or total error. However, low concentration clinical samples may fall below the LLOQ of the method, (i.e., the method lacks the required sensitivity). The best solution is to come up with a more sensitive method. Failing that, the values below the LLOQ but above the limit of detection (LOD) may be considered, bearing in mind the high variability in that region. To establish assay sensitivity, the assay background must be determined. Limit of background (LOB) is defined as a limit where the probability of a blank sample measurement exceeding the limit is 5% [18]. LOD is the lowest amount of analyte in a sample that can be detected with 95% or other stated probability although this may not quantify as an exact value. Therefore, for a given sample with an actual amount of analyte equal to LOD, there is a 5% probability that the measurement will be equal to or below LOB. LOD can be determined by making repeated measurements of samples with very low levels of analyte.

LOD is often used as the analytical "sensitivity" of the assay in a diagnostic kit. A common practice with diagnostic kits is the use of interpolated concentrations from a response signal of +3SD (or −3SD for a competitive assay) of the mean background signal from 30 or more blank samples. This practice is not recommended because the sampling size used can be too small, often without accounting for the type II error. Figure 6.8 illustrates the concept of LOB (type I error) and LOD (type II error) in blank matrix and low concentration samples, respectively, with normally distributed analyte concentrations. The National Committee for Clinical Laboratory Standards (CLSI) has presented an approach to determine LOD, which includes sufficient determinations of LOB from blank samples and LOD from very low concentration samples for statistical calculations [18,19].

If LOD is used for biomarker determinations, the user should be aware of the risk being taken with the higher variability at the LOD to LLOQ range, interpreting the data with caution.

6.3.5 Tests on Specificity and Selectivity

Specificity reflects the ability of the LBA to distinguish between the analyte of interest and other structurally similar components of the sample. Results from a nonspecific

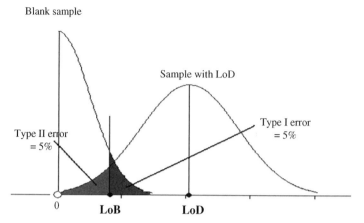

FIGURE 6.8 Limit of blank (LOB) and limit of detection (LOD).

assay can generate false-positives and/or an overestimation of the analyte concentration. Selectivity is the ability of the LBA to discriminate the analyte unequivocally in the presence of components that may be expected to be present in the sample and alter assay results. Lack of selectivity can result in binding inhibition or enhancement. In general, signal suppression (as from binding proteins) occurs more often than that of enhancement, resulting in a negative bias. Interference in an assay is the product of concentration of the interfering substance and the cross-reactivity (or binding inhibition). However, the concentration–response relationship of the LBA is typically nonlinear and often the magnitude of cross-reactivity (or inhibition) is not dispersed over the entire assay range. Therefore, the estimate of the extent of interference cannot be simply extrapolated across the entire assay range.

LBA specificity and selectivity are method-dependent. For example, if the reagent component is the target drug or its analog, the presence of the drug compound might itself interfere with the assay. In addition, biomarker homologs, precursors, or truncated forms may contribute to specificity problems. If reference materials of the analogs are available, specificity for the analyte of interest can be obtained by spiking the analogs into a VS sample. A "checker board" experimental design comparing various concentrations of VS against concentrations of the test compound ranging from below to 10-fold above the expected *in vivo* levels is typically adequate [20].

Demonstration of selectivity and specificity of an assay for a biomarker must be considered in the context of whether the assay is a definitive quantitative assay or a relative quantitative assay (see Section 1.2). It can be difficult to show absolute specificity and selectivity for a relative assay due to the uncertainty of the exact species being measured and unknown components of the matrix. At a minimum, reproducible measurements of endogenous samples with and without spiking of the reference analyte should be demonstrated. On the other hand, likely truncated forms of a well-characterized biomarker measured by a definitive quantitative assay can be tested for specificity, as in the following example.

TABLE 6.3 Whole PTH Specificity Test Against Peptide Fragments

	Control, No Addition (pg/mL)	% Bias from Control Fragment (3–84)		% Bias from Control Fragment (7–84)	
Spiked concentration (pg/mL)	0	75	750	500	5000
To QC at 15 pg/mL					
Kit A	12.4	34.11	87.90	27.98	NC
Kit B	16.5	0.79	0.92	0.81	0.95
Kit C	11.7	3.65	40.26	1.51	2.75
To QC at 75 pg/mL					
Kit A	96.9	2.01	11.46	4.57	NC
Kit B	75.9	0.93	0.94	0.97	1.00
Kit C	62.5	1.66	8.93	1.17	1.63
To QC at 750 pg/mL					
Kit A	799	1.10	2.33	1.39	NC
Kit B	703	1.00	1.00	1.02	1.03
Kit C	792	1.16	1.60	0.99	1.02

Data calculated from Ref. 21. NC: not calculable, value was above quantifiable limits.

6.3.5.1 Example Table 6.3 shows specificity testing with three human parathyroid hormone (PTH) commercial kits against PTH peptide fragments 3–84 and 7–84 [21]. In addition to the conventional cross-reactivity test using kit calibration solutions, the peptide fragments were spiked into QC at low and high concentrations to test for possible interference. This provides additional valuable information by including surrogates of clinical study samples in cross-reactivity assessments. For example, the cross-reactivity of fragment 3–84 was 139%, 0.6%, and 48% for kits A, B, and C, respectively. Spiking the QC showed that these peptides will not affect the quantification for kit C. Kit B may be useful when peptide 3–84 is present at low levels while kit A would not be an appropriate choice.

6.3.6 Parallelism and Dilutional Linearity to Evaluate Matrix Effects

For a majority of biomarker assays, standard calibrators are prepared in an analyte-free alternative matrix instead of the *de facto* sample matrix of patient samples. For such methods, it is crucial to demonstrate that the concentration–response relationship in the sample matrix is similar to that of the alternate matrix. Spike-recovery experiments with the reference standard may be inadequate to evaluate the matrix effect, as the reference standard may not fully represent the endogenous analyte. Instead, parallelism experiments are performed through serial dilutions of a high-concentration sample with the calibrator matrix. Multiple individual matrix lots ($\geq$3 lots) should be tested to compare lot-to-lot consistency. In the instance that the limited amounts of sample are available, a pooled matrix strategy can be used with caution as discussed by Lee et al. [15]. The samples can be serially diluted with the standard matrix (standard zero) with ≥ 3 dilution factors within the calibration range. Calculated concentrations (observed concentration corrected for dilution) from each sample should be evaluated for consistency across the dilutional range.

When parallelism cannot be performed, as when samples with sufficiently high concentrations of the analyte are unavailable, dilutional linearity should be tested in a manner similar to parallelism, with high-concentration spiked samples used in place of the endogenous samples. The test matrix sample is spiked with a concentration higher than or near the ULOQ and diluted in the standard matrix at ≥ 4 different dilution factors within the range of the calibration curve. Data are analyzed in a manner similar to parallelism studies, keeping in mind that the purpose and design of these experiments are different from those used in PK studies. In the latter case, the experiment often involves spiking concentrations above the ULOQ, and dilution within the dynamic range to demonstrate dilutional accuracy and precision, and the lack of a hook effect, often within one matrix lot. For biomarker experiments, samples at the high region of assay dynamic range should be chosen and tested undiluted and diluted inside the range, using at least three lots of matrix. One of the outcomes of dilutional linearity experiments is the determination of the minimum required dilution (MRD), which is the lowest dilution factor that alleviates the matrix interference sufficiently [17].

Depending upon the *a priori* goals of the study, failure to demonstrate parallelism need not invalidate the data from these efforts. Even if parallelism is not demonstrated, a method may still generate usable information on assay trends and has value in quasi-quantitative measurements. The following example is from the method qualification of a commercial kit for exploratory use. Standard calibrators were prepared by diluting the highest commercial kit calibrator (in protein-containing buffer) into normal human serum. Spike recovery in individual normal serum was acceptable but was not so for patient samples. Parallelism tests were conducted using patient samples. The typical result is shown in Fig. 6.9 where the patient sample was diluted separately in a protein buffer and in normal human serum to test for parallelism. A continuous response—concentration relationship was only demonstrable in the serum, but it was not parallel to the standard curve. Therefore, the method was categorized as a quasi-quantitative method.

6.3.7 Assay Qualification for a Quasi-Quantitative Ligand-Binding Assay Used in Exploratory Biomarker Studies

Quasi-quantitative assays traditionally include measures of enzymatic or ligand-binding activity, as in flow cytometry and anti-drug antibody assays [9]. One of the common characteristics of these assays is the lack of a true reference standard, where reference standards are poorly characterized, do not completely represent native protein, or differ from native proteins in terms of potency or immunoreactivity. As stated above, if the analytical response is continuous across the range in question, the analytical results can be expressed in terms of a characteristic of known test samples. The following is one example: an ELISA qualified as a quasi-quantitative assay because it could not be validated as a relative quantitative assay.

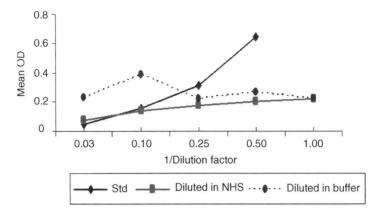

FIGURE 6.9 Parallelism test of a biomarker in buffer versus in normal human serum. A patient sample containing biomarker X was tested for parallelism by diluting in a protein-containing buffer and in normal human serum. The standard calibrator was prepared by diluting the highest commercial kit calibrator (in protein buffer) with normal human serum.

Cytokeratin (CK) is a family of intermediate filament proteins found primarily in epithelial cells. There are two main types of CKs: the acidic type I CK (e.g., CK18 and CK19) and neutral to basic type II (CK7 and CK8). CK filaments usually exist as heteropolymers consisting of both type I and type II forms bound in a 1 : 1 ratio [22,23]. CK7, CK8, CK18, and CK19 are found in carcinomas and can be detected in circulation with other tumor cell contents after tumor cell death [24]. Furthermore, CK18 is a proteolytic substrate for caspase-3 and -7. Proteolytic fragments can be detected in the circulation after the induction of tumor cell apoptosis. CK18 fragments are transiently increased in the serum of mice xenografted with Colo205 cells after treatment with an agonist anti-TRAIL receptor 2 antibody (Pan et al., unpublished data). Measurement of intact and cleaved CK18 in patient sera after treatment can be used as a biomarker of tumor cell death in clinical trials [25–29].

The M30-Apoptosense® ELISA (M30 ELISA) uses two mouse mAbs, M5 and M30, to detect a neoepitope on caspase-cleaved CK18 (Asp 396). M5, the capture antibody, detects a common epitope on both intact CK18 and caspase-cleaved CK18. M30 is used as the detection antibody in this assay (Fig. 6.10). The M30 ELISA standard is an *Escherichia coli* derived recombinant CK18 (rCK18) containing the M30 recognition motif [30].

During initial assay optimization and qualification, native serum CK18 immunoreactivity was shown to differ significantly from that of rCK18 in different matrices and assay configurations. Using different detection and capture antibody pairs, the data suggested that CK18 interacted with additional CK isoforms. Thus, CK18 might not be adequately represented by the rCK18 reference material. This conclusion was further supported by the absence of dilutional linearity and serum parallelism in the M30 assay (Fig. 6.11). Based on these data, the ELISA could not be qualified as a relative quantitative ligand-binding assay [7]. Assay sensitivity, precision, specificity, range, reagent stability, sample stability, and drug interference were assessed.

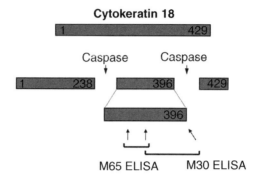

FIGURE 6.10 Schematic representation of the CK18 epitope map. Epitopes targeted by the antibodies used in the M30-Apoptosense and M65 ELISAs are shown. CK18 is cleaved at Asp238 and Asp396 by caspases during apoptosis. The M30-Apoptosense ELISA assay uses antibody M5 to capture CK18 and the antibody M30, which detects a neoepitope in CK18, formed after caspase cleavage at Asp396. The M65 ELISA uses M6 antibody to capture all CK18 fragments that contain epitopes in the 300–390 amino acid region of the protein and then M5 antibody for detection.

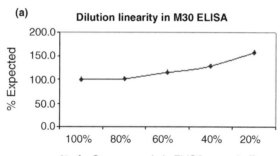

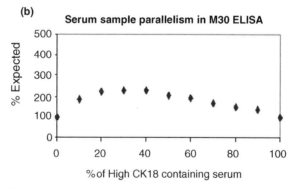

FIGURE 6.11 Testing assay dilutional linearity and parallelism in M30 ELISA. (a) Serum sample is diluted proportionally with ELISA assay buffer. Results were calculated using the detected OD result from each dilution to compare with expected OD at each dilution. (b) A high CK18 containing serum sample is proportionally mixed with a low CK18 containing serum. Detected OD result at each mix% was compared to expected OD result (b).

In addition, intradonor variation was measured among normal donors to provide an estimate of normal fluctuation of caspase-cleaved CK18. This quasi-quantitative assay was found to be acceptable for exploratory biomarker purposes. The aim of such a study was to compare the differences in serum caspase-cleaved CK18 in pre- and posttreatment samples from the same patient. Subsequently, the method was used in several clinical trials to explore the effectiveness of an apoptosis-inducing drug candidate. Similarly, another method employing an M65 ELISA, which measures total serum CK18, was also qualified as a quasi-quantitative assay for exploratory use in the same clinical studies.

6.4 METHOD DEVELOPMENT AND METHOD VALIDATION FOR ADVANCED APPLICATIONS

As described above, biomarker data can be used in "advanced applications" where the data are used in pivotal clinical studies or other critical decision-making scenarios that justify the additional effort and expense. The use of biomarker data to discriminate otherwise subtle, graded drug effects, monitor drug safety, or for submission to regulatory agencies for drug approval requires a higher degree of scientific rigor and regulatory compliance and validation efforts that are accordingly more expensive than exploratory validation. Similar to GLP validation, more extensive experiments are required to demonstrate method suitability and reliability, and greater documentation is pursued to allow traceability and reliability assessment for the data [7,15]. A workflow is depicted in Fig. 6.4, and examples are given in this section to illustrate the process.

6.4.1 Critical Reagent Characterization and Documentation

It is critically important to define and document the reference standard for an advanced application. For an established biomarker, a "gold standard" from a reputable organization (such as the World Health Organization) may be available, as with diagnostic kits. For most novel biomarkers, a "gold standard" is lacking. Characterization is thus often dependent upon supplier laboratories, be they commercial or in-house. Documentation, such as a certificate or other record of analysis, and a certificate of stability should be obtained. If these are not available, at least the source, identity, potency (or concentration), and lot number of the reference material should be documented. A consistent and sufficient supply of the same lot of reference material should be reserved and used for the duration of studies within a program.

If a lot change is required, experiments should be performed to qualify the new reference material. Standards prepared using the new lot should be compared against the previous lot within one run. A set of established VS should also be included in the run for assay acceptance. If differences are observed, the potency of the new reference lot should be adjusted to match the old lot. If existing reference material is depleted, a new lot should be qualified by comparison in multiple runs against a set of established VS. Sometimes there is a consistent bias of the VS results, indicating a systemic discrepancy of the new reference material against the old lot. Under such circumstances, a partial validation of accuracy and precision should be performed with a new set of standards and VS.

Similar to the reference material, documentation of the source, identity, potency (or concentration), and lot number of critical ligand reagents and their stability should be kept. If possible, the same lot of the capturing ligand should be used throughout a study. It is prudent to test for method robustness using multiple lots of reagents during advanced method validation. If a reagent change is required, qualification should be performed on the new reagents. For example, a qualification run can be made to compare the new lot against the previous one using a common set of VS and SC.

Variability of reagents and reference standards can be detected by tracking the assay performance of a common set of SC used within and between studies. The urinary NTx assay described above provides an example. A large pool of low and high SC was established during method validation and analyzed in more than 100 analytical runs in several clinical studies over 21 months. During this time, three changes in kit lots occurred. The SC data shown in Fig. 6.12 indicated a systemic negative shift of both low and high SC from the first kit lot to the second (bold arrow at run #40), even though the commercial kit met vendor release specifications. Only a slight positive bias was

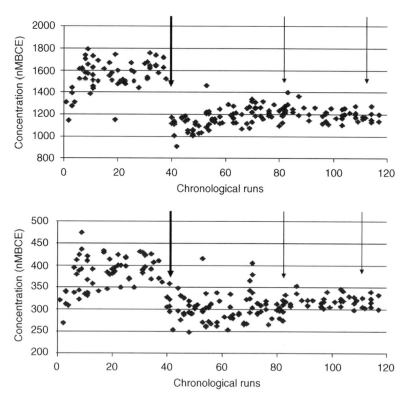

FIGURE 6.12   Urine NTx low and high endogenous pools data over a time span of 21 months. Upper panel: high pool. Lower panel: low pool. Vertical arrows: kit lot changes.

observed at the next lot change. SC data also allow assessment of the variability of the assay resulting from different kit lots, analyst-to-analyst variability, and analyte stability in urine.

6.4.2 Extension of Sample Integrity and Reagent Stability

More extensive stability data are necessary in advanced applications, closely mimicking a variety of clinical and environmental conditions that might conceivably be encountered in a large or otherwise complicated clinical trial. Sample collection vessel type and quality, matrix separation methods and conditions, sample temperature changes, and sample integrity/stability during bioanalytical processing (e.g. freeze–thaw stability) are critical points for consideration. For example, for a clinical study that lasts for several years, where the same reference material and assay reagents are used throughout, documentation of stability over time should be obtained. Documentation of chain of custody should be similar to that of a GLP or clinical PK study. In late-phase multisite studies, the use of a central sample repository offers numerous advantages in controlling this process.

6.4.3 Evaluation of Selectivity and Specificity for Clinical Studies

Biomarkers can reflect the dynamic changes in disease progression and response to therapy, but homeostatic and compensatory biological responses can alter the expected profile in response to drug treatment and concomitant therapies [31,32]. In the latter case, biomarker assay selectivity is a critical component for interpreting biomarker responses and clinical data, particularly when a concomitant therapy is a potential interferent in the assay. Table 6.2 illustrates the selectivity profile of an erythropoietin ELISA in samples drawn from a variety of patients of different tumor types and drug treatments. Treatment regimens included various cytotoxic and protein drug therapies. Also, sera from tobacco smokers and nonsmokers were examined for matrix effects. Aliquots of the serum samples from each individual were spiked with low and high concentrations of erythropoietin. Spike recovery results in Table 6.2 show that recovery in cancer patients was similar to that of the normal population, and no significant differences were seen between the smokers and nonsmokers, supporting assay selectivity in these sample types. A consistent, approximately 30% negative bias was determined to be due to the matrix difference of standards in buffer versus patient/donor samples.

Specificity for the biomarker in the presence of the drug under study should be tested. Samples from endogenous pools (such as the SC) can be spiked with the drug compound at concentrations spanning the expected therapeutic range. Figure 6.13 illustrates a specificity experiment for a target biomarker (upper panel) and its proximal biomarker (lower panel) each tested with three sample pools at pg/mL levels against various drug concentrations. As expected, at 10 ng/mL the test drug significantly inhibited quantification of the target biomarker. However, no effect was seen on a proximal biomarker, even at 10,000 ng/mL, demonstrating target selectivity.

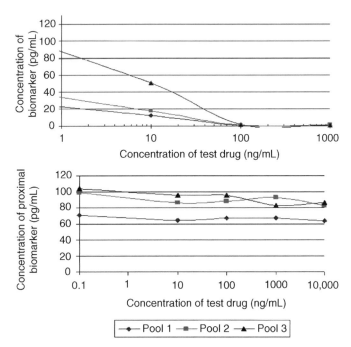

FIGURE 6.13   Specificity tests of two biomarkers against a drug compound. Samples were pooled to form three separate matrix pools, each represented by a different symbol. Upper panel: specificity of the target biomarker versus drug. The concentrations were 33, 50, and 123 pg/mL for pools 1, 2, and 3, respectively. Lower panel: specificity of a proximal biomarker versus the drug compound. The concentrations were 66, 85, and 93 pg/mL for pools 1, 2, and 3, respectively.

6.5   PARTIAL VALIDATION FOR CHANGE CONTROL

Changes in operators, assay equipment, reagent lots, and a variety of other unforeseen events can necessitate additional validation. The significance of the alteration in a method will determine the extent of validation necessary, leading to cross-validation, partial validation, or complete revalidation of an assay to control for changes during or between studies. Examples include changes in critical assay reagents (e.g., antibody lot or kit vendor), assay transfer from one site to another, changes in processes, instrumentation, or methodology (e.g., assay automation or detection systems). A validation plan should be prepared for even partial validations, describing the objective, scope, and experiments to be carried out to meet those objectives. An addendum report can be issued later as an appendix to the existing method. If the change is expected to be extensive, a new validation would be conducted according to the new analytical procedure, followed by a new validation report.

6.6   DOCUMENTATION, RECORD KEEPING, AND REPORTING

Validation data should be documented in an appropriate notebook in hard copy or in electronic format and retained according to applicable SOPs and regulations.

Determination of the appropriate level of documentation for an exploratory or advanced biomarker application is made by the organization or laboratory responsible for the biomarker study. In general, an analytical procedure and a validation memo containing the summary data should be adequate for exploratory application. For an advanced validation, the record keeping and reporting may be similar to that of the methods for PK support. The basic idea is that the data should be traceable and subjected to QC and QA review. The final method should be documented in an analytical procedure and the results presented in a validation report.

6.7 REGULATORY ISSUES

There is a general lack of regulatory guidance on what needs to be done to validate a biomarker assay. Routine and novel biomarkers are often performed in both bioanalytical and clinical laboratories. Bioanalytical methods for PK and toxicology studies follow the FDA guidance published in May 2001, which is often referred to as "GLP-compliant" [33]. Although biomarker laboratory analyses have many similarities to those studies, the variety of novel biomarkers and the nature of their applications often preclude the use of previously established bioanalytical validation guidelines. Assays for diagnostic and/or treatment decisions follow the standards, guidelines, and best practices required in the Clinical Laboratory Improvement Amendments (CLIA) of 1988, developed and published by Clinical and Laboratory Standards Institute (CLSI, formerly the National Committee for Clinical Laboratory Standards (NCCLS)) [34,35]. The CLSI/CLIA acceptance criteria are defined by the proven performance of the method, with adjustments over time using confidence limits [36]. For novel biomarker assays in early clinical development, where attrition of the clinical candidate and associated biomarker assays is high, the assay may only be used for a short period of time, precluding the establishment of appropriate confidence limits under these guidelines.

Biomarker development during discovery is not subjected to regulatory control by government agencies or GLP-compliant quality assurance (QA) units. When transitioning from preclinical to clinical development, assay objectives may shift. Goals may change from detecting only dramatic effects to quantifying graded trends in response to define exposure–response relationships. The rigor of the method validation usually increases from the exploratory phases to definitive studies. In general, data in exploratory or other early phases are not used for submission to government agencies in support of safety and efficacy. If the data are used for important business decision making, review by the internal QA may assure that the data are reliable for that purpose. On the other hand, biomarkers to support drug safety should be most similar to GLP compliant studies. Therefore, a "one-size-fits-all" mandate, such as the regulatory guidelines for PK support, is not suitable for biomarkers. Biomarker method development and validation should be "fit-for-purpose" so that assays could be successfully applied to meet the intended purpose of the study. In general, advanced validation should be performed in the spirit of GLP while exploratory validation is usually of research nature and non-GLP.

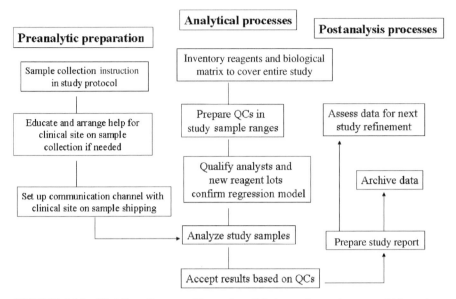

FIGURE 6.14   Workflow diagram of in-study validation and sample assay of biomarker.

6.8   IN-STUDY VALIDATION

The workflow for in-study validation is depicted in Fig. 6.14.

6.8.1   QC and SC Samples to Track Assay Performance and Stability

The performance of in-study assays is tracked by analyzing the performance of the assay using QC samples. Typically QCs at low, mid, and high concentrations of the analyte with at least two replicates at each level are included in each analytical run along with standards, SC, and the unknown samples. The number of QCs should be ≥5% of the number of study samples in the batch. Ideally, QCs used in the in-study sample analysis phase should be prepared identically to the low, mid, and high VS used in the prestudy validation phase, but this is not an absolute necessity. Where this is possible, it avoids the need to reassay and assign the target values. In addition, the determination and evaluation of SC in each run enables assay performance monitoring of authentic samples for trend analysis for stability and reagent consistency.

6.8.2   Kit Lot Changes

Sometimes a consistent supply of the same kit lot is not possible in a lengthy clinical study. Experiments should be performed upon a kit lot change to compare the new kit standard against the previous lot. If the previous kit standard lot is exhausted, charts of a common set of SC can be useful to detect lot differences, as shown in Fig. 6.12.

6.8.3   Acceptance Criteria

Assay acceptance criteria for biomarkers do not solely depend on the deliverable method accuracy and precision, as is the general rule in bioanalytical laboratories. Instead, the consideration should be on the assay suitability for the intended applications considering three major factors: (a) the intended use of the data during various stages of drug development, (b) the nature of the assay methodology and the type of data that the assay provides, and (c) the biological variability of the biomarker that exists within and between populations. Thus, the first factor helps shape the assay tolerance or acceptance criteria for biomarkers.

The acceptance criteria for a novel biomarker can initially be determined by assay performance in prestudy method validation. Data obtained from the in-study validation using subject samples can then be used to refine the initial acceptance criteria set during the prestudy validation. For example, an assay with 50% total error may still be acceptable for detecting a twofold treatment effect observed in a clinical trial. Setting acceptance criteria *a priori* may not be appropriate (or even possible) in an exploratory application of novel biomarkers, since the values seen in the incurred samples may not be what is expected or predicted.

For a quasi-quantitative method without standards (e.g., immunogenicity and enzyme activity), the accuracy of the method will not be determined. Instead, untreated samples (or a placebo control) are used to calculate % changes in the baseline. The QC precision data will be considered for method acceptance.

6.8.4   Stability

Long-term storage stability in the biological matrix can be updated during in-study validation.

6.9   CONCLUSIONS

This chapter describes the challenges and practical approaches to ligand-binding assays for biomarker quantification. The main points include (1) defining the purpose of the bioanalytical method application, (2) assay development using the appropriate reagents, (3) assay qualification and validation meeting the intended purpose of an assay, and (4) statistical treatments and interpretation.

A common primary goal for biomarker assays in drug development is to provide an early indication of drug exposure-related safety and efficacy, often aiding "go/no-go" decisions surrounding further drug development. For mechanism-based drug development, biomarkers are often used for different purposes. For example, a target biomarker for one drug candidate can be a proximal or distal marker for another drug candidate. Thus, the intended purpose(s) must be understood and defined before assay development for the biomarker begins.

The critical assay reagents for most ELISAs consist of the reference standard and capture and detection reagents. There is often a lack of knowledge of the chemical forms of the endogenous biomarker in the target populations. Due to the heterogeneous nature of many protein biomarkers, discrepancies may exist between the endogenous forms and the reference standard. In addition, there can be differences between standard curve blank control and the sample biological matrices. Parallelism is an important issue that has to be tested using authentic samples from the target population. Another important consideration is binding of the biomarker to endogenous binding proteins, receptors, and drugs, which may cause assay anomalies. Different methods may measure different forms of the biomarker, which often leads to confounding data. Exactly which form(s) of the biomarker is being measured in a given ELISA (e.g., bound or free) is beyond the scope of this chapter. For example, biophysical methods can be developed to investigate the protein interactions of the target and proximal biomarkers with the drug compound and other associated matrix proteins. ELISA reagents and procedures can be designed and manipulated to measure bound or free species of the biomarkers. A thorough understanding of the biology involved with the biomarker and the protein associations is required to identify which form(s) should be quantified to derive clinically meaningful data. However, this knowledge is often not available during the exploratory phase of drug development.

Statistical analysis of biomarker assay performance enables an assessment of whether the method will meet the study purpose before its application. Statistical data from in-study performance can continue to add information to the method appropriateness, especially data from the sample controls, which provide trends of authentic sample stability and reagent lot variability. Data from multiple exploratory and advanced biomarker studies, perhaps examining different drug candidates (from first-in-class to other drug candidates affecting related pathways), can contribute to the accumulation of knowledge surrounding a biomarker and aid its ultimate qualification. New "fit-for-purpose" development and validation methods thus need to evolve with accumulating knowledge.

ACKNOWLEDGMENTS

The authors are grateful to the Biomarker Subcommittee in the Ligand-Binding Assay Bioanalytical Focus Group of the American Association of Pharmaceutical Scientists for ideas and collaborations in the "fit-for-purpose" method validation concept. We also thank Binodh DeSilva, Yuling Wu, Jin Wang, and Feng Ca for contributions to the content and critical review of this manuscript, and Guang Chen for statistical support for CK18 assay qualification.

REFERENCES

1. FDA Mar 2004 Report. Innovation or Stagnation? Challenge and Opportunity on the Critical Path to New Medical Products. Available at www.fda.gov/opacom/hpview.html.

2. Bloom J.C., and Dean R.A. (eds) (2003) *Biomarkers in Clinical Drug Development.* Marcel Dekker, New York.

3. Biomarkers Definitions Working Group (2001) Biomarkers and surrogate endpoints: preferred definitions and conceptual framework. *Clinical Pharmacology and Therapeutics*, **69**, 89–95.

4. Bjornsson, T.D. (2005) Biomarkers applications in drug development. *European Pharmaceutical Review*, **1**, 17–21.

5. Wagner, J.A. (2002) Overview of biomarkers and surrogate endpoints in drug development. *Disease Markers*, **18**, 41–46.

6. FDA Guidance for Industry Exposure–Response Relationships—Study Design, Data Analysis, and Regulatory Applications. April 2003.

7. Lee, J.W., Smith, W.C., Nordblom, G.D., and Bowsher, R.R. (2003) Validation of assays for the bioanalysis of novel biomarkers. In: Bloom, J.C., and Dean, R.A. (eds), *Biomarkers in Clinical Drug Development*. Marcel Dekker, New York, pp. 119–149.

8. Lee, J.W., Weiner, R.S., Sailstad, J.M., Bowsher, R.R., Knuth, D.W., O'Brien, P.J., Fourcroy, J.L., Dixit, R., Pandite, L., Pietrusko, R.G., Soares, H.D., Quarmby, V., Vesterqvist, O.L., Potter, D.M., Witliff, J.L., Fritche, H.A., O'Leary, T., Perlee, L., Kadam, S., and Wagner, J.A. (2005) Method validation and measurement of biomarkers in nonclinical and clinical samples in drug development. A conference report. *Pharmaceutical Research*, **22**, 499–511.

9. Mire-Sluis, A.R., Barrett, Y.C., Devanarayan, V., Koren, E., Liu, H., Maia, M., Parish, T., Scott, G., Shankar, G., Shores, E., Swanson, S.J., Taniguchi, G., Wierda, D., and Zuckerman, L.A. (2004) Recommendations for the design and optimization of immunoassays used in the detection of host antibodies against biotechnology products. *Journal of Immunological Method*, **289**, 1–16.

10. Lambert, J.P., Ethier, M., Smith, J.C., and Figeys, D. (2005) Proteomics: from gel based to gel free. *Analytical Chemistry*, **15**, 3771–3787.

11. Washburn, M.P., Wolters, D., and Yates, J.R. (2001) Large-scale analysis of the yeast proteome by multidimensional protein identification technology. *Nature Biotechnology*, **19**, 242–247.

12. Stoch, S.A., and Wagner, J.A. (2007) Biomarker analysis as a decision-making tool in drug discovery and development: implications for peroxisome proliferator–activator receptors. *International Journal of Pharmaceutical Medicine*, **21**, 271–277.

13. Kummar, S., Kinders, R., Rubinstein, L., Parchment, R.E., Murgo, A.J., Collins, J., Pickeral, O., Low, J., Steinberg, S.M., Gutierrez, M., Yang, S., Helman, L., Wiltrout, R., Tomaszewski, J.E., and Doroshow, J.H. (2007) Opinion: Compressing drug development timelines in oncology using phase '0' trials. *Nature Reviews Cancer*, **7**, 131–139.

14. Lee, J.W., Figeys, D., and Vasilescu, J. (2007) Biomarker assay translation from discovery to clinical studies in cancer drug development: quantification of emerging protein biomarkers. In: Sikora, K. (ed.), *Genomics in Cancer Drug Discovery and Development. Advances in Cancer Research Hampton GM*, Elsevier, pp. 269–298.

15. Lee, J.W., Devanarayan, V., Barrett, Y.C., Weiner, R., Allinson, J., Fountain, S., Keller, S., Weinryb, I., Green, M., Duan, L., Rogers, J.A., Millham, R., O'Brien, P.J., Sailstad, J., Khan, M., Ray, C., and Wagner, J.A. (2006) Fit-for-purpose method development and validation for successful biomarker measurement. *Pharmaceutical Research*, **23**, 312–328.

16. Sweep, F.C., Fritsche, H.A., Gion, M., Klee, G.G., and Schmitt, M. (2003) Considerations on development, validation, application, and quality control of immuno(metric) biomarker assays in clinical cancer research: an EORTC-NCI working group report. *International Journal of Oncology*, **23**, 1715–1726.

17. DeSilva, B., Smith, W., Weiner, R., Kelley, M., Smolec, J., Lee, B., Khan, M., Tacey, R., Hill, H., and Celniker, A. (2003) Recommendations for the bioanalytical method validation of ligand-binding assays to support pharmacokinetic assessments of macromolecules. *Pharmaceutical Research*, **20**, 1885–1900.

18. Tholen, D.W., Linnet, K., Kondratovich, M., Armbruster, D.A., Garrett, P.E., Jones, R.L., Kroll, M.H., Lequin, R.M., Pankratz, T., Scassellati, G.A., Schimmel, H., and Tsai, J. (2004) NCCLS EP17-P Protocols for Determination of Limits of Detection and Limits of Quantitation: Proposed Guideline.

19. National Committee for Clinical Laboratory Standards (CLSI)—Document EP5-A: Evaluation of Precision Performance of Clinical Chemistry Devices: Approved Guideline. 1999; Document EP6-P: Evaluation of the Linearity of Quantitative Analytical Method: Proposed Guideline. 1986; Document EP7-P: Interference Testing in Clinical Chemistry: Proposed Guideline. 1986; Document EP9-A: Method Comparison and Bias Estimation Using Patient Samples: Approved Guideline. 1995.

20. Lee, J.W., and Ma, H. (2007) Specificity and selectivity evaluations of ligand binding assay of protein therapeutics against concomitant drugs and related endogenous proteins. *The AAPS Journal*, **9**, E164–E170.

21. Sukovaty, R.L., Lee, J.W., Fox, J., Toney, K., Papac, D.I., Thomas, A., Grover, T.A., and Wells, D.S. (2006) Quantification of recombinant human parathyroid hormone (rhPTH(1-84)) in human plasma by immunoassay: commercial kit evaluation and validation to support pharmacokinetic studies. *Journal of Pharmaceutical and Biomedical Analysis*, **42**, 261–271.

22. Fuchs, E., and Klaus, W. (1994) Intermediate filaments: structure, dynamics, function, and disease. *Annual Review of Biochemistry*, **63**, 345–382.

23. Prasad, S.P., Soldatenkov, V.A., Sprnivasarao, G., and Dristschilo, A. (1999) Intermediate filament proteins during carcinogenesis and apoptosis. *International Journal of Oncology*, **14**, 563–570.

24. Moll, L., Franke, W.W., Schiller, D.L., Geiger, B., and Krepler, R. (1982) The catalog of human cytokeratins: patterns of expression in normal epithelia, tumors and cultured cells. *Cell*, **31**, 11–24.

25. Einarsson, R. (1995) TPS—a cytokeratin marker for therapy control in breast cancer. *Scandinavian Journal of Clinical Laboratory Investigation*, **221** (Suppl.), 113–115.

26. Caulin, C., Salvesen, G.S., and Oshima, R.G. (1997) Caspase cleavage of keratin 18 and reorganization of intermediate filaments during epithelial cell apoptosis. *Journal of Cell Biology*, **138**, 1379–1394.

27. Cummings, J., Ward, T.H., LaCasse, E., Lefebvre, C., St-Jean, M., Durkin, J., Ranson, M., and Dive, C. (2005) Validation of pharmacodynamic assays to evaluate the clinical efficacy of an antisense compound (AEG 35156) targeted to the X-linked inhibitor of apoptosis protein XIAP. *British Journal of Cancer*, **92**, 532–538.

28. Cummings, J., Ranson, M., LaCasse, E., Ganganagari, J.R., St-Jean, M., Jayson, G., Durkin, J., and Dive, C. (2006) Method validation and preliminary qualification of pharmacodynamic biomarker employed to evaluate the clinical efficacy of an antisense

compound (AEG35156) targeted to the X-linked inhibitor of apoptosis protein XIAP. *British Journal of Cancer*, **95**, 42–48.

29. Olofsson, M.H., Ueno, T., Pan, Y., Xu, R., Cai, F., Kuip, K., Muerdter, K., Sonnenberg, M., Aulitzky, W.E., Schwarz, S., Andersson, E., Shoshan, M.C., Havelka, A.M., Toi, M., and Linder, S. (2007) Cytokeratin-18 is a useful serum biomarker for early determination of response of breast carcinomas to chemotherapy. *Clinical Cancer Research*, **13**, 3198–206.

30. Ueno, T., Toi, M., Biven, K., Bando, H., Ogawa, T., and Linder, S. (2003) Measurement of an apoptotic product in the sera of breast cancer patients. *European Journal of Cancer*, **39**, 769–774.

31. Heeschen, C., Dimmeler, S., Hamm, C.W., Boersma, E., Zeiher, A.M., and Simoons, M. L. (2003) Prognostic significance of angiogenic growth factor serum levels in patients with acute coronary syndromes. *Circulation*, **107**, 524–530.

32. Vural, P., Akgul, C., and Canbaz, M. (2006) Effects of hormone replacement therapy on plasma pro-inflammatory and anti-inflammatory cytokines and some bone turnover markers in postmenopausal women. *Pharmaceutical Research*, **54**, 298–302.

33. Code of Federal Regulations, Title 21, Vol. 1. Good Laboratory Practice for Nonclinical Laboratory Studies. Revised April 1, 2001.

34. National Committee for Clinical Laboratory Standards (CLSI)—Document EP5-A: Evaluation of Precision Performance of Clinical Chemistry Devices: Approved Guideline. 1999.

35. Code of Federal Regulations, Title 42, Vol. 3. Clinical Laboratory Improvement Amendment. Revised October 1, 2001.

36. Westgard, J.O. (2003) Internal quality control: planning and implementation strategies. *Annals of Clinical Biochemistry*, **40**, 593–611.

CHAPTER 7

The Use of Commercial Assay Kits for PK/PD Analysis in Drug Development

JOHN L. ALLINSON

ICON Development Solutions, Manchester, UK

JOHN D. CHAPPELL

ICON Development Solutions, Oxford, UK

7.1 INTRODUCTION

Commercial assay kits have been used widely in many laboratories around the world, most commonly in the field of diagnostics. In some countries, their use is highly regulated, sometimes including restrictions that only enable the use of approved assay kits for diagnostic purposes (e.g., requiring FDA approval for use in the United States). In other countries, the restrictions on use of assay kits in diagnostic procedures may mean that the clinical accountability is devolved to individual laboratories or even clinical scientists. However, it is the approval process of these assays that gives confidence to the user that the method is scientifically sound, is manufactured using products of defined quality, and is capable of performing to certain standards when a prescribed analytical method protocol is followed. This protocol and the method performance criteria are usually quoted in the product information provided with the kit.

This chapter will attempt to describe the various options available to validate commercial assays used in drug development appropriately to meet the expectations and requirements of each study in which they may be used. In particular, we will examine the use of commercial kits for pharmacodynamic (PD), efficacy and toxicity (biomarkers), and pharmacokinetic (PK) assessments. The PK assessment assays will focus on those molecules that are developed as therapeutic drugs, but which are also compounds that exist endogenously in humans. These drugs are often called new biological entities (NBEs) and examples include growth hormone, insulin, and erythropoietin.

Ligand-Binding Assays: Development, Validation, and Implementation in the Drug Development Arena. Edited by Masood N. Khan and John W. A. Findlay
Copyright © 2010 John Wiley & Sons, Inc.

The use of these assay kits in drug development is acceptable, provided the method protocol quoted is used without change and the method performance criteria are sufficient for each study's requirements. However, it is often the case that some of these methods require alteration in some way and it is here that problems can begin. Moreover, there are literally thousands of assay kits available from many manufacturers that are *not* approved for use in diagnostics but are supplied with instructions such as "for research and development use only." These are often for the quantitation of analytes that have grown in interest to scientists working in drug development and offer potential information of value to gain insight into a particular drug's safety, efficacy, or pharmacodynamic effects. Added to this is the possibility of also altering either the method protocol or some components of these kits, and this has resulted in different laboratories using different procedures to validate their assays—with little consensus—and, in the authors' experience, sometimes disastrous results.

One of the authors benefited greatly from spending many years in a diagnostic laboratory with excellent clinical and biomedical scientists in the UK's National Health Service, where the standard practice was to put every assay through a full validation exercise—basically reproducing all the experiments that the manufacturer performed and demonstrating that the laboratory could reproduce the performance criteria quoted in the product information provided with the kit. (Experiments for such criteria as antibody specificity are sometimes not reproduced in the laboratory using the kit due to various reasons.) This information was also produced for kits that had not been fully approved but were of interest at the time. These assays were carefully monitored over time to gain confidence that they could deliver a level of performance that would meet the needs of the day, which may have been additional information to a diagnostic procedure. Many of today's routine diagnostic assays were developed and refined in just this way—sometimes taking years to reach a level of performance that was robust enough to gain official approval.

This latter scenario is very similar to the one that exists within drug development today and the needs that scientists have for the assays that they use in the course of that development.

7.1.1 Definition of a Kit

For the purpose of this chapter, we include a wide range of reagents. These include fully accredited diagnostic kits, research and development kits (both with and without method protocols), reagent sets supplied as separate components to "build" or develop assays, and basic reagents that may be procured from a number of different manufacturers for the purpose of constructing a single assay method. We will also cover scenarios where an "approved" or "R&D" kit may require one or more component reagents to be replaced with the same, or similar, material from a different source.

Included in these components for possible change will be calibration standards and quality control (QCs) samples. A thorough understanding of how changing these parts of a kit may impact upon the results that a method may generate is required to avoid pitfalls or, at worst, potential misinterpretation of results. Moreover, we will also discuss scenarios of using a commercial kit for measurements in matrices or species other than those for which it was designed or checked for suitability.

7.1.2 History of Biomarker Assay Validation

By far the most amount of work conducted in the validation of biomarker assays has taken place within the diagnostics industry. This has led to there now being in place requirements for assay validation to meet approval by different regulators that are in use by every diagnostic manufacturing company.

Many, if not all, of these procedures have evolved over many years and with continuous feedback within the scientific communities around the world. Much of this has been conducted within an organization called the Clinical Laboratory Standards Institute (CLSI)—formerly known as the National Committee for Clinical Laboratory Standards (NCCLS). Many guidance documents are available from this organization's Web site (see below) that explain how some of the assay performance characteristics are established for the purposes of diagnostics. A number of these experiments are very similar to, or indeed the same as, experiments we conduct in validating biomarker assays for use in drug development and are listed in Table 7.1.

In addition to this organization, a number of professional bodies have been deeply involved in the evolution and development of laboratory services working in the clinical arena. In the United Kingdom, for instance, these include the Royal College of Pathologists (www.rcpath.org/), the Association of Clinical Biochemists (www.acb.org.uk/), and the Institute of Biomedical Sciences (www.ibms.org/)—formerly the Institute of Medical Laboratory Sciences, all actually international organizations based on their membership.

TABLE 7.1 Relevant Guidance Documents Available from the Clinical Laboratory Standards Institute (Formerly, National Committee for Clinical Laboratory Standards)

- EP05-A2 Evaluation of Precision Performance of Quantitative Measurement Methods
- EP06-A Evaluation of the Linearity of Quantitative Measurement
- EP07-A2 Interference Testing in Clinical Chemistry
- EP09-A2 Method Comparison and Bias Estimation
- EP10-A2 Preliminary Evaluation of Quantitative Clinical Laboratory Methods
- EP12-A User Protocol for Evaluation of Qualitative Test Performance
- EP14-A2 Evaluation of Matrix Effects
- EP15-A2 User Verification of Performance for Precision and Trueness
- EP17-A Protocols for Determination of Limits of Detection
- GP10-A Assessment of the Clinical Accuracy of Laboratory Tests
- ILA21-A Clinical Evaluation of Immunoassays
- ILA23-A Radioimmunoassays and Enzyme, Fluorescence, and Luminescence Immunoassays
- C24-A3 Statistical Quality Control for Quantitative Measurement Procedures
- C28-A2 How to Define and Determine Reference Intervals

In the field of drug development, the consensus on the validation of analytical methods has concentrated on drug assays typically used to produce pharmacokinetic data rather than on biomarker assays. Until the recently published paper from the AAPS LBABFG Biomarker Committee, there has been little in the way of consensus within the industry focused on biomarker methods [1,2]. Hence, we have a scenario where different laboratories may conduct biomarker assays differently, depending upon the technology used and whether the biomarker results are used for an indication of safety/toxicity or something else. One problem here is the essential requirement to ensure that the laboratory meets *all* of the requirements placed on the biomarker results data—and this includes *both* regulatory and clinical needs. Therefore, it is not surprising that in the validation of these assays, the experiments used to demonstrate analytical performance can often be a mixture of those used to validate drug (PK) and diagnostic assays.

7.2 VALIDATION DEFINITIONS THAT MAY BE INTERPRETED INCONSISTENTLY

The validation experiments conducted in the course of validating a commercial kit are the same as for any biomarker assay and the full list of possible experiments is given in Table 7.2.

It is not intended to describe the definitions of these in detail since this information can be found in other chapters of this book. It is important that attention is paid to these specific definitions since some terms may mean different things to different scientists, particularly those related to assay linearity and parallelism.

We describe the methods recommended to test for all of these components in the following sections. It is, however, perhaps useful to briefly cover those elements of these experiments or definitions that can cause the most confusion.

7.2.1 Analyte Stability

One of the most important matters to consider is that of analyte stability and for most analytes, manufacturers will rarely have stability data covering long periods of

TABLE 7.2 List of Experiments Utilized for the Validation of Biomarker Assays

- Accuracy
- Precision
- Sensitivity
- Linearity
- Parallelism
- Specificity
- Analytical range
- Analyte stability
- Standard and QC stability
- Reagent stability

time—especially if from the diagnostic arena, since most assays are typically conducted within a short time after collection (maybe up to 1 or 2 weeks at most). Moreover, for some biomarkers, it is important that the analyte concentration is sufficient to ensure that true stability can be evaluated on a statistical level when other components such as overall assay variability and batch-to-batch bias are taken into account. The author's laboratory routinely recommends that stability data are *never* generated from "spiking in" by using manufactured components since in many cases we have experience of demonstrating that the endogenous molecules do not necessarily have the same physical or functional properties. This is also an important consideration when purchasing commercially produced quality control material since they will not all have the same stability properties for the same biomarkers depending upon the source of the material used to manufacture them. If data are generated in this way, it must be used with great care and not accepted as being a true indication of the stability of the endogenous molecule when present in different biological matrices. It is good practice to apply this to all biomarkers—not just macromolecules.

7.2.2 Accuracy of Biomarker Assay Performance

Absolute accuracy in many biomarker assays may not be practical to demonstrate or determine. This is usually due to the degree (or lack of it) to which the primary calibration material can be characterized. This, however, is usually of reduced concern provided that other assay performance characteristics are adequate. Overall precision is by far the most important characteristic, since we are normally concerned with demonstrating relative changes in concentration of the biomarker over time (often considerably long periods). Therefore, although we can assess relative error (bias) in some cases, the ability to reproduce the same concentration results data over the "assigned" analytical range of the assay from the first batch through to the last in the projects for which the assay is used should be the overriding consideration as opposed to absolute accuracy when interpreting assay validation results.

7.2.3 Parallelism

Some workers will interpret this as the ability to reproduce calibration curves for a particular assay that are parallel to each other when plotted graphically—whether linear or nonlinear, as opposed to a demonstration of analyte recovery without bias, when sample matrix is diluted to assay samples whose concentrations lie above the analytical range of the method. Parallelism and other potential matrix effects should be investigated separately.

Since the matrices used for calibrators (and indeed QCs) may need to be different from the biological matrix of the samples to be analyzed, great care is required here—and especially when assays are expected to be used over long periods of time when calibrator and QC sample lots may necessarily change. Therefore, parallelism in terms of the biomarker assays described here is a relation of the biological matrix of interest to the calibrators—not a relation and acceptance of different calibrators to each other. While lot-to-lot change of calibrators is very important, this should not be confused with the evaluation of parallelism in the biological matrix of interest that is an *extremely* important, if not critical, component of assay validation.

Evaluation of parallelism for ligand-binding PK assays is very similar to that for biomarker PD assays since most PK assays that employ commercial kit methods are likely to be for endogenous compounds. This describes the dilution of incurred samples rather than dilution of spiked samples. The dilution of spiked samples is termed *dilution linearity* [3].

7.2.4 Dilution Linearity

Linearity has been described by some workers in a way which, by the current authors, would be interpreted as matrix parallelism, whereas others will use the term to describe the extent to which a calibration curve is linear in nonligand-binding assays. For the purpose of this chapter, the term linearity or "dilution linearity" is used to describe the results of experiments conducted using spiked samples to demonstrate the potential for high-concentration samples to be able to be diluted into the analytical range and read with acceptable accuracy and precision. It is often used to give an *indication* that matrix effects will not cause a problem upon sample dilution in circumstances where incurred or volunteer samples are not available with concentrations of analyte sufficiently high to conduct parallelism experiments.

7.3 VALIDATION EXPERIMENTS

7.3.1 Specificity

This can really be seen as being an assessment of analytical methods in the presence of four different types of components. It is particularly important, and most often challenging, in ligand-binding methods, which do, of course, form the majority of biomarker assays used in drug development today.

- First, in the field of diagnostics and, therefore, for many commercial assays, methods are assessed and information provided regarding specificity of the method to analyze samples that contain a number of other endogenous components commonly seen. This is because in diagnostic laboratories that handle specimens every day from patients suffering a wide range of diseases, there may be problems in the handling or collection of samples that can cause some physical deterioration in blood cells before plasma or serum may be separated from them. In addition, the fasting/nonfasting state of the patient can also cause difficulties. Hence, it is common to see method interference data on hemolysis and lipemia. Interference from bilirubin—elevated in cases of jaundice—is also commonly assessed, and this has been the case for many years.
- Second, with the advent of methods to measure such components as steroids, hormones, and cytokines, some manufacturers often now provide a significant amount of specificity data of the method to detect the specific analyte of interest

in the presence of other endogenous molecules that are structurally similar. Individual laboratories should consider whether further investigation of these or other molecules is required for their particular project.

- Third, in the field of drug development, it is also important to consider the potential method interference from the drug under development, and any potential metabolites that may be encountered in the biological samples to be analyzed.

- Finally, it is also important to consider comedication that is likely to be used in the patient population of interest for the later-stage clinical trials.

All of these interferences can be evaluated by spiking in the compounds of interest at concentrations that are likely to be encountered. The authors commonly test for up to two or three times these concentrations to allow some safety margin for possible specimens where they may be present at higher levels than expected.

It should be recognized that full specificity of LBA methods for macromolecules (e.g., proteins, oligonucleotides, etc.) can never be demonstrated for most assays because of a lack of knowledge of the structures and cross-reactivities/interferences of intermediate products of metabolism or the availability of these to test. Therefore, it is important for scientists working in this arena to appreciate the *full* range of challenges related to method specificity—some of which may not have been previously encountered within their analytical field of work.

7.3.2   Calibration

Commercial kits are usually supplied with calibration standard material. This may be in the form of a single vial of product from which a calibration curve can be constructed by serial dilution, or it may be a series of vials of ready-to-use standards with concentrations representative of the method's analytical range. For the purposes of assays used in drug development, it is often the case that the user will require a larger amount of calibration material, or a larger number of calibrator levels than is supplied. In the latter case, it is often possible to produce additional calibration standards from those provided either by dilution or by the mixing of those supplied.

It should be understood that in most cases, the calibration material provided may not be 100% pure (most are not supplied with a Certificate of Analysis). However, notwithstanding the recommendations below, this is often not a major issue since the majority of biomarker assays will, by definition, be *relative quantitative* assays that do not measure absolute concentration. In addition, in many assay kits, particularly more recent ones, the calibration material may not be well characterized or purified, or it may not be fully representative of the endogenous analyte to be measured. Therefore, we would recommend procuring material from at least one other third-party manufacturer against which concentrations can be checked to ensure consensus. If there is disparity, another source may be required. It is also a good idea to check with the kit manufacturer as to where they have sourced their calibration material, since they often do not manufacture it themselves. On more than one occasion with certain assays we have discovered that there may be very few sources of the required compound available, with different kit manufacturers all obtaining their calibration material from the same source.

It is also important for us to mention that the above proposition, while good practice, can be difficult. This is especially the case where concentration is expressed in arbitrary or poorly defined units, which may mean that it may even prove to be difficult to match and compare the concentrations of the different materials.

There will also be the need for consideration of the analytical range required. This point may also dictate the need for reoptimization of the assay if the required analytical range differs from that of the assay kit. This may only be possible in kits where components are supplied in a format that will allow it (e.g., antibodies supplied for plate coating such as R&D systems "Duo Sets" or those supplied for bead conjugation). The analytical range may require changes for a number of reasons, including reduction to focus on concentrations clinically relevant to a particular study or sensitivity issues where the quantitative range needs to be increased at low concentrations since the analyte to be measured may be expected to be reduced or suppressed by the drug under investigation.

7.3.3 Calibration Standard Matrix

This has been a subject of much discussion and debate. Many assay kits will be provided with calibration standards that have been prepared in a *surrogate* matrix. One example is protein-based buffer solution.

Surrogate matrix calibration standards can offer a number of benefits to the method. They usually increase the robustness of a method because they often display less variability batch to batch than calibrators in biological matrix. They are easier to prepare and usually more stable also. However, it is critically important to ensure that the matrix of the samples to be measured is thoroughly investigated using other experiments (spiked recovery followed by dilutional linearity and parallelism). In this scenario, it is also important to ensure that at least one, and preferably all, of the QC samples to be used is fully representative of the matrix of the samples wherever possible. (This may include using both unspiked and spiked matrix samples or pools, or mixing samples or pools of matrix with different analyte concentration to produce QC samples of differing and appropriate concentrations.)

Surrogate matrix calibration standards also mean that many methods can be used across many matrices (and even species) as long as the matrix-specific investigations are done via the experiments mentioned above and described in more detail later. This is why many approved diagnostic methods will be found with matrix specificity data for plasma containing different anticoagulants as well as serum or other biological fluids.

7.3.4 Calibration Curve Fit

Additional factors to consider in the calibration of the method are the curve fit of choice and possible weighting factors associated with the chosen model. The statistical basis for the selected algorithm is discussed in another chapter. The majority of assays have nonlinear calibration curves and this makes the choice of curve fit extremely important. Manufacturers will often recommend a curve-fit algorithm to use. However, it is common practice in the authors' laboratory to process the raw data responses from the calibration curves in the prevalidation batches by a variety of algorithms to assess the best curve fit from the analytical results obtained. These algorithms are commonly available on a variety of analytical platforms such as plate readers, LIMS, and some diagnostic analyzers (e.g., SoftMax-Pro and Watson LIMS). Users in the drug development environment should note that these software packages require validation before use on regulated studies. Weighting factors are a more complex issue, and we will leave it to the mathematicians and statisticians to describe the basis behind these elsewhere.

7.3.5 Quality Control, Statistics, and Acceptance Criteria

Quality control and acceptance criteria have also been topics of much debate. We will attempt to address the main points to be considered when using commercial assay kits here.

7.3.5.1 Quality Control Samples   First, many commercial kits come with quality control specimens. They will often have target values and acceptance limits provided in the documentation that comes with them. A number of points are worthy of consideration at this stage:

(a) What is the matrix of the QC samples? Is it the same as the matrix of the biological samples to be analyzed?

(b) Even if the matrix is the same (e.g., serum), the QCs may have been produced by spiking in analyte using either manufactured or endogenous materials.

(c) If spiking in has occurred, the source of the analyte material used for this may be very important, in terms of not only species but, potentially, also tissue. For example, some biomarkers that are present in multiple tissue types may have very different properties (physical as well as functional) when it comes to assessing them using different analytical methods or techniques.

(d) The source of the material used to prepare QCs may be the same as that used to produce the calibrators supplied with the kit and in these circumstances it is good practice to look for an alternative source.

(e) The acceptance ranges provided for the QCs may not be appropriate for the intended use, either because they do not reflect the analytical performance of the method and hence do not give sufficient information toward the assay being under adequate control, or because they are too wide to ensure that the results can be correctly interpreted from a clinical perspective when other issues are considered. (These will include physiological variability and assessment of clinical significance of either the degree of change over time, or the concentration itself in terms of clinical normality.)

TABLE 7.3 Examples of Quality Control Material

- Commercial QC material: assayed and unassayed. These may be lyophilized or liquid-stable preparations
- Incurred sample pools
- Commercially available matrix spiked with molecule of interest sourced from a third party supplier
- Surrogate matrix spiked with molecule of interest sourced from a third party supplier
- Commercially available matrix spiked with calibration standard material
- Surrogate matrix spiked with calibration standard material
- Spiking into matrix using another biological fluid (e.g., urine spiked with plasma/serum)
- Continuity QC samples: analyzing samples of low/medium/high concentration from previous batch to ensure consensus (*Note*: There are both regulatory and ethical issues to consider in this and pooling may be required.)
- Samples donated from normal volunteers under informed consent
- Samples from Bio-Banks

There are a number of alternatives to choose from when deciding which type of QC material is best for a particular method or project and a list of some examples is contained in Table 7.3.

7.3.5.2 *Quality Control Acceptance Criteria* Commercial assay kits that also have QC samples supplied will normally contain data on expected target value for each QC sample and usually also expected or acceptable ranges. The procedures used to produce these figures and reasoning behind them can vary widely between different manufacturers and so great caution is required, particularly with "R&D" type kits. It is common to find that these ranges do not have any connection to the actual performance of the assay from a statistical standpoint, and also that they are usually much wider than one may want to accept (or achieve).

Since we accept that the majority of biomarker assays will be relative (as opposed to absolute) quantitative methods, the main concern is one of reproducibility of the assay over the time course of the relevant study for which it is being used. Therefore, it is often common at the validation stage to set no accuracy acceptance criteria for the QC samples analyzed in the validation batches but to evaluate the intra- and interassay performance of the method using the QC sample results obtained therein. Thereafter, it can be assessed as to whether the assay's performance meets the requirement of the study and if so, acceptance criteria for the sample analysis batches can be set *a priori*.

For relative quantitative methods, one may then set "nominal" QC target values from the means of the results obtained in the validation batches. The interassay coefficients of variation (CVs) of the QC samples in those batches can then be used to calculate statistically relevant acceptance ranges. In the clinical diagnostics arena, these are usually taken as being 95% confidence limits (approximately, $2 \times CV$ or within ± 2 standard deviation (SD) of the mean). Using this type of quality control on an ongoing basis from validation is a good way of ensuring that the assay continues to perform as it did during the validation exercise and subtle changes in method performance can often be detected at an early stage. This type of data can be applied to individual batches for small number of samples, or multiple batches for large numbers of samples. In the latter case, more complex methods of QC result analysis may be warranted (e.g., in large phase 3 trials) such as Westgard Multi QC rules (see www.westgard.com/mltirule.htm).

Alternatively, a particular study may have less rigorous requirements from a method performance perspective, and this could be due to the fact that the assay results are to be used for early-stage decisions in the drug's progression, or it may be for a biomarker that has very marked responses to physiological effects. In these cases, it may be warranted to set an acceptance range based on a certain percentage relative error (bias), for example, within $\pm 20\%$ of the mean value.

In addition, one may wish to use a variation of the 4–6–x rule used in PK assays, or even a combination of some or all of the above.

Overall, it is the responsibility of the project team to decide what is appropriate taking into account all the requirements of the assay to enable adequate and valid clinical and statistical interpretation of the analytical results.

7.3.6 Planning of Validation Experiments

The degree of validation performed on any commercial kit should be no different from any other analytical method. It will be dictated by the use of the results data, defining the needs of the method and ensuring that the method is fit for purpose. This is described well in the AAPS LBABFG Biomarker Committee's white paper [1].

However, for some assay kits, a degree of benefit can be gleaned at an early stage from the manufacturer's quoted performance criteria. This information may also help in deciding other factors to be evaluated, such as optimum batch size and number of replicates required. This information can often replace some of the experiments that would be conducted in the method development/feasibility stage of a newly developed method. A note of caution is, however, worthy here. It is the authors' experience that the information received from different manufacturers may have been derived in quite different ways, using either different experiments or sample numbers/batches and may not be reproducible. That said, it has been our experience that performance criteria are often improved from those quoted by the manufacturer when assays are established in the investigator's own laboratory.

We do not intend to describe in detail the exact structure and content of the experiments below but will discuss the issues and concerns to consider when compiling them.

7.3.7 Acceptance of Validation Batches

Usually, the only criterion used to accept or reject validation batches should be the goodness of fit of the calibration curve. Calibrator results data can be viewed in different ways:

(a) The precision of replicate results for each standard.
(b) The relative error of each calibrator concentration when each result is back-calculated from the fitted calibration curve.
(c) The regression results of the curve fit that describes the goodness of fit.

7.3.8 Number of Replicates

Many biomarker assay kits (especially 96-well microplate-based assays) will have a recommendation to analyze calibration standards, QCs, and samples in duplicate. Some methods are so good that if reliable automated equipment is used for the assay protocol (e.g., dilutions, reagent additions, etc.), it may be possible to reduce this to a single replicate. On the other hand, if method performance requires improvement, then it may be necessary to increase the number of replicates, for example, to triplicates.

The use of triplicate analysis is also a useful tool when analyzing samples where there are no backup aliquots available and the analyte is unstable. Here, it will assist in avoiding failed results due to poor duplicate precision and inability to repeat the assay. Different *a priori* acceptance criteria will be required for individual sample results in this scenario. For instance, you may wish to use mean data if precision of the replicates is good, or two results that show best consensus where precision is poor, or even the median of the three results.

The number of replicates required can be assessed by conducting the validation batches as a replicate (two or three) assay and processing the data based on those replicates. In addition, process the data using only the first replicate of each standard, QC, or sample. Then compare the assay performance data from the perspective of precision and relative error for the different number of replicates. The results will easily enable you to decide if the performance remains good enough using single as opposed to duplicate, or duplicate as opposed to triplicate protocols. The authors have seen a number of assays over the years that would fall into all of these categories.

7.3.9 Sensitivity

Depending upon the study's needs, this could be the limit of detection (LOD), lower limit of quantification (LLOQ), or both. The limit of detection is the lowest concentration that a method is able to differentiate from zero with a certain degree of statistical certainty. This may be important if the absence of the biomarker of interest is clinically relevant (e.g., when a drug's action is used to switch off a metabolic pathway or feedback mechanism). It is usually determined by replicate analysis of either matrix or surrogate samples known to contain no analyte. The CLSI publication EP17-A in Table 7.1 can be referred to for this. It is common in the biomarker field to report results data with concentrations below this figure as "not detected." The LLOQ is the lowest concentration that the method can measure within acceptable accuracy and precision. The accuracy and precision that are appropriate need to be decided and a precision profile will assist greatly in determining the approximate value of the LLOQ that can then be interrogated in more detail by replicate analysis of validation or QC samples prepared with levels of analyte around that value. Sample results with concentrations below this level can be reported in different ways, for example, "BLQ" (below the level of quantification) or "<LLOQ" where the actual LLOQ is quoted (e.g., <10 mg/L). In addition, it may be required to report data in this area as the actual values obtained. The argument in favor of this is largely a statistical one and is therefore best left to statisticians to discuss further.

Because of these definitions, be cautioned that a manufacturer's quoted levels of sensitivity will rarely, if ever, be concentrations that can be quantified with acceptable precision and relative error.

7.3.10 Precision

This should be determined using validation samples, and it is ideal if these are the same samples that will be used as quality control samples in the sample analysis phases of the studies. Choice of the concentrations will be determined by the use of the assay and, as previously mentioned, assay kit components will usually need to be supplemented by additional QC samples, either due to different concentrations or specific matrix requirements. The concentrations may be driven by the analytical range of the method, or the clinically relevant range expected to be important when analyzing test samples, or both.

Typically, the number of individual validation/QC sample replicates required for the validation runs will be at least four, although we usually recommend a minimum of six, over between three and six batches. Depending upon the needs of the method, additional batches may be required if more experiments than usual are needed (e.g., additional specificity). What is important here is that the same numbers of replicates of validation samples are present in every batch. This provides analytical consistency throughout all validation batches. For really complex methods, the number of batches may rise considerably. This should not be an issue as long as all the results data are recorded in the method validation report and, indeed, it can often give a better insight into how the method will perform over a longer period of time or large number of batches.

Hence, it is important to ensure that sufficient validation/QC samples are prepared to cover all of the expected validation batches and, if possible, the study sample analysis batches also. For commercial QC material, this means obtaining sufficient material from the same manufacturer's lot number. Clearly, stability or shelf life may limit how long this material may be stored and used.

Intra- and interassay imprecision should be calculated from *all* of the validation batch data.

7.3.11 Accuracy

As previously described, most biomarker assays are relative quantitative methods and not absolute (sometimes called definitive) quantitative methods. These differences are solely related to how well defined the calibration standard material is, and how well it is characterized or represents the endogenous analyte to be measured.

Absolute accuracy is not a necessity for biomarker assays. Most biomarker studies address changes in concentration over a time course and this is why precision of the assay is far more important. Of course, it is important for the person interpreting the data to be fully aware of what the assay results mean, particularly if making a judgment on their clinical significance. If results are being compared to a clinical "reference range," then it is very important that each laboratory investigates and establishes the range using the method that will be used for the clinical trial and in a population that is relevant to the population being studied.

Therefore, accuracy or relative error (RE or bias) is often measured against a "nominal value" assigned to QC samples. Once this value is assigned, the continual ability of the method to obtain the same result for that sample within the defined limits of acceptance dictates whether or not the method is in control, stable, and robust.

The "assigned" value may be that of the manufacturer, or the mean observed during validation batches of prepared QC or validation samples, and if they are from spiking into biological matrix, will be the sum of both the spiked component and any endogenous biomarker present in the matrix. If well-characterized material is available for spiking into a matrix pool, then the amount of biomarker present in the pool can be assessed using the method of standard additions or replicate analysis of the pool itself. After accurate spiking with the material in solution, a value can be assigned from the observed pool concentration plus the added spiked concentration.

7.3.12 Parallelism

This parameter may be defined as a condition in which dilution of test samples does not result in biased measurements of analyte concentration. Thus, when a test sample is serially diluted to result in a set of samples having analyte concentrations that fall within the quantitative range of the assay, there is no apparent trend toward increasing or decreasing estimates of analyte concentrations over the range of dilutions.

Parallelism experiments are a very important component of assay validation that can demonstrate an effect that the matrix of interest may have on the assay performance. Some assays require that samples are diluted considerably before analysis, and in these cases this is usually less critical. However, it is important to fully understand the effects that the matrix exhibits and so these experiments should always be performed. Moreover, where parallelism is not observed, it is important to understand the significance that this may have on the method and its appropriate use. Parallelism experiment results may dictate the degree to which a sample *must* be diluted, the limitation as to what extent it *can* be diluted, or both.

Parallelism experiments also require samples that contain the analyte in sufficiently high concentration to demonstrate the property adequately. Thus, it may be impossible to determine this before incurred samples are available. It is also important to take into account the analytical error of the method when interpreting results.

Depending upon the biomarker and the analytical range of the method, dilutions of the matrix should be made and analyzed and assessed for "recovery" when results are back-calculated to account for the dilution factor. Dilutions can be made using different materials. Some assay kits will come with sample diluents or calibrator diluents, and these may be assessed. Physiological saline is often used for serum/plasma/urine also. If these do not demonstrate nonparallelism, it is fine, but if effects are seen, it may be necessary to use a sample of the same matrix. This should preferably have no analyte present or at least a very low concentration and different proportions of this sample and a high-concentration sample can be mixed to create a range of "dilutions" that have 100% of the same biological matrix. The recovery calculations must take into account the contribution from the "diluent" sample as well as the high-concentration sample if detectable biomarker is present in the diluent sample. Parallelism experiments are ideally conducted in at least three high-concentration samples, but this may be limited by available samples, and experiments can be continually conducted as more samples with higher and higher concentrations become available.

There are different methods of examining data graphically that aid interpretation and the reader is referred to the biomarker paper [1] mentioned above for examples of these.

7.3.13 Dilution Linearity

(This section also covers issues for PK/TK assays that are discussed later.)

This is a condition in which dilution of a spiked sample does not result in a biased measurement of the analyte concentration. Therefore, this gives an indication that samples can be diluted from above the assay range into the calibration range in a linear fashion. This is particularly important for ligand-binding assays (LBAs) where the range of quantification may be very narrow. The dilutional experiments should be based on the expected highest concentrations of study samples.

If possible, a linearity sample should be prepared at the highest concentration expected to be found in study samples. To do this, suitable analyte should be available to "spike" into the appropriate biological matrix. This linearity sample is serially diluted to result in a set of samples having analyte concentrations that fall within the quantitative range of the assay. The measured concentrations of the dilution samples should be plotted against 1/dilution using linear regression. It is recommended that the results should have a correlation coefficient (R^2) of >0.98 indicating that the analyte dilutes in a linear fashion. Alternatively, the demonstration that the accuracy and precision of the diluted samples are the same as for the assay performance within the calibration range observed during validation may suffice. This experiment may be possible even if the biological matrix has an endogenous component, as long as this concentration is toward the LLOQ of the method. Dilutions would be made with the same matrix to ensure that the endogenous concentration is consistent.

Dilution linearity is also normally monitored during the study sample analysis phase by using dilution linearity quality control (DLQCs) samples. These samples are prepared at concentrations above the assay range and then diluted into range at the same time as the study samples. The dilutions performed for these DLQCs should be representative of how the samples are diluted.

Dilution linearity can be performed using the kit standard material if required or appropriate. Here, the highest standard could be prepared as instructed in the kit insert and then a 9/10 dilution made. This may be used as the 100% value and 9/10, 8/10, 6/10,

4/10, 2/10, and 1/10 dilutions prepared (if appropriate, other dilutions could be made to check the complete range of the assay). The high standard, together with all dilutions, should be analyzed together in one run. Where possible, the dilutions should be made with the same matrix used for the reconstitution of the high standard. If this is not possible, dilutions should be made using physiological saline or other surrogate matrix, and this should be documented. Expected values should be calculated from the 100% result and the % difference between this and the observed results calculated. Graphs can be drawn of observed results against expected results and once again the linear regression analysis should be performed. For ligand-binding assays, the range of dilutions/concentrations evaluated should be such as to allow the detection of any "high-dose look effect" (paradoxical apparently similar response at two widely different analyte concentrations).

7.3.14 Recovery

For ligand-binding assays, this would be the same as accuracy in the context of the FDA Bioanalytical Guidance document (i.e., PK assays).

Recovery describes the ability of an analytical system response to quantitate an amount of analyte that has been spiked into sample matrix. It is usually conducted using several samples or pools and the spiked material may be either calibrator, QC, or another source of the biomarker to be measured.

Most immunoassays do not involve procedures such as extraction of analytes from the matrix using, for example, solvents. Therefore, whereas recovery may be an important indicator of method suitability for chromatographic assays in which procedures used to isolate the analyte from the interfering matrix components can result in a significant loss of analyte, in immunoassays this is not commonly the case and recovery experiments are of lesser importance.

However, spiked recovery can give insights into possible matrix effects. Moreover, many commercial assay kits quote recovery experiment results from the man-ufacturer's internal validation procedures and hence reproducing those experiments in the assay validation exercise is often useful in demonstrating that the assay is performing as expected by comparing results with the manufacturer's quoted data.

In addition to using spiked recovery, we have also found it useful to use samples that have very high concentrations for the spiking of samples that contain very low concentrations. This is really an experiment that also proves that endogenous analyte is not behaving differently from the calibration material and additionally confirms the suitability of the calibration material for the assay. When spiking into matrix, it is advisable to ensure that the final mixture retains at least 95% of the original sample matrix component. Therefore, if the material used for spiking is in a solution that is not the same as the matrix (e.g., buffer, ethanol, or other), then the volume contribution that this solution makes to the final mixture of the sample matrix and spike solution being tested should not be more than 5%.

When recovery experiments are conducted, the acceptance criteria may simply be to demonstrate that the results confirm the manufacturer's claims. Other acceptance criteria need to be established on a case-by case basis.

7.3.15 Correlation of Methods and Cross-Validation

Often, when using commercial assay kits, a laboratory may find itself in a position where it needs to establish the method in a number of different laboratories, if samples are being analyzed at several locations (e.g., one laboratory per continent, or maybe using different analytical service providers). Alternatively, a sponsor may have been using a kit in-house and then wants to establish the method in a Contract Research Organization (CRO). Other scenarios also exist where an established method needs to change to a different assay kit for the same analyte, perhaps due to method interference by certain anticoagulants that would complicate sample collection protocols, or where samples have already been collected using such an anticoagulant. Another possibility is where manufacturers cease to produce a certain assay kit midway through a clinical trial, perhaps due to manufacturing difficulties or problems with maintaining a specific antibody cell-line.

If a method is being established at more than one location, it is essential that it is adequately demonstrated that the method is performing the same at all locations. In addition, should a method need to be changed from one kit to another (maybe different manufacturers) or where major changes in kit components have been made (e.g., antibodies), then it is essential that besides revalidating the method, it is also demonstrated that it is producing the same analytical results as the previous method for continuity of the study.

Ideally, it is best to use incurred samples for method correlations and we like to use at least 50 different samples, and these should cover as much of the analytical range as possible. QC samples of all levels can also be used but care needs to be taken to ensure that these are behaving the same as the incurred sample for both methods since, depending upon how the QC samples have been prepared, this may not be the case for some biomarker assays because of the source and type of biomarker used for spiking. Moreover, high-QC samples may artificially skew the correlation of the sample data if the range of concentrations that the incurred samples represent is relatively small.

In PK assays, typically, methods are accepted as being correlated provided all analytical results are within a certain percentage of each other by the different methods (e.g., method 2 result = (method 1 result ± 10%). However, more complex procedures are often required for biomarker assays and such things as slope and intercept of the correlation are important, as is the correlation coefficient. It may also be useful to calculate the mean of each method's results over a range of samples.

In general, we prefer using well-established correlation equations that have been used for many years in clinical diagnostic laboratories and these include the following:

(a) *Altman–Bland and NCCLS EP9-A bias plots* visually show agreement between two methods, or against a reference method.

(b) *Passing–Bablok regression or Deming regression* to quantify the agreement (or accuracy) between two methods [4].

Once it has been established that methods *correlate* adequately, other actions may be required since there may still be systematic differences between methods, particularly when working with kits from different manufacturers or using different antibodies. Here, one can either use the regression analysis to recalculate all previously analyzed sample results to equate to the new method and then continue to analyze and report results from the new method or, alternatively, results from the new method can be adjusted to equate to the older method results as the new results are produced and this avoids changing any previously generated results data. This scenario is, thankfully, usually rare and only presented in the biomarker field (as opposed to PK). Some central laboratories that perform these adjustments describe the process as making results from two different assays for the same analyte "combinable."

7.3.16 Lot-to-Lot Changes

While some assay kits demonstrate little or no variability between lot numbers, this is not always the case, and it is good practice to evaluate an experimental batch to confirm that there are no significant differences with different manufacturing lot numbers. We find that the easiest and most reliable way of doing this is to run a batch using the new batch number kit and include in that batch all of the calibration standards and QC samples from the old lot number kit. For some manufacturers or kits, calibration and QC samples provided may have different lot numbers at different dates compared to the other reagent components so that, in some cases, for example, if calibration standards have the same lot number across two different kit lot numbers, there is clearly no requirement to conduct the analysis on the old kit standards since it is simply duplication.

The authors find that the best way of proving continuity of performance across different kit lot numbers is to use the same QC samples throughout the course of the study. Therefore, as previously mentioned, it is a good idea to ensure that sufficient material is available at the time of validation to construct QC samples for the whole study. Here, it is simply necessary to apply the same acceptance criteria across different lot numbers of reagent kits. Without these QC samples, confirmation of lot-to-lot performance just becomes more complex and time consuming to generate adequate data.

However, it is also good practice, particularly for larger studies that may also be run over longer periods of time and, hence, suffer from more lot number changes, to review QC performance on a continual basis and check for more subtle changes in performance between different lots, if such changes would be considered to potentially give rise to data that are different enough to warrant concern. Here, the user will find QC charts for such indicators as cusum plots to be highly sensitive to small systematic changes in performance. A reference to an application of this and other QC methods to clinical studies is supplied [5].

7.4 STABILITY

Although not necessarily considered by many to be part of an *assay validation,* stability does perhaps warrant a mention here.

(1) Manufacturers rarely have stability data for samples stored for long periods of time and hence the user will be required to generate such data in the matrix of interest to support the analysis of aged samples.

(2) For most biomarkers, we tend to use the approach of collecting samples and storing them at $-80°C$ within short period (e.g., 15 min) of collection on ice and centrifuged at $4°C$ as our baseline "zero time" samples. Some matrices will require different specific collection conditions to avoid any changes in the concentration of the biomarker occurring immediately after the specimen is collected and before it is stored in a state that will maintain the integrity of the analyte.

(3) We also tend to collect a volume that is large enough to provide all the aliquots to be stored at different temperatures and conditions, and then store those aliquots at the conditions required, placing the aliquots into the $-80°C$ freezer when each evaluation at the selected time period and temperature has been completed. Hence, we build up, over time, a stock of aliquots stored at $-80°C$ that have been potentially stored at $-80°C$, $-20°C$, $4°C$, room temperature, freeze-thaw cycles, and so on, and then thaw and analyze *all* these samples in one batch to reduce batch-to-batch variability. However, this also requires the analysis of the original sample before freezing as immediately as possible after collection. This is the "zero-time" sample, the concentration of which is the baseline value that future results of the various stored samples are measured against to prove stability.

(4) We *always* analyze our "zero-time" aliquot in triplicate (i.e., six replicates for a "duplicate" assay to give three results) to overcome any random errors and take into account standard analytical errors, since stability data are often critical in dictating study logistics.

(5) If data produced in this way show problems of stability at a critical temperature, it may be necessary to revert back to designing the experiments in a different way—possibly with real-time analysis rather than storage at $-80°C$ after exposure to the different conditions, although we have rarely found this to be required.

(6) It is important to use samples that have high enough concentrations to be able to interpret the results as being stable in the light of expected analytical variability (which can be gleaned from the validation interassay precision data). This may require the use of incurred samples if the analyte of interest is not normally present in high concentrations in normal individuals.

(7) We *never* accept stability data generated on manufactured/recombinant molecules spiked into matrix to be necessarily fully representative of the stability of endogenous analytes. It is not uncommon to find different commercially available QC material to have different stability properties for the same analyte because the source of the material spiked in may be different. For biomarkers, we believe that true stability data *can only* be derived from experiments using endogenous molecules in the matrix of interest. This, of course, is not the case for exogenously administered macromolecules.

(8) Provided samples with high enough concentrations are used, it is possible to conduct stability experiments on aged samples. Here, aliquots are made from the sample and then some of these are left at the different temperatures for whatever time period required, and placed in $-80°C$ storage as before—essentially the aged sample becoming the "zero-time" sample. Then the stability data results are generated by analysis as before and evaluated.

(9) Consideration of breakdown or conversion pathways need to be taken into account when interpreting these data since it is possible that what appears to be observed stability may actually be the result of the analyte of interest breaking down only to be replaced by more molecules from the results of interconversion from other substances that exist in the sample and that are part of the same metabolic pathway. A good example of this possibility is specific steroids in urine. Indeed, this can result in the production of higher levels of some analytes than were present in the sample when it was collected and is why correct storage and/or the addition of stabilizers may be required. A notable case in the public domain that was the result of this phenomenon was that of a British female athlete who was banned for failing a urine drugs test that showed a high concentration of a particular steroid. It was not until it was proven that this can occur in female urine that contains extremely small levels of this particular steroid when stored inappropriately from interconversion from other excreted steroids or precursors that the athlete was exonerated of any offence.

7.4.1 Stability in PK Studies

The assessment of stability in PK studies is usually performed by using spiked quality control samples that are representative of the biological matrix. At least two concentrations, that is, low and high, should be prepared using the analyte reference standard. The stability samples should be representative of the test article, since endogenous concentrations may have a different stability profile. If endogenous material is present, then this can be used to prepare samples using a "standard addition" approach, that is, by spiking material in addition to the endogenous material.

7.4.2 Different Species

(This section also covers issues for PK/TK assays that are discussed later.)

It is possible that some researchers will want to use an assay kit for a different species than the kit is intended to be used for. This is most likely to occur if a human diagnostic assay is used to measure animal samples. In drug development, all new chemical entities (NCEs) will be evaluated in preclinical studies, so relevant assays are required to support these studies, that is, TK/PK and PD analysis. There can be advantages of using the same analytical method across different species, for example, to enable comparability of data.

Even if a kit is not specifically designed for animal usage, or is specifically designed for a particular species, it is possible that the manufacturers have data to support the use of their kit with different species. Some suppliers do provide information on species cross-reactivity and some also provide a complete list of their kits that can be used in other species. When selecting a kit for different species, it may be advisable to search for a species-specific kit. The main reason for using a species-specific kit is that it ensures reactivity of the analyte with assay key reagent(s) and it is likely that there will be fewer problems with matrix effects. If a species-specific kit is not available, a search of the literature can be performed to investigate whether other researchers have used specific commercial kits, that is, to obtain information on potential cross-reactivity and so on.

Before selecting the analyte, the relevance of the molecule/analyte in the species needs to be investigated. In some circumstances it is not relevant to measure certain molecules in the intended species since different species have physiological differences. Working in the CRO industry, we have seen many examples of assays that have been used inappropriately, requests for analysis that are not appropriate, or for which certain assays will present challenges, both in analysis and interpretation of the resulting data across different species. These may be due to a number of reasons but common ones are as follows:

(1) Biomarkers that do not exist due to cross-species differences, for example, cortisol in rodents.

(2) Biomarkers that have different physical and/or physiological properties (e.g., histamine in dogs (high due to hypersensitivity) versus primates (extremely unstable analyte)).

(3) Biomarkers that have different sensitivities to physiological changes/toxicity in different species (e.g., Gamma GT)

As these problems are common in relatively routine biomarkers, it is likely that similar issues may be faced in the future with more novel, esoteric, or newly discovered biomarkers.

For PK assays, it may be the case that a human-derived molecule is being dosed to a different species. In this case, an assessment should be made of whether structurally similar molecules in that species are likely to cross-react. If the molecule does not appear naturally in the species, for example, a humanized monoclonal antibody, then the assay can be used for that species, but potential matrix differences have to be investigated and solved, that is, parallelism, dilution linearity, and so on.

7.4.3 Stability of Reagents

Commercial kits usually come with quoted dates of expiry and we believe that it is appropriate to observe this date as the last date for use of the kit. It is advisable, however, to check expiry dates of all components individually as this date should be for the shortest shelf-life component and all components may not necessarily have the same shelf life. Many kits have relatively long expiry after manufacture (usually at least months), unless they have very unstable components, such as radioimmunoassay kits, where the isotopic reagent is usually only stable for a few weeks at most before the method becomes unusable.

In addition, it is also clear that these assay kits do not suddenly expire with regard to their integrity at midnight of the date of expiry quoted. Therefore, we believe that as long as care is taken and procedures fully documented, it should not be considered that expired kits are unsuitable for use *per se*. Acceptance criteria should be used that are the same as for nonexpired kits. The QC samples, if properly used from a statistical standpoint, will indicate whether the method is still in control and hence still fulfill their intended purpose. This is one example where we believe that associating QC acceptance criteria with the expected performance of the assay as observed at validation is very important. Good, robust, and statistically sound QC procedures will give demonstrable confidence in the integrity of results data generated using expired kits.

7.5 REOPTIMIZING REAGENT CONCENTRATIONS

(This section also covers issues for PK/TK assays that are discussed later.)

The checkerboard approach is the common way a microtiter plate assay is developed and optimized. In terms of commercial kits, this approach could be used to change a kit component or, in the case of development kits (e.g., R + D systems "Duo Sets"), to optimize the assay range for the specific requirements of the program.

On a checkerboard, multiple concentrations of each reagent are added to a plate. Multiple replicates of a limited standard curve are added to the microtiter plate to see how the reagent concentration differences affect the assay range. If a very sensitive method is required, then the biggest difference between zero (blank) and the lowest standard would be required. The checkerboard should allow the assay developer to assess the ideal reagent concentration to obtain the required assay range. Checkerboards can also be run under various incubation conditions to compare the effect of these on assay response.

A checkerboard example that can be run for an ELISA is shown in Fig. 7.1. This is a sandwich ELISA using two antibodies against the analyte. Detection is achieved using an anti-species conjugate. Actual concentrations used should be at the discretion of the method developer.

The main points of this procedure are as follows:

(1) The initial coating levels are based on the binding capacity of the microtiter plate (1, 2, 5, and 10 µg/mL).

(2) The standard analyte concentrations are 0, low, medium, and high. The low standard concentration should be close to the required LLOQ.

(3) The second antibody concentrations are based on the manufacturer's suggested range of concentrations.

(4) The conjugate concentration is the suggested manufacturer's lowest and highest dilution.

	1	2	3	4	5	6	7	8	9	10	11	12
A	Blank	Blank	Blank	Blank	Blank	Blank	Blank	Blank	Blank	Blank	Blank	Blank
B	Low	Low	Low	Low	Low	Low	Low	Low	Low	Low	Low	Low
C	Medium	Medium	Medium	Medium	Medium	Medium	Medium	Medium	Medium	Medium	Medium	Medium
D	High	High	High	High	High	High	High	High	High	High	High	High
E	Blank	Blank	Blank	Blank	Blank	Blank	Blank	Blank	Blank	Blank	Blank	Blank
F	Low	Low	Low	Low	Low	Low	Low	Low	Low	Low	Low	Low
G	Medium	Medium	Medium	Medium	Medium	Medium	Medium	Medium	Medium	Medium	Medium	Medium
H	High	High	High	High	High	High	High	High	High	High	High	High

Note: Low, medium, and high refer to calibration standard analyte concentration.

Coating concentration			
1 μg/mL	2 μg/mL	5 μg/mL	10 μg/mL
Columns 1–3	Columns 4–6	Columns 7–9	Columns 10–12

Second antibody concentration		
1 μg/mL	2 μg/mL	5 μg/mL
Columns 1,4,7,10	Columns 2,5,8,11	Columns 3,6,9,12

Conjugate dilution	
1 in 1000	1 in 20,000
Rows A–D	Rows E–H

FIGURE 7.1   Example of checkerboard.

7.5.1 Edge Effects

(This section also covers issues for PK/TK assays that are discussed later.)

The phenomenon of edge effects is associated with microtiter plate based assays. The result of edge problems is to cause different responses (either higher or lower) between the wells of the plate edge and internal wells. Edge effects are particularly noticeable with replicate analysis, for example, when duplicate analysis is being performed.

Edge effects and other plate trends are investigated by a whole plate imprecision experiment (Fig. 7.2). This is done by placing the same solution of standard/quality control samples in all the wells of the plate. The standard/QC solution used should produce a reasonable response value in the assay, for example, >1.0 optical density (OD) for a colorimetric method. The OD response values for the whole plate, individual columns and rows are averaged and CVs calculated. Trends in the CV data indicate the potential for edge and other plate effects. In terms of acceptance criteria for whole plate precision, this will depend on the specific requirements of the study but a suggested criterion is a CV of less than 5%.

One potential reason for edge effects is that there can be slight differences between the plastic surface of the edge wells and that of the internal wells. This is caused when the surface area of the plastic is increased by irradiation. Lower coating

Whole plate imprecision																
Date					Method					Prepared by / Checked by						
Column / Row	1	2	3	4	5	6	7	8	9	10	11	12	Whole Plate Mean	Whole Plate Column CV (%)	Internal Plate Mean	Internal Plate Column CV (%)
A	3342	3371	2887	3293	3180	3246	3215	2974	3202	3389	3376	3927	3284	7.8		
B	2935	2648	2478	2666	2606	2584	2748	2943	2861	2972	3130	4066	2885	14.6	2762	7.5
C	2834	2530	2461	2551	2656	2748	2694	2739	2962	2853	2987	4085	2842	14.9	2718	6.5
D	2543	2451	2548	2690	2530	2675	2745	2802	3004	2906	3010	3979	2824	14.6	2736	7.2
E	2473	2498	2647	2614	2567	2685	2877	2839	2867	2786	3087	3928	2823	13.8	2748	6.4
F	2913	2629	2698	2615	2579	2674	2706	2860	2939	2948	3196	4043	2900	13.9	2784	7.0
G	3155	2971	2623	2612	2829	2331	2298	3233	2928	3280	3312	4181	2979	17.3	2842	13.1
H	3568	3382	3207	3275	3181	3356	3320	3558	3507	3802	3766	4159	3505	8.2		
Whole plate mean	2970	2808	2694	2790	2770	2782	2825	2994	3034	3117	3233	4046				
Whole plate row CV (%)	12.6	13.5	9.2	11.0	9.7	12.4	11.4	9.1	7.2	11.1	7.9	2.4				
Internal plate mean		2621	2576	2625	2633	2619	2678	2903	2927	2958	3120					
Internal plate row CV (%)		7.1	3.7	1.8	4.0	5.7	7.4	6.0	1.9	5.8	3.9					

Whole plate	Mean	3005	CV (%)	14.9		Internal plate	Mean	2765	CV (%)	8.1

Note: This figure clearly demonstrates a systematic difference in both mean and CV% of the whole plate versus the internal wells demonstrating edge effects. The precision (CV) improves from 14.9% to 8.1% by using the internal wells only.

FIGURE 7.2 Whole plate imprecision.

concentrations, for example, $<1.0\,\mu g/mL$, for a high-binding plate can exaggerate the slight differences in the plastic structure. Therefore, low coating concentrations should be avoided if possible. For ready-made kits, it is unlikely that the coating concentration can be changed and in these cases, the incubation conditions should be examined.

It is also possible that a slight temperature differential may occur between the outside (edge) and inside wells of a plate. This effect can be increased if evaporation occurs. To prevent evaporation, a good quality plate sealer should be used and the wells should be *fully* sealed. Placing the plate under conditions of high humidity can also help prevent evaporation. Humid conditions can simply be created by either placing the plate in a sandwich box together with moist tissue paper or by placing a beaker of water in the incubator.

Where edge effects exist that cannot be remedied, the only possible solution may be to only use the internal wells of the microplate. For a 96-well plate, this reduces the number of wells to 60 per plate.

7.6 THE USE OF COMMERCIAL KITS FOR PK AND TK ASSAYS

7.6.1 PK Validation History

The majority of kits are ligand-binding assays, for example, ELISAs. There is now consensus within the industry guidelines for validating LBAs for PK methods, as highlighted by the recent conference reports [3,6–9].

Assays supporting pharmacokinetic and toxicokinetic studies involve the measurement of the specific test article. Pharmacokinetic and toxicokinetic measurements are an important part of the drug development process since it is important to correlate the levels of drug in biological fluid with the dose.

Kit methods in general are only available for new drugs or NCEs if the compound itself is a form of an endogenous compound, for example, GM-CSF, erythropoietin, and others. The NCE may be a recombinant form or a highly modified macromolecule to increase potency or half-life, for example, a conjugated drug. The extent of modification may limit the use or suitability of commercial kits, depending on the epitopes that are recognized by the components of the commercial kit.

The kit will normally provide calibration standards. The guideline papers for validating PK assays suggest that a minimum of six nonzero standards should be used to construct a standard curve. Most commercial kits will not provide sufficient standards to comply with the guidelines. The more standards that are used to construct the calibration curve, the more consistent is the performance that can be achieved, which will aid the calibration curve modeling process. The main reason for this is that ligand-binding assay curve fits, in general, are nonlinear, and require for example four-parameter logistic (4PL) or five-parameter logistic (5PL) algorhythms to generate a suitable calibration curve. It is sometimes possible to dilute some of the kit standards to give additional standards depending on the volume provided and the availability of suitable diluents.

It is important to assess the relative differences between the test article and the kit standards. In most cases, there will be differences between the provided calibration standards and the test article. In this case it is advisable to replace the calibration standards with standards prepared from the test article and, in the authors' opinion, this is advisable in the majority of cases.

The next issue to resolve is in what matrix to prepare the standards, as most kits will use a surrogate matrix or buffer. However, the PK guidelines suggest preparing the calibration standards in the same matrix as the samples. This may not always be possible due to the endogenous levels of the compound that will affect the assay. However, in some cases the endogenous concentration may not be significant, depending on the expected concentration range in study samples and the analytical range for the PK Assay. In addition, the analytical range that the kit measures may not be suitable for measuring PK samples, due to massive concentration differences between endogenous concentrations and the expected plasma concentrations as a result of dosing.

If the decision is made to use the kit standards, then the assay should be controlled using quality controls prepared from suitable test article material. As in the case of the calibration standards, it is unlikely that sufficient quality controls will be provided in the kit to support a PK assay in terms of both number and volume.

If it is required to look at various forms of the same molecule, for example, native and different PEGylated forms of the same compound, then it is important to ensure that the assay has similar cross-reactivity to all forms. If different reactivity is observed, it may be necessary to calibrate each form individually.

Surrogate matrices that can be evaluated for use include buffer (normally with additive protein), affinity-purified, charcoal-stripped, and an alternative species matrix, for example, canine serum. The problem with surrogate matrices is that they may not be truly representative of the matrix, and chemically removing the analyte, for example,, by affinity purifying or charcoal stripping, can remove potential interfering factors. An alternative to stripping matrix of the analyte is to heat treat the sample if the analyte is known to be unstable in the matrix. This may be a case of simply storing the sample at room temperature for a few hours or actually heating the sample. Heating samples may also alter the matrix as it may denature proteins and can also affect potential interfering factors, so care needs to be taken when selecting the temperature to use for denaturation. Therefore, when developing assays with surrogate matrices, extensive matrix effects investigations are suggested, that is, parallelism, recovery, specificity and selectivity, and others. The advantage of surrogate assays is that they potentially can provide a more consistent matrix and this is emphasized by extensive use in kits for diagnostic purposes.

7.6.2   Economics Kit Versus Development Kit Versus Purchase Reagents

The purchase of kits to support a drug development program may not be the most cost-effective way of supporting a PK program. Kits are generally more expensive, since you are paying for the commercialization of the product. However, the kit is normally optimized and may be able to be used without major modification. If individual reagents, including development kits, are purchased, then an assay can be put together at a much cheaper cost than by purchasing a ready-made kit. The negative trade-off in developing an analytical method is that the scientists will have spent additional time developing the assay prior to the validation process. In addition, if a kit method requires extensive modification to be used for PK purposes, then a specific assay development program would seem to be an even more attractive option.

Most large pharmaceutical and biotechnology companies will invest in the development of a suitable assay to support their whole drug development program. It is important to ensure that, if reagents are obtained commercially, sufficient reagents are obtained to complete part of the drug development program. If it is not possible to obtain the same batch of materials to support the entire program, the potential impact of batch changes should be assessed. With kits designed for "R&D purposes only," it is more likely that batch changes could change the performance characteristics of the assay. It may be important to contact the kit manufacturers to discuss their internal QC procedures and how they ensure consistency between batches. From the authors' experience, novel kits can potentially give the biggest problems when batches of reagents are changed. There are, however, also examples of assays that have been used in drug development programs that have later been commercialized (e.g., NTPro-BNP).

The middle ground when wanting to avoid some of the pitfalls of method development is to use a commercially available development kit. Although most commercial kits will provide sufficient reagents for a single 96-well microtiter plate, with development kits you will normally be provided with sufficient reagents for 10 or more plates. The kit will contain matched antibody pairs, that is, for coating and detection. Although the kit will provide suggested concentrations and dilutions, it will not normally be optimized for use with biological matrix. This gives the developer flexibility to optimize the assay to the specific requirements of the drug development program. If reoptimization of reagent conditions is required, then the reader should refer to the section above that discusses these issues for biomarker assays as they are exactly the same for TK/PK assays.

7.7 MATRIX PROBLEMS

Matrix problems in ELISAs are caused by interaction of components of the biological fluid with reagents of the assay. This can result in either a positive or a negative effect on the recovery of an analyte from the matrix. Interacting factors include matrix proteins, such as immunoglobulins and binding proteins. The concentration of these potential interfering factors will differ between individuals and between different occasions in the same individual. In method development, the effect of matrix can be investigated by preparing curves in buffer, 1% matrix, 5% matrix, 10% matrix, 20% matrix, 50% matrix, and 100% matrix. These curves can be plotted on the same axis and the curves compared. In particular, the buffer curves should be compared to the matrix curves as, with no matrix effect, the curves should overlay (Fig. 7.3). This is also a good experiment for assessing the minimum dilution required to alleviate matrix effects. To investigate matrix problems further, selectivity and parallelism can also be run.

Matrix problems may be solved by dilution or by blocking. It is also sometimes the case that both approaches can be used to solve the problem. For example, a 1:100 dilution of the matrix is required to solve matrix problems but this compromises the sensitivity of the methodology. However, a 1:5 dilution of the matrix plus blocking with fetal calf serum combine to solve the matrix problem without affecting the methodology sensitivity.

7.7.1 Matrix Dilution

Solving matrix problems by dilution of the matrix into buffer to dilute out the interfering factor is a common solution to matrix problems. Common dilution factors used include 1:5, 1:10, 1:50, and 1:100. The minimum dilution required to alleviate

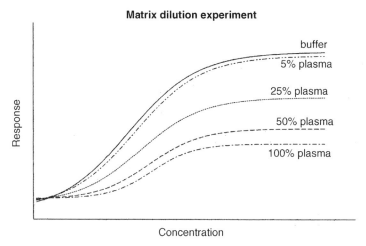

FIGURE 7.3 Matrix dilution.

matrix problems should be assessed. The main problem with matrix dilution is that it decreases the assay sensitivity. The dilution of the matrix can be performed as follows:

(a) The sample is diluted prior to assay and then the diluted sample is added to the microtiter plate.
(b) The dilution is performed as part of the assay procedure in the well, for example, adds $100\,\mu L$ assay buffer $+ 25\,\mu L$ matrix.

7.7.2 Matrix Blocking

The use of matrix blocking is another solution to the problem. As previously mentioned, this is particularly relevant if assay sensitivity will be an issue, that is, dilution of the matrix compromises the required sensitivity of the method. Thus, rather than diluting out the interfering factors, either consistent interference is imposed onto the assay or the interfering factor is adsorbed.

Serum (e.g., fetal or calf) or gamma globulins are good reagents for blocking out matrix effects. The blocking agents can be added at the blocking step or to the assay buffers. Adding these reagents to the conjugate solution to prevent nonspecific binding of the enzyme (conjugate adsorbed) is also possible.

7.8 CHANGING METHOD PROTOCOL

It is possible to switch kit reagents or change assay conditions if this suits the specific requirements of the study. Assay conditions, for example, incubation times, can be changed from the method supplied in the kit protocol to suit the drug development program.

Incubation time, if shortened, may have an effect on the assay range and may make the assay more likely to suffer from drift. Incubation times, if increased, may help with assay drift and improve the assay range. However, increasing the overall assay time can decrease the potential sample throughput. Incubation temperatures may affect the assay range and the assays robustness.

Under most circumstances, changing the primary or secondary antibody reagents in the kit is not advised. The most common example of a reagent change would be the detection reagents used to create the measured signal. The majority of kits still use a colorimetric end point, for example, TMB or p-NPP substrate, combined with an enzyme reaction, for example, horseradish peroxidase or alkaline phosphatase. It is possible, depending on the kit reagents, to substitute the colorimetric substrate with an alternative detection reagent. The most obvious change is to a fluorescent or chemiluminescent substrate, both of which can make the assay more sensitive and/or increase the dynamic range of the assay. If using a fluorescent or chemiluminescent substrate, a clear microtiter plate will not be suitable, that is, due to "cross talk." In this case, either the assay should be reoptimized using an opaque plate, for example, ideally black for fluorescent and white for luminescence. If reoptimizing on an alternative plate is not possible, then transferring the substrate onto a "read" plate prior to reading is an alternative approach.

7.9 CONCLUSIONS

This chapter describes a large range of potential analytical issues and describes possible ways to solve those issues. The authors have had many years experience (35 and 15) in using these methods in analytical procedures in both diagnostics and drug development, and most of what is written here is from hands-on experience throughout that time. Even so, we are still learning more each year as the subject is so complex, and new workers in this field need to be cautioned of the need to ensure that *all* potential issues related to these assays are addressed when proving they are fit for purpose via a method validation procedure specifically developed for a kit assay.

REFERENCES

1. Lee, J.W., Devanarayan, V., Barrett, Y.C., Weiner, R., Allinson, J., Fountain, S., Keller, S., Weinryb, I., Green, M., Duan, L., Rogers, J.A., Millham, R., O'Brien, P.J., Sailstad, J., Khan, M., Ray, C., and Wagner, J.A. (2006) Fit-for-purpose method development and validation for successful biomarker measurement. *Pharmaceutical Research*, **23**, 312–328.

2. Lee, J.W., Weiner, R.S., Sailstad, J.M., Bowsher, R.R., Knuth, D.W., O'Brien, P.J., Fourcroy, J.L., Dixit, R., Pandite, L., Pietrusko, R.G., Soares, H.D., Quarmby, V., Vesterqvist, O.L., Potter, D.M., Witliff, J.L., Fritche, H.A., O'Leary, T., Perlee, L., Kadam, S., and Wagner, J.A. (2005) Method validation and measurement of biomarkers in nonclinical and clinical samples in drug development: a conference report. *Pharmaceutical Research*, **22**, 499–511.

3. DeSilva, B., Smith, W., Weiner, R., Kelley, M., Smolec, J., Lee, B., Khan, M., Tacey, R., Hill, H., and Celniker, A. (2003) Recommendations for the bioanalytical method validation of ligand-binding assays to support pharmacokinetic assessments of macromolecules. *Pharmaceutical Research*, **20**, 1885–1900.

4. Passing, H., and Bablok, W. (1983) A new biometrical procedure for testing the equality of measurements from two different analytical methods. Application of linear regression procedures for method comparison studies in clinical chemistry. Part I. *Journal of Clinical Chemistry and Clinical Biochemistry*, **21**, 709–720.

5. Cull, C.A., Manley, S.E., Stratton, I.M., Andrew, H., Neil, W., Ross, I.S., Holman, R.R., Turner, R.C., and Matthews, D.R. (1997) Approach to maintaining comparability of biochemical data during long-term clinical trials. *Clinical Chemistry*, **43**, 1913–1918.

6. Viswanathan, C.T., Bansal, S., Booth, B., DeStefano, A.J., Rose, M.J., Sailstad, J., Shah, V. P., Skelly, J.P., Swann, P.G., and Weiner, R. (2007) Workshop/conference report—quantitative bioanalytical methods validation and implementation: best practices for chromatographic and ligand binding assays. *The AAPS Journal*, **9**, E30–E42.

7. Shah, V.P., Midha, K.K., Dighe, S., McGilveray, I.J., Skelly, J.P., Yacobi, A., Layloff, T., Viswanathan, C.T., Cook, C.E., McDowall, R.D., Pittman, K.A., and Spector, S. (1992) Analytical methods validation: bioavailability, bioequivalence and pharmacokinetic studies. *Pharmaceutical Research*, **9**, 588–592.

8. Shah, V.P., Midha, K.K., Findlay, J.W.A., Hill, H.M., Hulse, J.D., McGilveray, I.J., McKay, G., Miller, K.J., Patnaik, R.N., Powell, M.L., Tonnelli, A., Viswanathan, C.T., and Yacobi, A. (2000) Bioanalytical method validation: a revisit with a decade of progress. *Pharmaceutical Research*, **17**, 1551–1557.

9. Food Drug Administration (2001) *Guidance for Industry: Bioanalytical Method Validation*. U.S. Department of Health and Human Services, Food and Drug Administration, Center for Drug Evaluation and Research, Rockville, MD. Available at http: //www.fda.gov/cder/guidance/4252fnl.pdf.

CHAPTER 8

Development and Validation of Immunogenicity Assays for Preclinical and Clinical Studies

THOMAS H. PARISH

Procter & Gamble Pharmaceuticals, Norwich, NY, USA

DEBORAH FINCO

Pfizer Inc., Groton, CT, USA

VISWANATH DEVANARAYAN

Abbott Laboratories, Souderton, PA, USA

8.1 INTRODUCTION

Administration of biological protein therapeutics can lead to unwanted immunogenicity reactions in recipients of these products [1,2]. In contrast, a robust immune response is a desired response to most vaccines. The assessment of immunogenicity to understand the significance of such immune reactions, as they relate to patient safety, is now an integral part of a product development program for a biologic macromolecule. Thus, a well considered immunogenicity-assessment strategy, which includes a management plan for related adverse events and a bioanalytical testing strategy, is required [3]. Testing for anti-drug antibodies (ADAs) to biotechnology-derived therapeutic proteins and other macromolecules generally follows a tiered approach. Samples are initially screened for binding antibodies; presumptive positives are then confirmed in a confirmatory assay, and confirmed positives may be further characterized in a quasi-quantitative assay and, possibly, a neutralizing antibody (Nab) assay. Further characterizations, such as antibody isotype and subclass classifications, may be conducted, if needed. The generation of antibodies to drugs may affect pharmacokinetics (PK), pharmacodynamics (PD), bioavailability, efficacy, or safety.

Ligand-Binding Assays: Development, Validation, and Implementation in the Drug Development Arena. Edited by Masood N. Khan and John W.A. Findlay
Copyright © 2010 John Wiley & Sons, Inc.

Loss of efficacy is the most common consequence of immunogenicity resulting from ADA binding drug, either by neutralizing drug activity or by increasing drug clearance. In patients treated with interferon beta products for multiple sclerosis, the presence of neutralizing antibodies was correlated to a loss of efficacy and relapse in multiple sclerosis [4]. These patients may initially develop binding antibodies that later on become neutralizing antibodies. Neutralizing antibodies are of particular concern for mimetic therapeutics to an endogenous protein. If the Nabs cross-react with endogenous proteins (that do not have redundant biological pathways) a total loss of both protein and drug functionality could be catastrophic for the patient. This situation was observed in patients treated with a recombinant human erythropoietin approved for treatment of anemia. Anti-human recombinant erythropoietin antibodies, which neutralized not only the recombinant protein but also native erythropoietin, led to the absence of red cell precursors in the bone marrow (pure red cell aplasia) of patients, rendering them to be transfusion dependent [5].

This chapter will deal primarily with undesired immunogenicity; however, approaches to design and validation of assays for evaluation of immune response to protein therapeutics where one desires to stimulate an immune response (e.g., vaccines) may be similar. This chapter will provide an overview of immunogenicity risk, the current regulatory environment, and recommendations for immunogenicity assessment in nonclinical and clinical studies. Current recommendations for optimization and validation of immunogenicity assays (total binding ADA assays and Nab assays), with the primary focus on ligand-binding assays, will be described, as well as an assessment of technical challenges associated with these assays.

8.2   IMMUNOGENICITY RISK-BASED STRATEGY

When reviewing a drug application, the FDA has two major concerns that are paramount for approval: (1) whether the drug is safe and (2) whether the drug is efficacious. Therefore, a risk assessment analysis [6–8] should be performed by the sponsor on each macromolecule drug to develop an appropriate strategy for evaluating immunogenicity. In developing a strategy, it is critical to consider the risk of generating an immune response, the potential severity of a response, and overall risk/benefit of the candidate therapeutic to the target population. From a bioanalytical perspective, this assessment may have implications on timing and frequency of sample collection, total and neutralizing antibody assessment, qualitative or quasi-quantitative measurement, as well as other considerations. The assessment may drive decisions as to whether a neutralizing antibody assay is warranted for nonclinical toxicology studies and at what phase of a clinical program this may be needed. Additionally, the risk assessment, as well as the mode of action (MOA) of the therapeutic, may drive the selection of the assay type used to assess antidrug antibodies.

Unfortunately, no specific FDA recommendations have been issued regarding the use of risk assessments or how to use the information obtained from characterizing an ADA response. The current EMEA guideline for immunogenicity [9] recommends using a risk-based strategy and notes that applicants should take into consideration both the risk of developing an unwanted immune response and the potential clinical consequences. Further complicating the application of a risk assessment plan is the fact that the immunogenicity of each protein drug must by evaluated on a case-by-case basis.

In a recent publication on risk-based strategy [3], a general approach was proposed for assigning immunogenicity risk levels and risk level-based "fit for purpose" bioanalytical schemes for investigation of ADA in nonclinical and clinical studies. Risk assessment was divided into three variables: (a) those that affect the incidence of ADA, (b) those that affect the risk of consequences of ADAs, and (c) those that have an impact on the patient. Biological drug products are then classified into three distinct risk categories: low, medium, and high. Finally, using these risk categories, a bioanalytical strategy for animal and human studies is proposed.

Care must be employed when extrapolating ADA results from animal studies to humans, as the potential therapeutic compound may have poor homology to the related protein or the compound's target in animals. Thus, the ADA response may identify and bind to completely different epitopes than would be seen by the immune system in humans. A humanized protein may readily be seen as "foreign" by an animal's immune system. However, the detection of ADA may help explain unexpected observations such as an accelerated clearance of the drug. If the drug is related, or equivalent, to an endogenous compound found at very low levels, for example, a cytokine, then further evaluation of the ADA response to determine the presence and characteristics of neutralizing antibodies may be justified.

It is suggested that, for low-risk products in clinical studies, the characterization of titer and relative concentration of ADA is sufficient, and Nab may be explored as necessary. For medium-risk products, it is proposed that characterizing the binding epitopes of the ADA response may be beneficial. Cell-based or competitive ligand-binding (CLB) assays may be used, while the use of a cell-based assay to evaluate Nab against an endogenous protein should be considered. For higher risk products, one may consider using both a cell-based and a CLB assay. Furthermore, it is suggested that, when a Nab assay is not available, epitope mapping of the binding site(s) of ADA may shed some light on the neutralizing potential of an antibody; however, this is not a commonly accepted approach. Highly sensitive ADA and Nab assays are essential, as antibodies to low-level endogenous compounds can be both present in low concentrations and be of low affinity [10].

8.3 REGULATORY GUIDANCE

A number of current regulatory guidances advocate the need for immunogenicity testing in nonclinical and clinical studies, but do not recommend which types of assays should be used or when and how testing for binding and neutralizing antibodies should be carried out. The ICH Topic S6 guidance *Preclinical Safety Evaluation of Biotechnology-Derived Pharmaceuticals* [11] specifies that the "measurement of antibodies associated with administration of these types of products should be performed when conducting repeated dose toxicity studies to aid in the interpretation of these studies. Antibody responses should be characterized (e.g., titer, number of responding animals, neutralizing, or non-neutralizing), and their responses should be correlated with any pharmacological and/or toxicological changes." Since assessments of the neutralizing capabilities of antibodies are not implicitly stated as a requirement, companies have different interpretations of whether or not neutralizing antibody assays should be part of the regulatory toxicity studies.

The EMEA Guideline on *Comparability of Medicinal Products Containing Biotechnology-Derived Proteins as Active Substance: Non-Clinical and Clinical Issues* [12] indicates that antibody titers, cross-reactivity, and neutralizing capacity should be determined as part of nonclinical toxicity studies. For clinical studies, the immunogenicity of a similar biological medicinal product (a biological product claiming to be similar to another biological medicinal product already marketed) must always be investigated. Specifics regarding the assays indicate that sensitive screening assays should be used, with neutralizing antibody assays available for further characterization of antibodies detected by the screening assay.

Another guideline from the EMEA, *Guideline on the Clinical Investigation of the Pharmacokinetics of Therapeutic Proteins* [13], has a section on immunogenicity, which stresses the importance of correlating antibody responses to drug exposure or relevant PK parameters.

The EMEA issued *Guideline on the Immunogenicity Assessment of Biotechnology-Derived Therapeutic Proteins* [9], was effective from April 2008. The guidance references ICH S6 [11] with respect to nonclinical immunogenicity assessment. Furthermore, it states that, in cases where there is the potential for antibodies to a therapeutic to cross-react with an endogenous protein, there may be value in understanding the impact of such antibodies and their potential consequences when conducting animal studies. Nab assays are generally described as bioassays, although it was noted that, if neutralizing cell-based assays are not feasible or available, CLB assays or other alternatives may be suitable if they demonstrate neutralizing capacity/potential in an appropriate manner.

Currently, the various regulatory documents recommend the need for immunogenicity assessment, but the recommendations on Nab assays may vary between documents. Due to the lack of detail or clarity of intent for immunogenicity assessment, different companies may have different interpretations of the expectations for immunogenicity testing, leading to different approaches between companies.

8.4 ASSAY DESIGN

A consequence of the challenges involved in developing ADA assays has been the considerable progress made in the field of identifying, quantitating, and characterizing unwanted immunogenicity. A consortium of members of the American Association of Pharmaceutical Scientists (AAPS) has formulated recommendations for optimization and development of ADA assays, following extensive discussion on procedures and practices undertaken by the industry for assessment of antibodies to biotherapeutic drugs during preclinical and clinical development. This led to publication of several papers. One of these papers describes the design and optimization of immunoassays for detection of host antibodies [14], while the other describes the design and optimization of cell-based assays for detection of neutralizing antibody responses elicited to biotechnology products [15].

8.4.1 Assay Formats/Methodologies

The current, most practical approach for testing unwanted immunogenicity is the detection, measurement, and characterization of antibodies generated using ligand-binding assays (LBAs). New methods and platforms for immunogenicity assessment are continually being exploited to increase the ability to detect antibodies. For a majority of biotherapeutics, an initial assessment of immunogenicity typically involves the use of a two-tiered approach: a screening assay complemented by a confirmatory step (e.g., immunoblotting, antigen depletion, etc.), which may then be supplemented by an assay for quasi-quantitation of the amount of antibody present. Additionally, antibodies may be further characterized for their binding epitopes, isotype, or neutralizing capacity [16]. Most commonly, the assay utilized to evaluate and characterize ADA neutralizing activity is derived from the cell-based assay used to determine the potency of the drug. The exact testing scheme will be part of the risk assessment strategy and can vary depending upon the nature of the product and its stage in product development [3].

8.4.2 Screening, Confirmatory, and Characterization Binding Assays

Screening assays are used to determine the presence (or absence) of antibodies based on the ability of the antibodies to recognize the relevant antigenic determinants in the therapeutic protein. Such assays are based mainly on immunochemical procedures, such as enzyme-linked immunosorbent assays (ELISAs; direct, indirect, or bridging), electrochemiluminescence (ECL), radioimmunoprecipitation assays (RIPA), or bio-sensor-based methods such as surface plasmon resonance (SPR) [17]. Each of the currently available assays has distinct advantages and disadvantages. Solid-phase immunoassays can be conducted using a variety of formats. These include direct, indirect, and bridging formats that, depending upon the assay platform, may use different types of detection reagents, for example, enzymatic/colorimetric, radioactive, fluorescent, chemiluminescent, or electrochemiluminescent. These assays can provide quasi-quantitative data on antibody concentration in unknown samples, provided an appropriate validation is performed. However, since no true reference standard for a given ADA response is available and no reference standard selected from a specific nonclinical species is representative of each and every sample tested, these concentrations are relative and may not reflect actual ADA concentrations in patient samples. More importantly, due to the differences in affinity, epitopes recognized, and so on, demonstration of adequate parallelism between the dilution of a reference standard and the dilution of study samples is often not possible. For this reason, the criteria for identification and confirmation of positive samples are derived using assay response units, and further characterization of antibody binding is carried out using end point titers rather than concentration levels.

Confirmatory assays are used to demonstrate that a positive result from the screening assay is truly positive and not due to nonspecific binding of the antibodies in the sample to an epitope unrelated to the drug. Many scientists choose to modify the screening assay to evaluate specificity of the ADA response in the sample. Typically, the sample containing the suspected ADA is preincubated with a high concentration of the drug and subsequently reevaluated in the screening assay. The extent of the response change (typically inhibition of response) is then used to evaluate whether the ADA is specific to the drug. It should be noted that this demonstrates specificity of the response; however, it may not confirm that the response is due to ADA. For example, in bridging assays, bridging in the assay from soluble ligand (e.g., a soluble receptor) may result in a false-positive result for the presence of an ADA. Competition with drug would inhibit this response, but would not confirm that the response is due to immunoglobulin. For this reason, some companies may also use an Ig removal confirmatory step to confirm that a detected response is due to antibody. This approach is only applicable if the drug or drug candidate is not a monoclonal antibody.

Once an ADA-positive sample has been shown to be specific in the confirmatory assay, typically the next step is to determine the titer of the sample. Often, the titer is determined in the screening assay, using the same approach used initially to determine positive samples. Serial dilutions of the sample are made prior to analysis.

Assay formats vary in suitability between different proteins and are very often dependent upon the class of therapeutic protein (e.g., a therapeutic cytokine or a monoclonal antibody). Furthermore, if the assay format requires labeling of drug as capture (e.g., ECL) and/or detection reagents, critical epitopes may be impacted by such labeling and this may lead to erroneous results. There are distinct advantages and disadvantages with each of the various platforms. Therefore, should the initial assay of choice not meet desired expectations (e.g., give poor sensitivity or a high background), more than one assay may need to be developed and used for detection of antibodies. In fact, different assay formats may need to be developed for preclinical versus clinical studies due to the nature of the drug; for example, the activity of the drug may be specific to only humans. While the drug molecule may appear to be completely foreign to the animal(s) used in preclinical studies, to human subjects the drug may resemble an endogenous molecule (e.g., beta interferon). Hence, a more sensitive assay and/or an assay able to detect specific epitopes may be required for clinical studies, as antibodies elicited in humans may have a lower affinity and different specificity for the drug compared to those elicited in animals.

In a ligand-binding assay, one must assess whether the selected assay format allows for appropriate epitope exposure and detection of antibodies with different on rates and off rates. If certain assay formats are incapable of recognizing antibodies, alternative approaches may be considered for antibody detection [18,19]. While it is desirable to have the most sensitive and specific assay available, it is also advisable to keep the method as simple as possible. Sometimes rushing to use the most advanced technological method available can result in disaster if the vendor subsequently goes out of business or no longer supports the product on which the immunogenicity strategy was based.

8.4.3 Enzyme-Linked Immunosorbent Assays

ELISAs are the most prevalent methods used for detecting antibodies. These assays can be conducted using a variety of approaches, which include direct, indirect, bridging, and competitive inhibition formats (Fig. 8.1). These assay formats offer high throughput, are easily automated, use simple technology, require low capital investment, and enjoy comparatively short method development times. A major

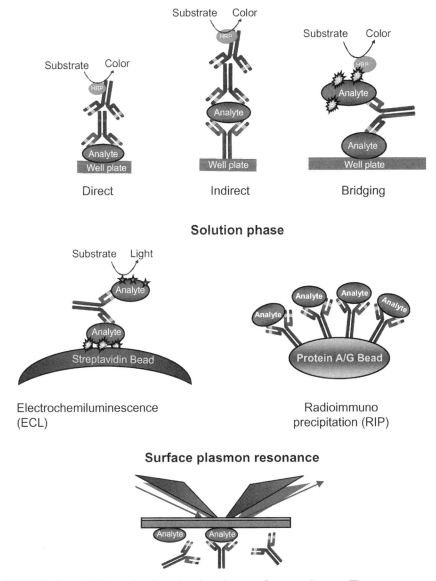

FIGURE 8.1   ELISA and other plate-based assay formats. *Source*: Figure courtesy of Ref. [52].

limitation of the ELISA method is that some antibodies, particularly those with "low affinity," which tend to dissociate rapidly, may be washed off during this procedure and their presence not detected. Moreover, these assays can be susceptible to significant inhibition due to soluble/circulating therapeutic present in the sample. The most commonly used ELISA formats include direct or sandwich ELISA, indirect ELISA, and bridging ELISA.

8.4.3.1 *Direct or Sandwich ELISA*

The direct format represents the most simplified ELISA system. In this assay, serum or plasma samples are incubated with the antigen (usually the drug), which has been previously immobilized directly onto well surfaces of microtiter plates. The bound antibody is detected using an enzyme-labeled anti-immunoglobulin reagent of appropriate specificity.

Pros: High throughput, simple, low cost.

Cons: Immobilization of the antigen can alter its conformation and/or mask epitopes such that these may not be recognized by the host's antibody response [18].

8.4.3.2 *Indirect ELISA*

In this format, a capturing agent (e.g., a monoclonal antibody specific to the drug or streptavidin to capture drug conjugated to biotin) is immobilized onto the surface of the plate. The bound ADA is then detected using an enzyme-labeled anti-immunoglobulin reagent of appropriate specificity. This allows for better and specific exposure of available epitopes on the antigen (drug) to binding by the ADA in sample [18].

Pros: Improved and controlled presentation of available epitopes on the drug molecule to antibodies in the sample.

Cons: Require species-specific reagents, which can present problems in terms of suitable assay controls, particularly when using an animal serum as a positive antibody control for the assay. May suffer from nonspecific binding.

8.4.3.3 *Bridging ELISA*

In the "bridging ELISA" format, antibody is captured by immobilized antigen and detected using the same labeled antigen. This is often the screening method of choice. Generally, drug is used as a capture reagent and is also the labeled detection reagent.

Pros: The use of this format overcomes the nonspecificity issue and the requirement for species-specific reagents associated with in direct assays. This method has high specificity (antigen must be recognized twice by antibody for detection).

Cons: This format can result in false-positive results if there are other factors in the serum beside anti-drug antibody that may form a bridge between the capture and detection reagents. The bridging assay is affected more by free drug interference than the sandwich or indirect assays.

8.4.4 Electrochemiluminescence (ECL) Assays

The availability of ECL technology from instrument providers such as Meso Scale Discovery (MSD) has enabled practical applications of electrochemiluminescent assays. The MSD platform uses carbon electrode plates that are available uncoated or coupled with biotin or streptavidin. Thus, the platform may be used with direct, indirect, and bridging formats.

Pros: High throughput, increased sensitivity over ELISA, less susceptibility to free drug interference, enable the development of assays without wash steps, and allow for multiplexing. Solution-phase incubations are possible.

Cons: Dependent on single proprietary technology. Multiple reagents need to be conjugated for use.

8.4.5 Radioimmunoprecipitation Assays

In this assay format, serum is incubated with radiolabeled drug and the drug–antibody complexes that form are precipitated through the addition of an appropriate reagent (e.g., immobilized protein A, G, or L or antiglobulin or PEG), followed by centrifugation. The precipitate is then assessed for antibodies by counting the radioactivity present in the drug–antibody complex. A modification of this approach, in which serum is preincubated with protein A and specific antibodies are detected using radiolabeled antigen, has been successfully used for detection of antibodies in sera of rheumatoid arthritis (RA) patients treated with infliximab and adalimumab [20].

Pros: These assays can be very sensitive and have been shown to be useful for detection of antibodies against erythropoietin [5,21]. Solution-phase incubations are possible.

Cons: Prone to artifacts. The radiolabeling process can mask or denature epitopes recognized by antibodies.

8.4.6 Biosensor-Based Immunoassays

This platform has gained immense popularity in recent years for detection of antibodies. This is because, unlike other methods, it allows monitoring of antigen–antibody interaction (antibody on and off rates) in real time and does not require the use of a labeled secondary reagent. Several types of biosensor instruments that differ to some extent in technical principles are now available. A majority of published biosensor-based assay data, however, cites the use of BIAcore instruments (e.g., Biacore 2000 and Biacore 3000) for monitoring the immune response during product development and in clinical trials. An advantage of the Biacore 3000 instrument is compliance with the 21 CFR Part 11 requirements, which facilitates its use under conditions of regulatory scrutiny.

The Biacore utilizes surface plasmon resonance to detect a change in refractive index at the surface of the sensor chip following the binding of an antibody to an antigen immobilized on the sensor chip. This change in refractive index is directly proportional to the amount of antigen-binding antibody present in the serum sample being tested. Specificity confirmation can be obtained by sequential injection of a species-specific antibody. The ability of the instrument to monitor the interaction in "real time" and provide a continuous signal of the events occurring on the sensor surface enables detection of rapidly dissociating or "low-affinity" antibodies if these are present in the sample [10].

It is important to detect low-affinity antibodies as they can neutralize the therapeutic product and may predict the generation of a later mature immune response, as shown in a recent study [19]. In this study, the SPR assay, despite its lower sensitivity (capable of detecting 1 µg/mL of positive-control antibody) and lower tolerance to competition from the administered therapeutic agent, detected antibodies in a higher percentage of patients (4.1%) as compared to the more sensitive (capable of detecting 10 ng/mL positive-control antibody) bridging ELISA (0.3%). Additionally, the SPR assay identified patients who developed neutralizing antibodies that were not recognized by the ELISA assay. Antibody characterization in terms of affinities, antibody class and subclass can also be performed easily and rapidly [19]. Furthermore, evidence from studies in which sequential assessment of samples has been undertaken suggests that antibodies may be detected at earlier time points following administration of the therapeutic macromolecule by SPR than by ELISA [22]. Despite their attributes, SPR assays are generally less sensitive in comparison with ELISA and require extensive development and optimization for evaluation of suitable immobilization conditions and regeneration strategies that are critical parameters for assay performance. However, in some cases, SPR has been shown to be more effective than ELISAs at detecting low-affinity ADAs, thus illustrating the fact that no single assay should be assumed to be the "right" detection method for any given drug program.

> *Pros*: Full automation capability, more effective at detecting low-affinity antibodies than ELISA, measures antibody on and off rates, and minimal reagent labeling.
>
> *Cons*: Very expensive (capital and reagent/supplies), low throughput compared to ELISA.

8.4.7 Neutralizing Antibody Assays

Once samples are identified as positive in the binding assays, one generally wants to further characterize these antibodies as to whether they are neutralizing or not. To assess the presence of neutralizing antibodies (Nabs), the test sample is preincubated with the therapeutic and, if Nabs are present, the therapeutic is unable to bind to its target or it can bind but is no longer bioactive, resulting in an attenuated assay response. Test systems based on ligand-binding assays or cell bioassays are the most common platforms currently in use [9,15,23].

Nab assays determine the *potential* to neutralize *in vivo*. However, these *in vitro* assay systems are static systems that do not take into consideration the dynamic interactions that occur *in vivo* (e.g., clearance of ADA-drug immune complexes, equilibrium/affinity between drug/antibody/target). There are examples of Nab (even to endogenous protein) that have no/minimal impact on drug efficacy, pharmacodynamics, or adverse events [24,25]. Thus, one should keep in mind that when Nab assays are used, the results must be evaluated in the context of other clinical end points to determine their significance.

8.4.7.1 *Competitive Ligand-Binding Assays*

In a CLB Nab assay format, a microtiter plate coated with target (receptor or ligand) is incubated with a defined concentration of the drug added to patient sample and binding of the drug to target is assessed directly (labeled therapeutic) or indirectly (detection reagent to therapeutic) using enzymatic, radiochemical, fluorometric, chemiluminescent, or electrochemiluminescent end points. Biacore technology may also be employed for CLB assays.

Generally speaking, the CLB Nab assay format is the simplest and most sensitive approach for assessing Nabs, since it utilizes a standard LBA technique such as an ELISA. Optimization of immunoassays is a well-defined and efficient process that examines plates, buffers, blocking reagents, coating concentrations, drug concentrations, detection reagents, incubation times, and temperature [26,27]. For CLB Nab validation, white papers or regulatory guidance are not available; however, the recommendations by Mire-Sluis et al. [14] for validation of ADA assays can be used.

CLB assays can be used instead of a cell-based bioassay in certain situations [9]. In particular, a CLB could be used when the drug is an antagonist, since the mode of action involves inhibiting binding of the drug to its target. Further, some scientists may prefer to use a CLB assay for an agonist in early stages of a clinical program and then switch to a bioassay when the program is more advanced. Finally, in some cases, it may not be possible to develop a bioassay with desired sensitivity and performance and a CLB assay may be the only option, as described in the EMEA guidance [9].

8.4.7.2 *Cell-Based Bioassay*

For a cell-based Nab bioassay, treated cells respond directly or indirectly to the drug in a concentration-dependent manner. Possible biological responses of the cells to drug treatment include cell proliferation, apoptosis, phosphorylation, chemokine release, and expression of proteins or genes [15,22,28–30]. These responses may by quantitated by techniques such as immunoassay, multiplex assays [31], flow cytometry [23], and gene expression profiling [32].

In contrast to the CLB assay format, cell-based bioassays are more complex, time, consuming, costly, and often are less sensitive. However, it is important to note that this methodology is a functional assay and, thus, demonstrates neutralization of a biological response. It is argued by some that a functional end point more closely mimics *in vivo* physiological responses [15].

Recommendations for the design, optimization, and qualification of Nab bioassays have been published [15] and provide a good starting point for assay development and understanding the potential challenges that may be encountered.

Currently, there are no published recommendations for the validation of Nab bioassays; however, Gupta et al. [15] described assay qualification criteria similar to those proposed by Mire-Sluis et al. [14] for optimization/validation of ADA assays.

8.5 OPTIMIZATION AND VALIDATION: TOTAL BINDING ANTIBODY ASSAYS

The optimization and validation of immunoassays for immunogenicity (ADA) testing has been described in detail in several publications [9,14,33,34]. In this section, we will describe the evaluation of relevant performance characteristics (validation parameters) that require the most effort. Some of these are different from the validation of traditional bioanalytical pharmacokinetic (PK) methods for macromolecules [35–37]. Precision, specificity, robustness, and ruggedness are determined similarly between ADA and PK methods. However, recovery/accuracy, sensitivity, stability, linearity, system suitability controls, and selectivity are treated differently between these two types of assays.

8.5.1 Minimum Required Dilution

Prior to beginning the formal validation exercise of an ADA method, the minimum required dilution (MRD) should be determined. MRD is defined as the dilution that results in adequate reduction in background without compromising unacceptably on assay sensitivity [14]. Data from at least 10 drug-naïve samples at different levels of dilution (for example; 1:1, 1:2, 1:5, 1:10, 1:20, 1:40, and 1:80) are needed for determining the MRD. At each dilution level, the percent reduction in background should be determined. To determine an approximate level of sensitivity at each dilution level, a surrogate measure such as the Z' factor can be calculated using the formula

$$Z' = \frac{[\text{mean}(S) - 3 \times \text{SD}(S)] - [\text{mean}(B) + 3 \times \text{SD}(B)]}{\text{mean}(S) - \text{mean}(B)}$$

where S refers to signal of the diluted samples and B refers to signal of the assay diluent or buffer. The mean and standard deviation (SD) are determined from the 10 or more drug-naïve samples used in this evaluation. The values of Z' factor range from 0 to 1. Values closer to 1 are more desirable as they represent a more optimal separation between signal and background after taking into consideration the variability. The dilution level at which both the percent reduction in background and Z' factor are optimal is then chosen as the MRD.

For certain assay formats such as ECL, the signal of the diluent (reagent blank) samples is usually greater than the signal of the matrix blank samples. In such cases, the percent reduction in background is irrelevant. So the MRD is simply the dilution level that results in an optimal fold change between the diluted samples to matrix blank, without compromising much on variability, that is, the dilution level that optimizes the Z' factor.

8.5.2 Accuracy/Recovery

Accuracy is applicable to PK assays while *recovery* is associated with ADA methods. The majority of ADA assays do not use a standard curve because a well-characterized reference standard is not obtainable. In addition, ADA responses are usually hetero-geneous and differ from subject to subject, such that calculating accuracy is not relevant. Thus, recovery is employed to demonstrate that the matrix does not interfere with the detection of the ADA. In practice, the response for the maximum dilution (titer) of matrix that has been spiked with ADA versus matrix without ADA is evaluated and should remain within an acceptable range. The acceptance ranges for recovery are usually expressed in response values rather than concentration units (accuracy). The ADA used in recovery experiments may be obtained from one subject, a pool of subjects, or even from a different species than the test subjects and thus does not necessarily reflect the ADAs in the study samples.

8.5.3 Screening Cut Point

The screening cut point is defined as the level of assay response at or above which a sample is defined to be "reactive" for the presence of ADA (also called "potentially positive"), and below which it is probably negative. The cut point value is determined statistically from the analysis of serum or plasma samples from naïve subjects. Typically, for clinical studies, samples from approximately 50 or more subjects are used to set the screening cut point. For practical considerations, samples from 15 or more subjects may suffice for preclinical studies. More subjects are required for clinical studies because their responses tend to be more variable than the genetically similar animals commonly used in preclinical studies. These samples should be analyzed in six independent runs, preferably by two or more analysts/instruments if multiple analysts/instruments will be utilized during the in-study phase for screening subject samples. A "balanced" experimental design that allows reliable assessment of potential sources of variability is recommended [34]. It is recommended that these naïve samples come from subjects disease-matched to the test group. If such samples are not available, healthy donors may be used, but should be compared later on to the relevant disease population samples to ensure that the distribution of the data is similar.

Three types of screening assay cut point may be used depending on the character-istics of the data from these samples. They are (1) fixed cut point, (2) floating cut point, and (3) dynamic cut point [34].

(1) *Fixed Cut Point*: If the same cut point determined during prestudy validation is used for screening samples during the in-study (bioanalysis) phase, it is defined as a fixed cut point. This cut point should be revalidated when there are critical changes in the assay (change in critical reagents, different instruments, laboratory, etc.). The cut point value can be fixed within a given study, for a target population, or across studies and multiple target populations. To use this approach, the means and variances of the data from multiple runs should not be

significantly different. If the data from multiple runs for each instrument are similar, but data from individual instruments are different, then an instrument-specific fixed cut point may be used during the in-study phase. If the means are different between runs, then the use of a floating cut point should be investigated.

(2) *Floating Cut Point*: If a cut point is calculated by adding or multiplying a correction factor (determined from the prestudy validation data) to the biological background from each plate/run during the in-study phase, this is defined as a floating cut point. The addition or multiplication of the correction factor depends on whether or not log transformation is used for the data from the validation samples (Fig. 8.2). The biological background may be represented by the negative control (pool of matrix from subjects that are negative for anti-drug antibody), the assay diluent, or the predose subject sample (subject-specific cut point). A floating cut point may be plate-specific, unique for each run (common for a number of plates within a run), or unique for each subject (using the subject's pretreatment/"baseline" sample result). If a subject-specific floating cut point is used, then the pretreatment and post-treatment samples should be tested in the same plate (or at least in the same run). To use the floating cut point approach, the variability of subject samples between assay runs should not be significantly different (means can be different). This is because the correction factor used in the determination of the floating cut point for each plate/run of the in-study phase uses the variation estimate from the prestudy validation data.

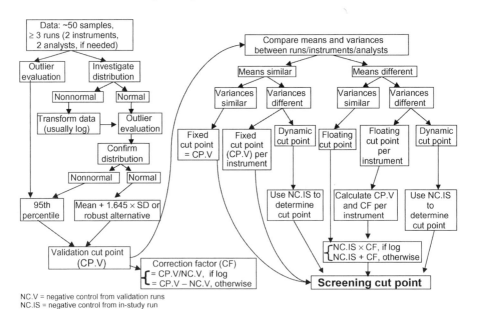

NC.V = negative control from validation runs
NC.IS = negative control from in-study run

FIGURE 8.2 Scheme for evaluating cut point samples and calculating screening cut point. *Source*: Figure courtesy of Ref. [34].

(3) *Dynamic Cut Point*: A cut point that is evaluated separately for each plate/run/ study and does not use the data from prestudy validation is defined as a dynamic cut point. A practically limiting factor is that a significant number of samples are needed in each plate/run to compute this cut point. When differences between runs (means and/or variances) are encountered, an investigation of the source of such differences is recommended. For example, if these differences were primarily due to analysts or instruments, then one should consider the appropriateness of analyst or instrument specific fixed or floating cut points before instituting a dynamic cut point approach.

Occasionally, naïve samples are encountered with preexisting or high levels of ADAs. If a confirmatory test shows that the ADA response is specific to the drug, such samples should be excluded from the cut point calculations. In addition, samples that are identified as outliers using appropriate statistical criteria [34] should also be excluded or down weighted in the analyses. If a substantial number of naïve samples are positive from the relevant disease population, it is acceptable to include samples from a healthy or non-diseased population for determining the cut point. For example, if the distribution of the data of outlier-removed samples is not statistically different between healthy and disease-matched subjects (i.e., means and variances are not significantly different), then the cut point evaluation can be made from a collection of samples where half the samples are from healthy subjects and the other half are from the relevant disease population.

A series of assessments are required for calculating the appropriate screening cut point, as shown in Fig. 8.2. First, the distribution of drug-naïve matrix sample results should be tested for normality. If the distribution is not normal, appropriate data transformation (usually logarithm) should be selected to ensure approximate normality, and the outliers should be evaluated in the transformed scale. Then the mean plus 1.645 times the standard deviation of these data (or suitable, robust alternatives) defines the cut point from these validation data. If transformation of the data does not result in approximate normality, or if a nonparametric approach is preferred for other reasons, then the 95th percentile of the data can be used to define the cut point of these validation data, but the outliers should be evaluated in the original (untransformed) scale of the data. Next, the assay run means and variances should be compared using appropriate ANOVA-based statistical methods. The results from these analyses will then determine the suitability of a fixed or floating cut point, or the need for a dynamic cut point. If a floating cut point is to be used for testing clinical samples, then an additive or multiplicative correction factor should be determined from these data, depending on whether or not the data had to be transformed (Fig. 8.2). See Appendices 2A–C of Shankar et al. [34] and Appendix 8.A for further details on these calculations.

8.5.4 Confirmatory Cut Point

The confirmatory cut point, sometimes referred as specificity cut point, is also derived from response units, typically expressed as percent inhibition of samples spiked with study drug relative to original (unspiked) samples, and confirms whether the ADAs identified from the screening assay are specific to the drug or cross-reactive to an unrelated component of the assay. The validity of the confirmatory cut point for distinguishing specific binding versus nonspecific binding of ADA to the study drug is critical and must be determined objectively. The use of subjective criteria, such as 50% inhibition of signal, should be discouraged. This is particularly important for samples that are slightly above the screening cut point (low ADA positives) because a minor decrease in signal of a drug-spiked sample may result in a 50% or greater decrease relative to the unspiked counterpart (or coated well), possibly leading to a false-positive assessment. Furthermore, the signal may only be reduced down to the assay background, but not lower, which might be less than 50% of the signal of the uninhibited sample; in such cases, false-negative results could occur. If the variability of the percent inhibition values is not taken into consideration, a subjective 50% inhibition criterion can be too conservative or too liberal, with uncertain implication on the false-positive error rate. High ADA-positive samples are generally not prone to this problem when excess drug is used for inhibiting the signal. Therefore, the confirmation of ADA-reactive (potentially positive) samples from the screening assay should be determined by an objective experimental approach, in the context of assay variability near the low-positive range of the assay, as described below.

To determine the confirmatory cut point, the amount of drug to be added to the ADA-reactive samples from the screening assay should first be determined. Typically, a high level of positive control (most likely of animal origin) is added to the sample matrix to obtain a response signal near the upper limit of the dynamic range of the instrument. This sample is first preincubated with various levels of drug and subsequently analyzed in the screening assay. The level of spiked drug that reduces the response to just below the screening cut point is noted. These experiments are then repeated using lower levels of the positive control to demonstrate that the inhibitory concentration of drug is reproducible. To ensure this inhibition of the response in the ADA-positive patient samples, an elevated level of drug (i.e., 10-fold higher than the amount determined above) is then used during validation to set the confirmatory cut point by spiking the same samples used for setting the screening cut point.

The confirmatory cut point is then set by statistical analysis of the percent inhibition of the responses of the drug-spiked and unspiked samples [34]. This analysis and calculation is similar to the procedure described above for the screening cut point, the primary difference being that these analyses are based on the ratio of drug-spiked to unspiked samples or percent inhibition data (see Appendix 3 of Shankar et al. [34] for further details).

8.5.5 Sensitivity

Unlike fully quantitative methods that utilize the reference standard curve to estimate the analyte levels in the study samples, sensitivity of ADA assays *per se* is not a critical validation characteristic. This is because, for the reasons described in Section 8.2, the screening, confirmation, and characterization of ADA-positive samples are based on the assay response unit rather than the ADA concentration levels. In addition, sensitivity of an ADA assay is highly dependent on the positive-control reagent(s) used to characterize it, assay format, number of wash steps, minimum dilution, and the screening cut point. In addition, the activity of the positive control directly influences the sensitivity of the assay. Despite these caveats, assay "sensitivity" is typically determined and reported in concentration units (e.g., ng/mL) and is generally requested by the regulatory agencies. It is particularly useful during assay development for choosing an optimal ADA detection method (comparisons between methods during initial development) and for the determination of a low-positive control for validation.

To determine assay sensitivity in concentration units during validation, polyclonal ADAs in the positive control will require some type of affinity purification or monoclonal antibodies may be used. While the initial ADA-positive control can be developed by hyperimmunizing animals with the drug and is appropriate at the beginning of a drug's preclinical program, pooled ADA serum from positive study subjects should be used whenever possible by the time the clinical program begins. Use of sera from hyperimmunized animals at this stage may lead to overestimating the actual sensitivity of the ADA method. An ADA from hyperimmunized animals normally consists of high-affinity antibodies that may misrepresent the true affinity of ADAs encountered later on in actual studies, resulting in an inaccurate assessment of the assay's sensitivity. Determining when to use hyperimmune ADA sera will depend on what and how much actual ADA sera are available. A highly conserved protein drug may only elicit a very low and infrequent response during preclinical evaluation, so ADA obtained from hyperimmunized animals may be the only available option.

The recommended sensitivity for ADA screening assays at the preclinical stage is 500–1000 ng/mL and 250–500 ng/mL for clinical assays [14]. In addition, the sensitivity of any ADA assay should be justified using the results of the risk assessment analysis. Sensitivity of ADA assays is defined [34] by the lowest concentration at which a positive-control antibody preparation *consistently* provides a signal above the assay screening cut point (ADA positive). This may be the concentration of the control antibody at which the assay result is expected to be above the screening cut point at least 95% of the time, or just 50% of the time, depending on the level of consistency preferred. Experimentally, we suggest preparing five or more serial dilutions of the positive-control spanning the screening cut point. The dilutions should be prepared in pooled drug-naïve matrix and tested in at least six assay runs by more than one analyst/instrument if multiple analysts/instruments will be used during clinical sample analysis. Each of these dilution curves should be fitted by an appropriate regression model to interpolate the dilution at which the screening cut point is reached. For 50% level of consistency, the mean of the interpolated dilution levels corresponding to the results from these assay runs defines the sensitivity of the assay. For 95% level of consistency, the mean and standard deviation of these interpolated dilution levels are used to define the sensitivity of the assay as mean $+ t_{0.05,df} \times$ SD, where $t_{0.05,df}$ is the critical value determined from the t-distribution corresponding to a 5% false-positive rate and "df" is the degrees of freedom that depends on the number of samples and runs used in the calculation. See Appendix 4 of Shankar et al. [34] for further details.

8.5.6 Control Range

Data for the control range are collected during validation, are set after validation, and are generally expressed in response units or titers. Response units are usually dictated by the type of instrument used to detect the ADA binding (e.g., optical density (OD) for microplate readers or relative light units (RLU) for SPR). Typically, two positive-control levels are prepared: a low control near the cut point and a high control in the upper range of the measurable response. The lower range of the high and low controls and the upper range for the low control are routinely determined statistically, while an upper range for the high control is not always determined. The same pool of ADA-positive serum can be used to prepare both of these controls. The negative control is often prepared from a pool of drug-naïve samples used for establishing the cut point. System suitability criteria [34] can be defined based on the negative control, low-positive control and high-positive control. The response of the low-positive control should be defined objectively such that it is neither too low nor too high comparative to the cut point. For example, it can be a concentration at which 1% of the samples can be expected to be negative (signal below the screening cut point), and can be determined using the same data from the sensitivity evaluation experiment, as described by Shankar et al. [34]. To define the acceptance criteria for the controls, data for each control from at least three runs and two analysts and the same number of replicates as intended for study samples are needed. For a 1% failure rate of the negative control, the upper limit of the negative control is the mean signal $+ t_{0.01,\mathrm{df}} \times$ SD, where the mean and SD are derived from this experiment. For the low- and high-positive controls, if both upper and lower limits are defined, then the acceptance range would be the mean response $\pm t_{0.005,\mathrm{df}} \times$ SD, where $t_{0.005,\mathrm{df}}$ assumes a 1% failure rate with respect to the lower or high extremes. If a lower failure rate is preferred, then the thresholds can be raised accordingly. A set of titration controls in titration assays to confirm dilutional linearity of a positive control may also be helpful. In addition, it is acceptable to have overlapping acceptance limits for the negative control and low-positive control, as long as these limits were derived based on objective error rate thresholds as described above.

Alternatively, if a floating cut point approach is used for the screening cut point during the in-study phase, the acceptance criteria can be defined for the ratio of low-positive control to low-negative control, and the ratio of high-positive control to high-negative control, using similar statistical formulae as above (log transformation might be necessary). Even if the individual controls fall outside the limits, as long as all the results across controls vary in a similar direction such that the ratios of the controls are within the system suitability limits, the use of a floating cut point approach will help to ensure the validity of the assay.

8.5.7 Selectivity/Specificity

This tests the ability of the assay to detect the analyte in matrix without interference from cross-reacting or unrelated analytes. For ADA assays the major cross-reacting substance can be the drug itself, as high concentrations could inhibit ADA binding, resulting in false-negative assay results. Thus, it is important during validation to determine the maximum amount of drug that can be tolerated in a sample without triggering false-negative results. This information along with knowledge of the half-life of the drug can then be applied to determine the appropriate "drug free" time points for sampling during preclinical and clinical trials. During multidose studies, this information will be especially important to avoid detecting false-negative results. The macromolecule may also affect assays differently, depending on the assay, assay format or type, and the characteristics of the ADA.

If interference occurs, the impact may be evaluated by assessing the amount of antigen required to reduce the antibody signal (positive) to background for a range of antibody concentrations. Other approaches, for example, acid dissociation of immune complexes [38], removal of the excess biological by solid-phase adsorption, and/or use of an assay that allows sufficient sample dilution to avoid this problem, may be considered. Such approaches need to be validated for effectiveness and adopted on a case-by-case basis.

Issues such as potential interference (specificity) in the assay from comedications, dosing regimen (e.g., potential for product to be present in the sample), and/or disease-specific issues (e.g., presence of rheumatoid factor) also need to be considered during validation. It may be possible to assess interference by spiking drug-naïve patient samples with an antibody preparation of known concentration, such as the ADA control used for the sensitivity measurement, and assessing recovery by measuring its response over a range of concentrations. This should provide some indication of whether factors in the matrix can interfere with the ability of the ADAs to bind to the antigen. Comparisons should also be made by conducting a similar experiment using sera from healthy subjects. Such "recovery" experiments will determine if the effects observed are due to substances present only in the patient matrix. These samples should be investigated over the full range of expected sample dilutions. In some cases, this may limit the final dilutions that can be validly assessed. However, one must remember that the selectivity/specificity determined here was established with a positive control that may not be representative of all ADA responses since each ADA may be unique.

8.5.8 Linearity

This does not apply to ADA assays as there is no standard curve or reference standard to interpret results. However, it is important to demonstrate that a linear relationship occurs between the amount of ADA in a sample and the response as demonstrated by decrease in response with increasing dilution of sample. It is also important to determine if large concentrations of ADA would produce a prozone or "Hook" effect that, if present, would result in a false-negative or low-titer value. An acceptable approach to investigating linearity involves spiking various concentrations of ADAs into the matrix as well as spiking in a high amount of ADAs, serially diluting the sample, and observing if there is a positive dose–response relationship.

8.5.9 Stability (Freeze–Thaw Cycles, Storage Temperature, and Storage Time)

This may be assessed for the positive-control samples but, due to the variable nature of ADAs, this will only be an estimate of a sample's true stability. In addition, it is also important to determine the stability of any of the critical reagents used in the method. These may include, but are not limited to, second antibody–enzyme conjugates, coated plates, biotinylated drug, and so on. Most antibodies are stable at $-70°C$ for extended periods. Preparing and freezing multiple aliquots of samples will minimize the number of freeze–thaw (FT) cycles the ADAs are exposed to and reduce the possibility of inactivating the ADAs present in the sample or enzymes coupled to the secondary antibody–enzyme conjugates in key reagents. In general, IgG is very stable and can be frozen and thawed many times. IgMs may be more susceptible to precipitation upon multiple FT cycles.

8.5.10 Precision

Precision is a quantitative measure of the random variation between a series of measurements from a method. Approaches for determining precision of data from the screening assay (assay response), specificity confirmation assay (percent inhibition), and titration assay (titers) are described below.

8.5.10.1 Screening Assay   Precision of the screening assay can be determined using data from at least six independent assay runs of the assay controls (negative control and low-positive and high-positive controls). The intra-run precision and intermediate (inter-run) precision of the assay response data at each of these controls should be reported. These values can be determined using standard statistical formulae similar to those described for the concentration data in a recent publication [30]. If analyst-specific cut points are used for testing study samples, then the inter-analyst CV should also be determined.

8.5.10.2 Confirmation Assay   The objective of precision assessment for the specificity confirmation assay is to test the reproducibility of signal inhibition when spiking a positive sample with drug. To calculate % inhibition, the low- and high-positive control samples from at least six independent runs should be spiked with the appropriate level of drug, as determined during the confirmatory cut point experiment. The percent inhibition data can then be analyzed to determine the intra-run precision and intermediate precision, in the same way as the assay response data are analyzed to determine the precision of the screening assay.

8.5.10.3 Titration Assay   Using a dilution profile of an ADA-positive sample, titer is defined by the reciprocal of the dilution of the sample that corresponds to the screening assay cut point (interpolation method). Alternatively, instead of interpolation, it is sometimes defined by the reciprocal of the lowest dilution whose signal falls below the screening assay cut point. In these evaluations, it is important that the concentration of serum/plasma remains constant in the sample; otherwise, the response may be skewed, resulting in inaccurate results.

In either approach, if the goal is to compare close titer values (such as eightfold difference between titers of two ADA samples), it is important to apply the interpolation method to determine the titers, or if a noninterpolation method is used, the serial dilutions should be narrowly spaced (ideally twofold or less). In addition, an objective method is needed for determining the ability of the assay to differentiate titers (titer precision). This titer precision is defined by the minimum significant ratio (MSR), which is the smallest fold change between the titers of any two ADA-positive samples that can be considered as significant. For example, MSR = 5 means that at least a fivefold difference in the titer results between any two positive samples will be required to conclude that they are statistically different. Evaluation of MSR is mostly relevant when comparison of samples with close titers is of interest.

The determination of MSR for titer precision requires dilution profile data of at least five high-positive mock samples, diluted past the screening cut point, from at least three independent runs by two or more analysts (if relevant). The mock positive samples are drug-naïve samples from individual donors spiked with a high concentration of the ADA-positive control. The titer results of all these mock positive samples from different runs should be log transformed and analyzed to obtain the overall standard deviation. This estimate of overall SD is then used to determine the MSR of the titer results, where $MSR = 10^{[2^* sqrt(2)^* SD]}$, assuming that base 10 was used in the log transformation of the titer results. In addition to the practical usefulness of the MSR concept in this application, an attractive feature is that it applies to any range of titer results. This is because the variability in log scale tends to be quite similar across the entire range of titer results.

The following points should be noted in the evaluation of MSR: (1) because the mock positive samples will generally have different characteristics from the real ADA-positive patient samples, the MSR determined from this approach may not be a fully accurate reflection of the variability of patient titer results and (2) the use of mock positive samples rather than a pooled positive control is stressed here due to the relevance of both the biological and analytical variability in the interpretation of MSR.

Refer to Table 8.1 for solutions to common problems observed with development of ADA assays using LBAs.

8.6   OPTIMIZATION AND VALIDATION: NEUTRALIZING ANTIBODY ASSAYS

Within the pharmaceutical industry and regulatory agencies, the role of CLB assays versus bioassays for assessing Nabs is debated. The EMEA guidance primarily advocates the use of bioassays for both nonclinical and clinical studies for all biologics; however, it does also state that a CLB may be used if a bioassay is not feasible. In terms of safety, Nabs are of greatest concern for drug mimetics of endogenous proteins because of the possibility of cross-reactivity of the ADA with the endogenous molecule.

TABLE 8.1 LBA Method Development Troubleshooting Guide

Problem	Probable Cause	Possible Solution
High background response	Poor blocking of solid phase	Evaluate alternate blocking materials (e.g., Tween-20, BSA, OVA, fish gelatin)
	Denaturation of coating material	Adjust concentration of coating material or investigate using an indirect coating approach (e.g., MAb capture)
	Poor specificity of anti-ADA signal molecule	Evaluate signal molecules from other vendors (e.g., affinity purified Abs)
	Matrix contains nonspecific binding antibodies.	Look at obtaining naïve matrix from several vendors. Human serum is especially variable across vendors
	Inappropriate or incorrect concentration of surfactant in wash solution	Adjust concentration of surfactant in wash solution or evaluate alternate surfactants
Poor precision	Washing process may be too robust	Adjust pressure and frequency of washing process
	Poor pipetting technique	Increase volume of sample and detection solution. Use electronic pipettors whenever possible. Compare precision across analysts
	Poor affinity of anti-ADA signal molecule	Evaluate signal molecules from other vendors
Low sensitivity	Low numbers of drug bound to the solid phase	Evaluate different coating buffers, ionic strengths, and pH. Also investigate using an indirect coating approach (i.e., MAb capture)
	Poor affinity of anti-ADA signal molecule	Evaluate signal molecules from other vendors. Evaluate complexes that can amplify the signal such as avidin/biotin. Evaluate other platforms (i.e., ECL or SPR)

TABLE 8.1 (*Continued*)

Problem	Probable Cause	Possible Solution
	Low-affinity positive control	Evaluate several different positive-control preparations. Try increasing the incubation time of each of the reagents
	Interference from matrix	Compare sensitivity in buffer versus matrix. Look at diluting matrix further before analysis
No or poor inhibition observed in confirmatory assay	Reactive epitopes on drug (captured or spiked) are blocked to ADA binding	Evaluate indirect coating or alternate assay format (e.g., RIPA)
	Captured drug on solid phase is denatured	Investigate alternate capture chemistry to solid phase or assay format

As discussed in Section 8.5, the recommended parameters for validation of anti-drug antibody assays include minimal required dilution, cut point, sensitivity, precision, drug interference, positive-control stability, recovery, and robustness [14]. While the focus of Mire-Sluis et al. [14] was on total ADA assays, these same criteria are applicable to validation of Nab assays. These, and the recommendations for assay qualification by Gupta et al. [15], should be used as guidance for validating Nab assays in the absence of validation-specific recommendations. For Nab assays, utilizing a concentration–response curve (common for reporting amount of drug neutralized) and evaluation of linearity, parallelism, accuracy, precision, and regression analysis are additional validation considerations that may be unique to these types of assays. If Nab assays are designed using concentration–response curves, accuracy and precision should be determined within the linear range of the assay. Although the intent of this book is to discuss the use of ligand-binding assays, in the context of immunogenicity, one would be remiss if bioassays were not also discussed to some extent. The reader is also referred to the Gupta et al. [15] publication for a more detailed description of optimization considerations for bioassays.

8.6.1 Optimization

Bioassays are more difficult and time-consuming to develop because the assay system requires the use of a cell line, which also needs to be examined for parameters such as optimal cell culture conditions, viability, and maintenance. The recommendations by Gupta et al. [15] are a useful guide for developing cell-based Nab assays. Competitive ligand-binding assays are similar in some respects to total binding immunoassays and are generally easier to optimize and validate than bioassays.

8.6.1.1 Cell Line Identification and Assay Format/End Point Selection (Bioassays)
The first and, perhaps most critical, step in designing a Nab bioassay is identifying an appropriate cell line. This may not be an easy process for novel targets, for small drugs such as peptides and aptamers, and because of intellectual property rights. Understanding the mechanism of action, target, and effector pathways of the drug are all critical components for identifying a suitable assay system and end point. In general, biological therapeutics function as either agonists or antagonists. Agonistic biologicals such as cytokines, growth factors, hormones, or some monoclonal antibodies (mAbs) work by binding directly to target cell-surface receptors and activating a signaling pathway, while antagonistic biologicals, such as soluble receptors and some mAbs, work by blocking receptor–ligand binding by binding their ligand either in solution or at the cell surface.

If available, a potency assay developed for the batch release of the biological is a good starting point because it can often be adapted for use as a Nab bioassay. For example, a neutralization assay for GM-CSF can be a modification of the proliferation assay used for potency assessment for GM-CSF. This approach is advantageous, as optimization of cell line maintenance and culture conditions had already been performed. However, this assay needs to be tailored for use as a neutralization assay, as it may not be adequately sensitive for the purpose in its original format. Therefore, the performance of the potency assay in the presence of test sample (appropriate species serum) and response to the therapeutic to yield a sufficiently sensitive assay requires validation. Ideally, the cell line should yield a functional end point upon treatment with the therapeutic protein, the assay should be simple to perform, and the biological end point should be tolerant of the test sample matrix and perform adequately over a range of concentrations.

If a potency assay is not available, it is often necessary to evaluate several cell lines for biological responsiveness to the therapeutic. Stable cell lines are preferred over primary cells because of availability, reliability, and convenience. The human cell line TF-1, derived from an erythroleukemic patient, proliferates in response to several cytokines such as granulocyte-macrophage colony stimulating factor (GM-CSF), IL-3, erythropoietin (Epo), and IL-5 [39]. This cell line has been used successfully for deriving data related to neutralization activity of GM-CSF-induced antibodies [40]. Similarly, the subclone of the human erythroleukemic cell line, UT7/Epo, that is highly responsive to Epo provides an excellent assay for the determination of neutralization potential of Epo-induced antibodies [41]. Anti-CD40 therapeutic stimulation of the Burkitt lymphoma cell line, Daudi, results in upregulation of CD54 cell-surface expression and is a useful cell line for assessing neutralizing antibodies to anti-CD40 therapeutics [23].

For cell-based Nab bioassays, it is critical to assess the stability of the cell line over time (passages) and through cryopreservation. Stability assessment should be performed by comparing assay controls such as concentration–response curves or neutralizing capacity of the positive control (PC). Additional parameters, such as cell growth, appearance, and viability may also aid in stability assessment. Further, monitoring receptor expression by a method such as flow cytometry may also be valuable.

After cell line identification, extensive optimization of assay conditions is often necessary to maximize the biological response. Multiple assay end points, sample incubation times, cell seeding density, cell viability, and the need for cell culture conditions, such as culture media, supplements, passaging, and fetal calf serum, are all conditions that may need to be assessed. For the anti-CD40 therapeutic Nab bioassay, Baltrukonis et al. [23] found assay robustness was significantly impacted by the source of culture media and lots of fetal bovine serum.

8.6.1.2   *Matrix Interference (Bioassays and CLB Assays)*   The effects of individual patient sample matrix need to be assessed on the optimized test system. If feasible, it is recommended that sample matrix be examined concurrently during cell line identification and assay optimization. Therefore, determination of the appropriate dilution of sample matrix is important during assay optimization, as this will dictate the test sample dilution and, in turn, the assay sensitivity. The effect of sample matrix on the ability of the cells to respond to the product should be evaluated at multiple concentrations and the highest matrix concentration that has a minimal effect on the cellular response selected and further evaluated using a positive-control antibody spiked into sample matrix. It is important that the assay detects the antibody and differentiates it from assay matrix components, for example, complement, coagulation factors, soluble receptors, lipids, and coadministered medications that are likely to be present in the sample. Where possible, implementation of strategies (such as for overcoming problems with matrix effects, assessing specificity of the antibodies for minimizing interference) should be defined to provide sound scientific data. Since sera are heterogeneous in their content of interfering substances, multiple individual sera are needed to define the effects of the assay matrix. If possible, the selected cell line (if several are available to choose from) should be able to tolerate serum from the different species used in the product development program. Matrix interference may be especially problematic for bioassays. Additionally, one should consider both normal serum and disease-state serum as a component of optimization and validation depending on patient population for clinical studies.

8.6.1.3   *Drug Concentration (Bioassays and CLB Assays)*   Selecting and optimizing a concentration of the drug for use in the neutralization assay is essential. For CLB assays, availability of the target or ligand is a critical consideration often encountered for novel targets. Whether it is commercially available or needs to be produced in-house, and whether it is stable in solution are important questions. In a CLB or bioassay, a typical standard curve for a biological consists of a dose range (5–10 points) with at least four concentrations in the linear portion of the curve. It is important to evaluate this dose–response curve and select a dose capable of yielding 70–80% of the maximal response with good discrimination between signal and noise in the assay matrix. The selected concentration should provide a reliable and robust response and be adequately sensitive to detect clinically relevant neutralizing antibodies. If an assay requires a high concentration of drug to elicit a suitable assay signal, the amount of antibodies needed to neutralize a response may not be at physiologically relevant levels. A very high dose of the biological may compromise the detection of

neutralizing antibodies, but a low dose will not allow valid discrimination between signal and background; both of these situations should be avoided. It is necessary to assess the performance of the assay by assessing the observed signal to background ratio of the cellular response to the product and the variability associated with it. Assays showing less than a fivefold change in response to product in serum may not provide an assay response that is adequate for observing an inhibitory effect due to neutralizing antibodies.

Drug concentration may be fixed or variable depending upon the assay format selected. When using a variable drug amount, the serum concentration is usually kept constant and a series of drug concentrations are combined with serum to generate a drug curve. EC_{50} readouts of the drug curve are commonly used, and changes in EC_{50} values are indicative of neutralizing antibody response.

8.6.1.4 *Positive Controls (Bioassays and CLB Assays)* Finding suitable neutralizing controls can be a major challenge. Some companies try various vaccination protocols to try to have a greater chance of generating a neutralizing antibody, but there are situations where such cannot be identified and this creates a major challenge regardless of whether assays are bioassays or CLB assays.

8.6.2 Validation

8.6.2.1 *Validation Parameters* Cut point, sensitivity, precision, assay specificity, drug interference, stability, and confirmation assays should be considered as validation parameters. As a general guide, the validation parameters described in Section 8.5 for total binding assays can be applied to CLB assays and, in some cases, to bioassays. Members of the American Association of Pharmaceutical Scientists Ligand-Binding Assay Bioanalytical Focus Group are currently working on a bioassay validation white paper, with anticipated publication in 2009.

As mentioned previously, greater sensitivity and ease of development are generally achieved with CLB Nab assay formats as compared to functional, cell-based assays. Using both assay formats, Baltrukonis et al. [23] compared Nab and CLB results for serum samples from a 3-month toxicity study in monkeys treated with an agonistic CD40 antibody drug and observed a significant correlation between the results. In this case, both the bioassay and the CLB assay had similar sensitivities. Caras [25] reported comparisons in sensitivity between three bioassay end points (STAT phosphorylation, cell proliferation, cytokine production) and a competitive binding end point. The competitive binding end point had sensitivity in the 100 ng/mL range while the bioassay sensitivities ranged from 600 to 5000 ng/mL. Thus, even in cases where similar sensitivity between bioassays and CLB assays can be achieved, the bioassay may not always offer an advantage. Furthermore, where sensitivity of the CLB assay format is superior to that of a bioassay, the CLB assay format may be able to provide data that are more meaningful.

8.6.2.2 *Specificity (Bioassays and CLB Assays)* Inclusion of an approach for establishing specificity is useful in determining the presence of interfering substances and for assurance that the inhibitory response is attributed to specific

neutralizing antibodies rather than matrix effects. This strategy should be implemented simultaneously with the neutralization antibody assay. In their recommendations for Nab bioassay optimization, Gupta et al. [15] advocate the use of four possible matrix interference assays (confirmatory assays): alternative stimulus, sample-induced inhibition, immunodepletion, and immunocompetition. These approaches may be used independently or in combination, depending on the dynamics of the test system and immunogenicity testing strategy employed.

a. *Alternative Stimulus Assays*: In the alternative stimulus assay, another irrelevant stimulus (at a concentration capable of inducing a similar cellular response to that of the therapeutic in the cell line used for assay) is included in the assays. For example, if ligand A and ligand B both can stimulate cell proliferation in a cell line and the therapeutic was to ligand A, ligand B could be used as an alternative stimulus to demonstrate that the neutralizing antibodies were specific for ligand A. This strategy has been described for detection of neutralizing Epo antibodies [28].

b. *Sample-Induced Inhibition*: This approach involves testing the samples in both the absence and presence of the therapeutic. This allows for both the determination of interference/background inhibition and whether there is therapeutic present in the sample that could affect the assay. Baltrukonis et al. [23] implemented testing study samples without the addition of drug to assess whether circulating drug remaining in the sample was at a level that could cause potential assay interference. A unique cut point was established for this as well as a cut point established to discriminate positive from negative response in samples that had drug added as part of the assay.

c. *Immunodepletion*: The samples can be pretreated with an absorbing resin, for example, protein G, which binds immunoglobulin molecules resulting in immunodepletion (or removal of the antibody molecules). Both the pre- and posttreatment samples are then assessed for neutralization activity [45]. Thus, immunodepletion (removal of Ig) may be used to demonstrate that a response is due to immunoglobulin and not due to other factors in the serum.

d. *Immunocompetition*: This step is equivalent to specificity testing in total ADA assays. The technique is not as applicable to Nab assays, since it requires the addition of excess drug, which would induce a biological response in the cells in bioassays, or result in additional drug binding to the target in the CLB assay, thus disrupting the controlled test system. However, there are examples of its use in Nab bioassays [28].

8.6.3 Technical Challenges for Nab Assays

In general, bioassays have more technical issues due to serum effects on cells, greater variability and sensitivity. Additionally, both bioassays and CLB assays are complicated by interferences from drug and/or endogenous proteins that may be difficult to overcome.

8.6.3.1 Drug Interference   Depending on the dose, regimen (single versus multidose), route of administration, sample collection time points, and the half-life of the drug, the presence of the drug in the test sample may be unavoidable and poses a significant challenge for Nab assays. The response of the Nab bioassay is usually defined to a single concentration of drug. Most Nab bioassays cannot detect neutralizing antibodies in the presence of high drug levels in the test sample [19]. This problem can sometimes be overcome by incorporating an acid-dissociation strategy combined with an affinity adsorption step for removing the drug from test samples.

8.6.3.2 Endogenous Protein Interference In addition to assay interference caused by drug in the test sample, interference may be encountered from endogenous proteins behaving similarly to excess drug in the test sample. Some endogenous proteins are present in the serum at mg/mL concentrations and may make the practicality of a Nab assay infeasible. For example, apolipoprotein A-I (apoA-I) is the primary apolipoprotein component of high-density lipoprotein (HDL) in normal human serum at concentrations in excess of 10 mg/mL [42]. A naturally occurring variant of apoA-I termed apoA-I Milano was discovered in Italy in approximately 40 individuals with the unusual combination of low levels of HDL-cholesterol, long life spans, and less atherosclerosis. It has been hypothesized that increasing nascent HDL particles by infusing apoA-I Milano will lower the risk of coronary events [43,44]. Recombinant biotherapeutic mimetics of apoA-I Milano are currently under development as potential biotherapeutics [43]. In this situation, could a Nab assay for antibodies to the drug, given that such ADA may also cross-react with endogenous protein, be developed to provide reliable results in the presence of systemic apoA-I concentrations in the milligram per milliliter range? Such an assay would probably not be needed, in light of the likely saturation of any ADA elicited by the high level of endogenous protein. Thus, the value of doing Nab assessment for such situations is questionable.

8.7 ASSAYS AND RISK ASSESSMENT

8.7.1 Qualitative Versus Quasi-Quantitative LBA Assay Formats

The data from quantitative ADA assays can be difficult to interpret. In the past, some scientists have used a monoclonal antibody "standard" to construct a dose–response curve that was then employed to interpolate concentration results. However, since most ADA responses are polyclonal and, thus, heterogeneous in nature, the comparison of this response to a monoclonal antibody calibration curve can be misleading, as the sample response is an average of all the ADAs present in the sample. The specificity and affinity of these ADAs may also be different from the ADA standard, leading to false assumptions and inaccurate results. Using a monoclonal antibody standard may also lead to less sensitive assays, resulting in the reporting of false-negative results due to the high affinity of the monoclonal antibody for the drug.

It is a regulatory expectation that the sensitivity of the assay will be determined in concentration units, (i.e., ng/mL). Thus, an approximate concentration of antibody can be assumed for a ADA positive sample, noting that the ADA used in determining the sensitivity may not be representative of each sample tested. A confirmatory assay should subsequently be run to evaluate the specificity of the ADA for the drug. Once specificity is established, the ADA-positive samples should be analyzed in a titration assay for reporting the relative titers as described in Section 8.5.

8.7.2 Qualitative Versus Quasi-Quantitative Nab Assay Formats

Depending on the risk-based strategy employed by the investigator, the Nab assay may be either qualitative or quasi-quantitative. In the qualitative assay format, samples are incubated at the minimal required dilution with a fixed concentration of the drug and added to the test system. Some investigators may use a fixed concentration of serum and varying concentrations of drug, but this is generally less common. The sample is reported as either positive or negative for Nabs depending on whether the test sample crosses the cut point of the assay.

For the quasi-quantitative format, there are three distinctive approaches that may be used: end point titer, amount of drug neutralized per milliliter of serum, or amount of serum required to neutralize the biological activity induced by a constant amount of drug. The end point titer is perhaps the most common approach in which samples are serially diluted into a negative control matrix to maintain the minimal required dilution. The negative control matrix is often a pool of individual matrices used in determining the cut point. These serial dilutions are incubated with a fixed concentration of the drug and then added to the assay test system. The dilution of the test sample that intercepts the assay cut point is the end point titer in the assay. This value or the value interpolated at the assay cut point from regression analysis is reported as the reciprocal of the dilution or log (reciprocal of the dilution) [15].

The methodology for reporting data as amount of drug neutralized per milliliter of serum requires a full drug concentration–response curve as a standard curve. Sample response data are graphed against the standard curve to determine the corresponding drug concentration. This value is then subtracted from the concentration of drug used in the test system and adjusted for the minimal required dilution to determine the amount of drug neutralized per milliliter of serum.

Alternatively, results may be reported as the "amount of serum required to neutralize the biological activity induced by a constant amount of the antigen" [40]. For example, for GM-CSF, the volume of serum required to neutralize the activity of 10 IU of cytokine can be calculated using serum ED_{50} responses obtained by fitting common asymptotes and slope for all sera analyzed. This approach can also be used to analyze responses to different GM-CSF preparations/products and can be applied to other biologicals.

One of the difficult issues associated with assays for antibody detection is the interpretation and evaluation of the results obtained. The usual approach for evaluation of antibodies is firstly the classification of the sample as positive or negative for antibodies in a preliminary screening assay followed by confirmation of positives, and secondly a careful and thorough quantitation of the amounts of antibodies (if present) in the relevant biological sample and further characterization by testing for neutralization, antigen specificity, isotype analysis, and so on. The results obtained and the analysis will depend on the type of assay, the assay design used, and the issue being considered, for example, a yes/no screening assay or a classification approach or a more useful quantitative assay.

8.7.3 Nonclinical

In nonclinical studies, it is not uncommon to have a high incidence and level of antibodies to human, humanized or chimeric proteins, fusion proteins, or peptides. Generally, total-binding antibody assessment is employed in nonclinical studies. While comparing animal to potential human responses is not always predictable, data from nonclinical studies may be helpful in evaluating whether changes to the production process of the drug, route of administration, or formulation affect immunogenicity [9]. Nonclinical study results may also help in understanding the potential immune response differences between reference and comparator products.

The need for routine neutralizing antibody assessment in nonclinical studies is controversial with respect to whether such data are needed to interpret toxicity and the toxicokinetic data. Currently, no guidance unequivocally requires neutralizing antibody assessment for nonclinical toxicology studies. ICH Guidance S6 [11] states that immunogenicity should be evaluated (e.g., titer, number of responding animals neutralizing or nonneutralizing) and appearance of antibodies should be correlated with any pharmacological and/or toxicological changes. Several publications have discussed strategic approaches for testing for neutralizing antibodies in nonclinical studies and when such may be justified [2,3].

Currently, the extent to which neutralizing antibody assessment is performed may range from the evaluation of PK/PD/biomarker data to the need for performing competitive ligand-binding or cell-based bioassays. In general, Nab assays are generally not performed in animal studies, unless the study served as the primary study supporting safety of a product for humans [2]. Determination of Nabs from nonhuman primate studies may need to be considered on a case-by-case basis depending on a variety of factors, such as type of drug and mechanism of action, antibody incidence, observed toxicity, and availability of relevant and sensitive biomarkers as well as PK data. The type of assay potentially used for assessment of neutralizing antibodies is an additional area of contention for both nonclinical and clinical studies. Some advocate using only a functional bioassay to assess for neutralizing antibody activity while others deem ligand-binding assays sufficient. Shankar et al. [3] state that "given that nonclinical immunogenicity data do not predict safety in humans, if neutralizing antibody testing is deemed necessary, it could be either a target binding–inhibition immunoassay or cell-based assay, irrespective of risk." In the context of the nonclinical setting in which antibody data are used to interpret toxicity and toxicokinetic data, the need for neutralizing antibody data in addition to total binding data is debatable. Thus, at this time, different companies have different policies regarding the need for Nab assays during nonclinical development, and these may or may not be based upon risk-based assessments.

8.7.4 Clinical

The extent and frequency of immunogenicity testing with both total binding and Nab assays may be evaluated during the risk assessment. The frequency of sample collection may be, in part, dependent on extrinsic factors such as frequency and route of administration, formulation, and immune status of the patient. Other factors, such as half-life of the drug or biodistribution, will also dictate ADA assessment frequency. Intrinsic factors, such as homology with an endogenous protein, may require the use of a very sensitive assay, as well as lengthy follow-up, post study, to confirm that the subject did not generate a potentially dangerous Nab response to the drug.

Investigators tend to have their own in-house policies regarding their implementation of Nab assays, based on the risk level and/or development phase of the product. Some companies conduct neutralization assays for both nonclinical and clinical programs, while most others implement them at various phases of the clinical program, after considering the risk of immunogenicity and potential safety and/or efficacy implications associated with antibody generation for a particular product. With respect to neutralizing antibody assays, the type of assay used may be either a cell-based assay or a CLB assay. The type of assay may vary depending upon the mode/mechanism of action of the drug and/or the development stage of the program (e.g., FIH versus Phase III). It should be pointed out that there are ongoing and completed clinical trials with biotherapeutics in which total binding antibody data were deemed satisfactory, and neutralizing antibody assessment was not done. However, most companies generally have neutralizing antibody assays in place by the Phase III development stage.

As was described for nonclinical programs, the value of Nab assay data for protein therapeutics without endogenous counterparts can be debated. When PK data demonstrate decreased drug exposure in conjunction with total ADA, is there additional value in having an *in vitro* neutralizing antibody assay? Furthermore, if there are good biomarkers for pharmacodynamics, one could further argue that Nab data will not provide additional information to interpret the efficacy and safety of the drug. Thus, the use of Nab assays in clinical studies needs to be driven by risk assessment approaches, and a single approach should not be advocated for all therapeutic proteins.

There are therapeutic drugs, such as interferon beta for treating MS patients, in which the Nab results provided meaningful data regarding impact on efficacy of the drug and patient relapse [4]. These data could not be ascertained from the ADA binding data alone. Because of the substantial body of evidence that correlated Nab with patient relapse, controversial recommendations have been established to remove patients from further treatment after twice testing positive for Nab antibodies of a certain titer [46]. Goodin et al. [47] state that "although the findings of sustained high-titer Nabs are associated with a reduction in the therapeutic effects of IFN-beta on radiographic and clinical measures of MS disease activity, there is insufficient information on the utilization of Nab testing to provide specific recommendations regarding when to test, which test to use, how many tests are necessary, and which cutoff titer to apply." They advocate that further trials and long-term Nab data analysis are needed to ascertain clinical impact.

Thus, there are some instances in which Nab results may provide data that, with ADA and PK data alone, are not sufficient for risk management of a patient. For the treatment of conditions in which a PD marker is not available and clinical end points may not be as clear-cut, neutralizing data may provide critical data to make decisions regarding discontinuation of treatment or other intervention. However, for other therapeutics, the detection of ADA alone in conjunction with PK and/or PD data may be sufficient to assess the efficacy and safety of a therapeutic protein. In a study conducted in 15 patients who had highly reactive rheumatoid arthritis who received human anti-TNF-alpha mAb, 87% of the patients developed antibodies to the drug and 69% had decreased efficacy [48]. In this study, total binding antibody titers, with no neutralizing antibody data, in combination with other clinical end points were used and correlated with drug efficacy and adverse events. This illustrates that, in some cases, Nab assays may not be needed to interpret data adequately, although there still may be regulatory expectations to test for neutralizing antibodies. It should be noted that the patient population reported in the study had a much greater incidence of immunogenicity than was originally reported for the product in studies supporting approval, in which the incidence in patients receiving the drug for 5–12 months was reported as approximately 5% of neutralizing antibodies [49]. In Gaucher disease patients receiving enzyme-replacement therapies, the generation of neutralizing antibodies has been described, although the presence of Nab antibodies as detected in an *in vitro* assay did not always correlate with a decrease in clinical efficacy [50]. Furthermore, when dosing was continued for 24 months or greater, a number of patients were no longer antibody positive and were tolerated to the therapeutic. Thus, although Nab assessment was performed, it did not appear to be essential to interpret drug safety and efficacy.

As described by Shankar et al. [3], there is no single approach for testing neutralizing antibodies that should be advocated for nonclinical and clinical studies. Depending on a risk assessment strategy, different therapeutic proteins will have different needs in terms of type and level of immunogenicity testing and Nab testing in particular to assess the efficacy and safety of a particular drug.

Due to the limited number of patients exposed to drug in clinical studies, such studies may not accurately predict the ADA incidence and the degree of neutralizing antibody generation for that subsequently observed in postapproval stages involving larger numbers of patients. Thus, regulatory guidelines have indicated that monitoring for ADA and Nab in particular may be necessary post approval as part of a pharmacovigilance surveillance [9]. The need to do this as a general practice is controversial. Postmarketing immunogenicity commitments should also be risk-based and should not necessarily apply to all approved biological therapeutics.

8.8   APPLICATION AND INTERPRETATION OF DATA

The FDA recommends "real-time" immunogenicity testing for clinical trials of drugs that are considered higher risk [6], since timely immunogenicity data may prove useful in determining whether to continue therapy or intervene, due to the impact of neutralizing antibodies on efficacy and patient safety. In general, for most biological compounds that are considered of low or medium risk, real-time immunogenicity testing is generally not employed.

To obtain the desired number of patients, many trials today are global in scope and, hence, operational delays can occur, resulting in the receipt of samples weeks after their collection. Samples are first analyzed in the screening and confirmatory assays before they are scheduled for Nab analysis. Thus, neutralizing antibody data are usually available some time after patients have produced such antibodies. Typically, other assessments of efficacy may point to neutralizing activity of ADA without having actual ADA and Nab data. It is important to note that both neutralizing and non-neutralizing antibodies can influence the pharmacokinetics of the product. Therefore, correlation of antibody characteristics (binding versus neutralizing) with clinical responses requires a comparison of data generated from antibody assays with results from pharmacokinetic assays as well as PD and other clinical end points. In some cases, it might be difficult to identify a sufficiently sensitive clinical end point to establish the impact on clinical outcome directly, and adoption of a surrogate measure of response may be the only option. *In vivo* comparison of patients' clinical responses to a product before, and following, antibody induction can provide information on the correlation between antibody development (and antibody characteristics) and clinical responses. This can be achieved either by intra-group analysis (response in patients before and after occurrence of antibodies), or by comparison with patients within the study who do not show an immune response. The most common approach for reporting the results from total binding assay analysis is as a titer value.

Depending upon the drug, Nab data may be used to manage risk, as has been recommended by the European Federation of Neurological Societies Task Force for Interferon-Beta [46]. It also is possible that Nab data could be used to make recommendations for dosing in patients with ADA to induce tolerance. In other cases, Nab data may be correlated with total ADA, PK, and biomarker end points to confirm observed *in vivo* effects, although the value of the additional Nab data may be disputed. Furthermore, Nab data may provide a "diagnostic tool" to explain an observed clinical event such as the pure red cell aplasia (PRCA) incidence with erythropoietin. In this case, the demonstration of neutralizing antibodies in patients who developed PRCA explained the cause of the observed clinical outcome. Additionally, patients on erythropoietin who are not responding to treatment are advised to be tested for neutralizing antibodies and have bone marrow biopsies. Treatment should be discontinued in patients who develop antibody-mediated PRCA [51]. With some low-risk drugs and some drugs that do not have endogenous counterparts, the need for a Nab assay may be questionable, and Nab data may not provide any additional information to evaluate the actual *in vivo* efficacy and safety of a therapeutic compared to that obtained with total ADA, PK, and biomarker data. The value of Nab data and how these data are used may vary on a case-by-case basis.

8.9 CONCLUSIONS

The consequences of an immune response to biological therapeutics are diverse, and often range from a transient appearance of antibodies without any clinical significance to severe adverse "anaphylactoid" or life-threatening reactions. Often antibodies that recognize epitopes on the protein that are not linked to activity have less clinical impact. However, these antibodies can influence pharmacokinetics and, as such, indirectly influence efficacy. Neutralizing antibodies interfere with biological activity by binding at, or in proximity to, the active site, or by induction of conformational changes, and can induce loss of clinical efficacy. Discrimination between neutralizing and non-neutralizing antibodies is a regulatory expectation and the assays used should be able to discriminate accordingly. However, it is important to note that both neutralizing and non-neutralizing antibodies can influence the pharmacokinetics of the product. Thus, it is critical to use appropriately validated assays and, based upon risk assessment strategies, to apply assays appropriately in the nonclinical and clinical settings. Correlation of antibody characteristics (binding versus neutralizing, if needed) with nonclinical/clinical responses requires a comparison of data generated from antibody assays with results from pharmacokinetic assays as well as tests designed to assess clinical responses.

The positive control is the sole basis for verifying whether the ADA assay developed is appropriate for its intended purpose, even though this control may not completely reflect the characteristics of the antibodies elicited *in vivo*. Thus, as a biological therapeutic moves through the clinical development process, it is important to periodically compare the specificity of this control to confirmed positive clinical samples and determine its relevancy to what was observed in the clinic. Pooling of clinical samples to improve or modify the positive-control preparation may be necessary to reflect these new ADA specificities. While this new control will require assay re-validation, the resulting positive control will lead to a more robust assay.

The decision on which type of method to use for the ADA screening/confirmation assays will depend upon the structure of the drug and conclusions from the risk assessment. The most common and first approach is to use an ELISA-based LBA method, which offers quick development times, high throughput, and low cost. However, more complex method platforms (possibly more sensitive) such as, ECL or SPR assays may need to be developed if the ELISA platform does not meet the program's needs. While not commonly used, RIPA methods can provide many of the positive attributes of the ELISA with increased sensitivity.

The development, use, and type of Nab assay employed will also be dependent on the nature of the drug and results from the risk assessment. While the CLB format is simpler to develop and less time-consuming to run, more often a cell-based bioassay is required due to the drug's mode of action. Depending on the biological output from the target cell, neutralization could be quantitated using an immunoassay, multiplex assay, flow cytometry, or gene expression profiling.

While the procedures and the parameters evaluated during the validation for each ADA method may be different, each of them must be able to distinguish a positive from a negative response in a complex milieu. Without appropriately validated anti-drug antibody assays, the relevance of ADA on safety and efficacy in the context of nonclinical and clinical studies cannot be determined.

APPENDIX 8.A   ILLUSTRATION OF SCREENING CUT POINT EVALUATION

Assay response data from 51 disease-matched subject samples in duplicate were available from six runs (two analysts, three runs each). A balanced experimental design (Table 8.A1) was used for this evaluation. Since a reportable result for a subject sample during the bioanalysis phase is the average of the response from duplicate samples, all analyses for these validation data were carried out on the average of the duplicate samples.

Appendix 8.A.1   Evaluation of Distribution and Outliers

The process outlined in Fig. 8.2 was used in the determination of the screening cut point. First, the distribution of the assay response data was assessed. Since the data were relatively more symmetric in the log scale than in the original scale, analyses

TABLE 8.A1   Balanced Experimental Design

Analyst	Assay Run	Assay Plate	S_1-S_{17}	$S_{18}-S_{34}$	$S_{35}-S_{51}$
			\multicolumn{3}{c}{Validation Serum Samples}		
A_1	R_1	P_1	X		
		P_2		X	
		P_3			X
	R_2	P_1		X	
		P_2			X
		P_3	X		
	R_3	P_1			X
		P_2	X		
		P_3		X	
A_2	R_4	P_1	X		
		P_2		X	
		P_3			X
	R_5	P_1		X	
		P_2			X
		P_3	X		
	R_6	P_1			X
		P_2	X		
		P_3		X	

This table illustrates an experimental design that is balanced for the key assay variables considered such as the analyst, assay run, plate testing order, and sample groups tested. In this scenario, each of the two analysts conducts three assay runs, testing 51 drug-naïve matrix samples in each run such that three groups of 17 samples are tested in each of three plates. Note that all samples are tested in each run and each sample group is tested in every plate testing order by each analyst. Such a balanced design ensures that the difference between the levels of a factor (say, between assay runs) is not confounded by the effect of another factor (say, sample groups), thus providing a more reliable assessment of key assay variables. The plate testing order here refers to the order in which the plates are tested within a run (assumed to be P_1, P_2, and P_3).

were carried out on the log-transformed data. Outliers were identified based on the studentized residuals from the mixed effects model on log transformed assay response data. The mixed effects model included analyst as fixed effect, and assay runs and samples as random effects. Samples with |studentized residuals| > 3 were considered as statistical outliers, and were therefore excluded from the cut point analysis. Three subject samples were identified as biological outliers, with results from all runs excluded from the cut point determination. In addition, results for two other samples were deleted as analytical outliers from assay run six. Therefore, the number of subject

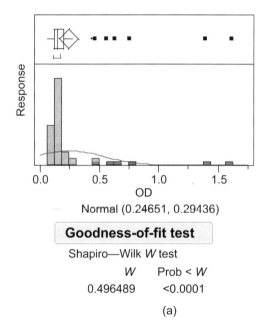

Normal (0.24651, 0.29436)

Goodness-of-fit test

Shapiro—Wilk W test

W	Prob < W
0.496489	<0.0001

(a)

FIGURE 8.A1 Distribution of the drug-naïve matrix sample results. Using JMP outlier box-plot, the distribution of the drug-naïve matrix sample results is plotted in both the original scale of the reported optical density results (panel a) and logarithmic scale (panel b). The ends of the box correspond to the 25th and 75th percentiles, also called the quartiles (Q1 and Q3). The difference between these quartiles is the interquartile range (IQR). The line across the middle of the box indicates the median. The center of the diamond indicates the sample mean, and its length corresponds to the 95% confidence interval. The dashed lines extend from both ends of the box to the outermost data point that falls within the distances computed as (Q3 + 1.5 × IQR) and (Q1 − 1.5 × IQR). The bracket along the edge of the box identifies the shortest half, which is the densest 50% of the observations. The normal density curve estimated using the data is displayed. Since the distribution of the original data is highly skewed to the right, logarithmic transformation is considered and the outliers are evaluated in this log-transformed scale. The outliers can be identified from either the box-plots of the reported results provided in this figure, or using the studentized residual plots from the ANOVA. The outlier box-plot individually lists the outlier points, as evident from these figures. Among these points, the smallest one was not identified as an outlier by the studentized residual plots.

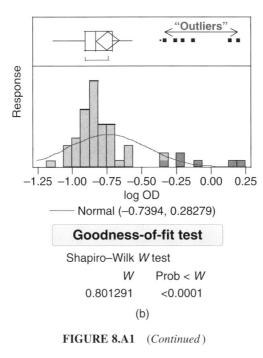

Normal (−0.7394, 0.28279)

Goodness-of-fit test

Shapiro–Wilk W test

W	Prob < W
0.801291	<0.0001

(b)

FIGURE 8.A1 *(Continued)*

samples that were used for all further analysis was 48, 48, 48, 48, 48, and 46, respectively, for the six runs. See Figs 8.A1 and 8.A2 for the distribution of the untransformed and log-transformed data with and without the outliers.

Appendix 8.A.2   Evaluation of Cut Point Based on the Validation Data

Since the distribution of the log-transformed data after removing these outliers satisfied the Shapiro–Wilk normality test (Fig. 8.A2b), the cut point determination for these validation data was made using the parametric method (i.e., mean $+ 1.645 \times$ SD). The threshold 1.645 for normally distributed data ensures 5% false-positive rate. This cut point of the log-transformed values of the sample replicate means was determined for each analyst, each assay run, and for all the data combined (Table 8.A2).

Appendix 8.A.3   Comparison of Mean and Variances Across Assay Runs and Selection of Appropriate Type of Screening Cut Point

The difference of the log assay response between the assay runs was assessed using a one-way analysis of variance (ANOVA) with assay runs as fixed effect (Fig. 8.A3). This analysis showed that the run means were not statistically significantly different

($p = 0.3068$). In addition, the variability across six assay runs using Levene's test was not significantly different ($p = 0.6565$). These results suggest that a fixed cut point can be used during the in-study (bioanalysis) phase. However, due to possible analytical variations during the in-study phase, a floating cut point approach was chosen as a safer alternative for this assay. The floating cut point during the bioanalysis phase is determined by adding or multiplying a correction factor determined from these validation data to the average of the negative control samples from each plate/run. Therefore, the final step in this screening cut point evaluation is to determine this correction factor.

Appendix 8.A.4   Determination of Correction Factor for Screening Cut Point Evaluation

Because the distribution of the log-transformed data is relatively less skewed than the untransformed data as described previously, the cut point correction factor should be additive in the log scale, and thus multiplicative in the original scale. The additive

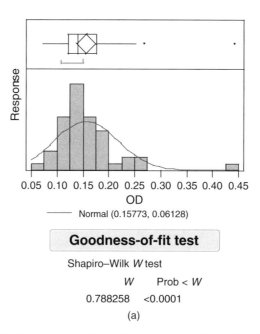

FIGURE 8.A2   Distribution of the drug-naïve matrix sample results without the outliers. These data are similar to Fig. 8.A1a and b, without the outliers. After excluding the outliers identified from the box-plot approach, data in the logarithmic scale (panel b) is closer to a normal distribution and is confirmed by the Shapiro–Wilk test for normality. The p-value of 0.1316 suggests that the distribution of the log-transformed data is not significantly non-normal.

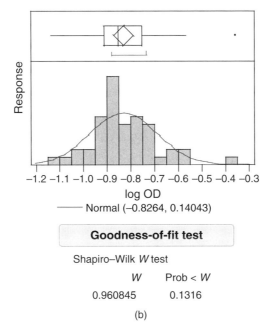

Normal (−0.8264, 0.14043)

Goodness-of-fit test

Shapiro–Wilk *W* test

W	Prob < *W*
0.960845	0.1316

(b)

FIGURE 8.A2   (*Continued*)

TABLE 8.A2   Illustration of the Screening Cut Point Calculation

(a)

Assay Number	Analyst	Log$_{10}$-Transformed Estimates			Sample Absorbance Cut Point
		Biweight Mean	Biweight SD	Sample Cut Point	
1	A	−0.892	0.222	−0.527	0.297
2	A	−1.098	0.210	−0.753	0.177
3	A	−1.082	0.202	−0.750	0.178
4	B	−1.154	0.200	−0.824	0.150
5	B	−1.151	0.173	−0.866	0.136
6	B	−1.064	0.204	−0.730	0.186
Pooled intra-assay	A	−1.024	0.212	−0.676	0.211
	B	−1.124	0.193	−0.807	0.156
	Combined	−1.074	0.202	−0.741	0.182
Interassay	Combined	−1.076	0.219	−0.716	0.192

(*continued*)

TABLE 8.A2 (*Continued*)

(b)

Assay Number	Analyst	Log$_{10}$-Transformed Estimates			Absorbance Multiplicative Normalization Factor
		Negative Control Mean	Sample Cut Point	Additive Normalization Factor	
1	A	−1.1531	−0.5266	0.6255	4.231
2	A	−1.2924	−0.7528	0.5396	3.464
3	A	−1.2697	−0.7503	0.5194	3.306
4	B	−1.2234	−0.8242	0.3992	2.507
5	B	−1.1807	−0.8661	0.3146	2.064
6	B	−1.1612	−0.7296	0.4316	2.701
Pooled intra-assay	A	−1.2384	−0.6763	0.5621	3.648
	B	−1.1884	−0.8069	0.3815	2.407
	Combined	−1.2134	−0.7408	0.4726	2.969

Table 8.A2a and b provides an illustration of the screening cut point calculation based on log transformed data values during the validation phase where each of two analysts test drug-naïve matrix samples in three runs each (total of six assay runs). Fifty-one samples were assayed for the cut point determinations in Table 8.A2. Three samples were identified as biological outliers, with results from all runs excluded from the cut point determination. In addition, results for two other samples were deleted as analytical outliers from assay run 6. Therefore, the number of samples was 48, 48, 48, 48, 48, and 46, respectively, for the six runs. This differing sample size across runs was taken into consideration when calculating the pooled cut points. Log transformation ensured approximate normality of the data. The assay run means were not significantly different, and the variances were fairly similar. While a fixed cut point is justified, a floating cut point was preferred as a safer choice for this assay because of possible analytical variations during the in-study (bioanalysis) phase. The calculations described in Appendix 8.A are summarized in Table 8.A2a. The calculation of normalization (correction) factor to be used for floating cut point in the bioanalysis phase is illustrated in Table 8.A2b. Note that because the cut point calculation is performed on the log-transformed data, the normalization factor is additive in the log scale, and multiplicative in the untransformed scale. During the in-study (bioanalysis) phase, one would multiply the mean of the negative control mean from each run by the multiplicative factor from Table 8.A2b to derive the floating cut point for that run. Given the differences between the multiplicative factors from each analyst, it may be preferable to use the analyst specific multiplicative factor, and hence the analyst-specific floating cut point in this scenario.

correction factor in the log scale was first determined by calculating the mean assay response (in log scale) of the negative control samples and then subtracting this result from the cut point (in log scale) determined for the validation samples using the parametric method as described above. This was carried out for each analyst and each assay run, and for all the data combined. The multiplicative correction factors in the original scale were then determined by taking the antilog of these additive correction factors in the log scale. See Table 8.A2a and b for a summary of these results. Given the

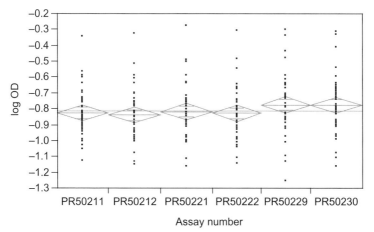

Analysis of variance

Source	DF	Sum of squares	Mean square	F ratio	Prob > F
Assay number	5	0.1678996	0.033580	1.2058	0.3068
Error	256	7.1292630	0.027849		
C. total	261	7.2971626			

Tests that the variances are equal

Test	F ratio	DFNum	DFDen	Prob > F
O'Brien[.5]	0.5465	5	256	0.7409
Brown–Forsythe	0.6740	5	256	0.6435
Levene	0.6569	5	256	0.6565
Bartlett	0.9101	5	.	0.4732

FIGURE 8.A3   Comparison of assay run means and variances. This illustrates the comparison of optical density readings in log scale (represented by log OD in the vertical axis) between six assay runs. Each point represents the result from a drug-naïve matrix sample. The vertical span of the diamonds represents the 95% confidence interval for the corresponding run mean. The horizontal lines near the top and bottom of the diamonds are useful for pair wise comparisons of the assay runs. As evident from this figure, and as confirmed by the ANOVA F-test, the assay run means are not statistically significantly different ($p = 0.3068$). Also, the Levene's test for the equality of variances among assay runs indicated that the variances are not significantly different ($p = 0.6565$). This justifies the use of a fixed cut point for the in-study phase, or the use of a floating cut point if preferred.

differences between the multiplicative factors from each analyst (3.648 and 2.407), it may be preferable to use the analyst-specific multiplicative factor, and hence the analyst-specific floating cut point in this scenario. However, since other analysts were expected to be involved during the in-study phase, a combined multiplicative correction factor (2.969) and thus a common floating cut point was preferred for the in-study phase.

Appendix 8.A.5 Evaluation of Screening Cut Point During the In-Study Phase

The floating cut point for each plate/run in the bioanalysis phase will thus be determined by multiplying this common multiplicative correction factor, 2.969, to the average of the negative control results from each plate/run in the bioanalysis phase. Similarly, the screening cut points for sensitivity and other experiments performed during the validation of this assay was determined using this same method (multiplying 2.969 to the negative control average from each plate/run).

REFERENCES

1. Baert, F., Noman, M., Vermiere, S., Assche, G.V., D'Haens, G., Carbonez, A., and Rutgeerts, P. (2003) Influence of immunogenicity on the long-term efficacy of infliximab in Crohn's disease. *New England Journal of Medicine*, **348**, 601–608.

2. Koren, E., Zuckerman, L.A., and Mire-Sluis, A.R. (2002) Immune responses to therapeutic proteins in humans: clinical significance, assessment and prediction. *Current Pharmaceutical Biotechnology*, **3**, 349–360.

3. Shankar, G., Pendley, C., and Stein, K.E. (2007) A risk-based bioanalytical strategy for the assessment of antibody immune responses against biological drugs. *Nature Biotechnology*, **25**, 555–561.

4. Giovannoni, G., Munschauer, F.E., and Deisenhammer, F. (2002) Neutralizing antibodies to interferon beta during the treatment of multiple sclerosis. *Journal of Neurology, Neurosurgery, and Psychiatry*, **73**, 465–469.

5. Casadevall, N., Nataf, J., Viron, B., Kolta, A., Kiladjian, J.J., Martin-Dupont, P., Michaud, P., Papo, T., Ugo, V., Teyssandier, I., Varet, B., and Mayeux, P. (2002) Pure red cell aplasia and anti-erythropoietin antibodies against human erythropoietin in patients treated with recombinant erythropoietin. *New England Journal of Medicine*, **346**, 469–475.

6. Worobec, A., and Rosenberg, A.S. (2004) A risk-based approach to immunogenicity concerns of therapeutic protein products. Part 1. Considering consequences of the immune response to a protein. *Biopharm International*, **17**, 22–26.

7. Rosenberg, A.S., and Worobec, A. (2004) A risk-based approach to immunogenicity concerns of therapeutic protein products. Part 2. Considering host-specific and product specific factors impacting immunogenicity. *Biopharm International*, **17**, 34–42.

8. Rosenberg, A.S., and Worobec, A. (2005) A risk-based approach to immunogenicity concerns of therapeutic protein products. Part 3. Effects of manufacturing changes in immunogenicity and the utility of animal immunogenicity studies. *Biopharm International*, **18**, 32–36.

9. Guideline on Immunogenicity Assessment of Biotechnology-Derived Therapeutic Proteins. Committee for Medicinal Products for Human Use (CHMP). Adopted 13 December 2007. Available at http://www.emea.europa.eu/pdfs/human/biosimilar/1432706enfin.pdf.

10. Thorpe, R., and Swanson, S.J. (2005) Assays for detecting and diagnosing antibody-mediated pure red cell aplasia (PRCA): an assessment of available procedures. *Nephrology Dialysis Transplantation*, **20**, (Suppl. 4), iv16–iv22.

11. Guidance for Industry. S6 Preclinical Safety Evaluation of Biotechnology-Derived Pharmaceuticals. International Conference on Harmonization (ICH). July 1997. Available at http://www.ich.org.

12. Guideline on Comparability of Medicinal Products Containing Biotechnology-Derived Proteins as Active Substance: Non-Clinical and Clinical Issues. Committee for Medicinal Products for Human Use (CHMP). June 1, 2006. Available at http://www.emea.europa.eu/pdfs/human/biosimilar/4283205en.pdf.

13. Guideline on the Clinical Investigation of the Pharmacokinetics of Therapeutic Proteins. Committee for Medicinal Products for Human Use (CHMP). July 31, 2007. Available at http://www.emea.europa.eu/pdfs/human/ewp/8924904enfin.pdf.

14. Mire-Sluis, A.R., Barrett, Y.C., Devanarayan, V., Koren, E., Liu, H., Maia, M., Parish, T., Scott, G., Shankar, G., Shores, E., Swanson, S.J., Taniguchi, G., Wierda, D., and Zuckerman, L.A. (2004) Recommendations for the design and optimization of immunoassays used in the detection of host antibodies against biotechnology products. *Journal of Immunological Methods*, **289**, 1–16.

15. Gupta, S., Indelicato, S.R., Jethwa, V., Kawabata, T., Kelley, M., Mire-Sluis, A.R., Richards, S.M., Rup, B., Shores, E., Swanson, S.J., and Wakshull, E. (2007) Recommendations for the design, optimization, and qualification of cell-based assays used for the detection of neutralizing antibody responses elicited to biological therapeutics. *Journal of Immunological Methods*, **321**, 1–18.

16. Koren, E., Smith, H.W., Shores, E., Shankar, G., Finco-Kent, D., Rup, B., Barett, Y.C., Devanarayan, V., Gorovits, B., Gupta, S., Parish, T., Quarmby, V., Moxness, M., Swanson, S.J., Taniguchi, G., Zuckerman, L.S., Stebbins, C.C., and Mire-Sluis, A. (2008) Recommendations on risk-based strategies for detection and characterization of antibodies against biotechnology products. *Journal of Immunological Methods*, **333**, 1–9.

17. Swanson, S.J., Ferbas, J., Mayeux, P., and Casadevall, N. (2004) Evaluation of methods to detect and characterize antibodies against recombinant human erythropoietin. *Nephron Clinical Practice*, **96**, c88–c95.

18. Brickelmaier, M., Hochman, P.S., Baciu, R., Chao, B., Cuervo, J.H., and Whitty, A. (1999) ELISA methods for the analysis of antibody responses induced in multiple sclerosis patients treated with recombinant interferon-beta. *Journal of Immunological Methods*, **227**, 121–135.

19. Lofgren, J.A., Dhandapani, S., Pennucci, J.J., Abbott, C.M., Mytych, D.T., Kaliyaperumal, A., Swanson, S.J., and Mullenix, M.C. (2007) Comparing ELISA and surface plasmon resonance for assessing clinical immunogenicity of panitumumab. *Journal of Immunology*, **178**, 7467–7472.

20. Bartelds, G.M., Wijbrandts, C.A., Nurmohamed, M.T., Stapel, S., Lems, W.F., Aarden, L., Dijkmans, B.A.C., Tak, P.P., and Wolbink, G.J. (2007) Clinical response to adalimumab: relationship to anti-adalimumab antibodies and serum adalimumab concentrations in rheumatoid arthritis. *Annals of the Rheumatic Diseases*, **66**, 921–926.

21. Tacey, R., Greway, A., Smiell, J., Power, D., Kromminga, A., Daha, M., Casadevall, N., and Kelley, M. (2003) The detection of anti-erythropoietin antibodies in human serum and plasma. Part I. validation of the protocol for a radioimmunoprecipitation assay. *Journal of Immunological Methods*, **283**, 317–329.

22. Rini, B., Wadhwa, M., Bird, C., Small, E., Gaines-Das, R., and Thorpe, R. (2005) Kinetics of development and characteristics of antibodies induced in cancer patients against yeast expressed rDNA derived GM-CSF. *Cytokine*, **29**, 56–66.

23. Baltrukonis, D., Finco-Kent, D., Kawabata, T., Poirier, M., and LeSauteur, L., (2006) Development and validation of a quasi-quantitative bioassay for neutralizing antibodies against CP-870893. *Journal of Immunotoxicology*, **3**, 157–164.

24. Wagner, C.L., Schantz, A., Barnathan, E., Olson, A., Mascelli, M.A., Ford, J., Damaraju, L., Schaible, T., Maini, R.N., and Tcheng, J.E. (2003) Consequences of immunogenicity to the therapeutic monoclonal antibodies ReoPro and Remicade. *Development in Biologicals*, **112**, 37–53.

25. Caras, I. (2007) Evaluation of immunogenicity for pre-clinical and clinical investigations. In: Lyscom (ed.), *Immunogenicity to Biologics*, Biopharm Knowledge Publishing, UK, pp. 81–95.

26. Crowther, J.R. (2001) *The ELISA Guidebook. Volume 149. Methods in Molecular Biology*, Humana Press, Inc., Totowa, NJ.

27. Law, B. (1996) *Immunoassay: A Practical Guide*, Taylor and Francis, Inc., Bristol, PA.

28. Wei, X., Swanson, S.J., and Gupta, S. (2004) Development and validation of a cell-based bioassay for the detection of neutralizing antibodies against recombinant human erythropoietin in clinical studies. *Journal of Immunological Methods*, **293**, 115–126.

29. Bertolotto, A. (2004) Neutralizing antibodies to interferon beta: implications for the management of multiple sclerosis. *Current Opinion in Neurology*, **17**, 241–246.

30. Yu, Y., Piddington, C., Fitzpatrick, D., Twomey, B., Xu, R., Swanson, S.J., and Jing, S. (2006) A novel method for detecting neutralizing antibodies against therapeutic proteins by measuring gene expression. *Journal of Immunological Methods*, **316**, 8–17.

31. Indelicato, S.R., Bradshaw, S.L., Chapman, J.W., and Weiner, S.H. (2005) Evaluation of standard and state of the art analytical technology-bioassays. *Development in Biologicals*, **122**, 103–114.

32. Bertolotto, A., Sala, A., Caldano, M., Capobianco, M., Malucchi, S., Marnetto, F., and Gilli, F. (2007) Development and validation of a real time PCR-based bioassay for quantification of neutralizing antibodies against human interferon beta. *Journal of Immunological Methods*, **321**, 19–31.

33. Geng, D., Shankar, G., Schantz, A., Rajadhyaksha, M., Davis, H., and Wagner, C. (2005) Validation of immunoassays used to assess immunogenicity to therapeutic monoclonal antibodies. *Journal of Pharmaceutical and Biomedical Analysis*, **39**, 364–375.

34. Shankar, G., Devanarayan, V., Barrett, Y.C., Bowsher, R., Finco-Kent, D., Fiscella, M., Gorovits, B., Kirschner, S., Moxness, M., Parish, T., Quarmby, V., Shores, E., Smith, H., Smith, W., Zhong, J., Zuckerman, L., and Koren, E. (2008) Recommendations for the validation of immunoassays used for detection of host antibodies against biotechnology products. *Journal of Pharmaceutical and Biomedical Analysis*, **48**, 1267–1281.

35. DeSilva, B., Smith, W., Weiner, R., Kelley, M., Smolec, J., Lee, B., Khan, M., Tacey, R., Hill, H., and Celiniker, A. (2003) Recommendations for the bioanalytical method validation of ligand-binding assays to support pharmacokinetic assessments of macromolecules. *Pharmaceutical Research*, **20**, 1885–1900.

36. Viswanathan, C.T., Bansal, S., Booth, B., DeStefano, A.J., Rose, M.J., Sailstad, J., Shah, V. P., Skelly, J.P., Swann, P.G., and Weiner, R. (2007) Quantitative bioanalytical methods validation and implementation: best practices for chromatographic and ligand binding assays. *Pharmaceutical Research*, **24**, 1962–1973.

37. Validation of Analytical Procedures: Text and Methodology Q2(R1). International Conference on Harmonization of Technical Requirements for Registration of Pharmaceuticals for Human Use (ICH). 2005. Available at http://www.ich.org.

38. Patton, A., Mullenix, M.C., Swanson, S.J., and Koren, E. (2005) An acid dissociation bridging ELISA for detection of antibodies directed against therapeutic proteins in the presence of antigen. *Journal of Immunological Methods*, **304**, 189–195.

39. Kitamura, T., Tange, T., Terasawa, T., Chiba, S., Kuwaki, T., Miyagawa, K., Piao, Y.F., Miyazono, K., Urabe, A., and Takaku, F. (1989) Establishment and characterization of a unique human cell line that proliferates dependently on GM-CSF, IL-3, or erythropoietin. *Journal of Cellular Physiology*, **140**, 323–334.

40. Wadhwa, M., Bird, C., Fagerberg, J., Gaines-Das, R., Ragnhammar, P., Mellstedt, H., and Thorpe, R. (1996) Production of neutralizing GM-CSF antibodies in carcinoma patients following GM-CSF combination therapy. *Clinical and Experimental Immunology*, **104**, 351–358.

41. Kelley, M., Cooper, C., Matticoli, A., and Greway, A. (2005) The detection of anti-erythropoietin antibodies in human serum and plasma. Part II. Validation of a semi-quantitative 3*H*-thymidine uptake assay for neutralizing antibodies. *Journal of Immunological Methods*, **300**, 179–191.

42. Iwaoka, M., Obata, J., Abe, M., Nakamura, T., Kitta, Y., Kodama, Y., Kawabata, K., Takano, H., Fujioka, D., Saito, Y., Koybashi, T., Hassebe, H., and Kugiyama, K. (2007) Association of low serum levels of apolipoprotein A-I with adverse outcomes in patients with nonischemic heart failure. *Journal of Cardiac Failure*, **13**, 247–253.

43. Nissen, S.E., Tsunoda, T., Tuzcu, E.M., Schoenhagen, P., Cooper, C.J., Yasin, M., Eaton, G.M., Lauer, M.A., Sheldon, W.S., Grines, C.L., Halpern, S., Crowe, T., Blankenship, J.C., and Kerensky, R. (2003) Effect of recombinant ApoA-I Milano on coronary atherosclerosis in patients with acute coronary syndromes. A randomized controlled trial. *The Journal of the American medical Association*, **290**, 2292–2300.

44. Dullens, S., Plat, J., and Mensink, R. (2007) Increasing apoA-I production as a target for CHD risk reduction. *Nutrition, Metabolism and Cardiovascular Diseases*, **17**, 616–628.

45. Menetrier-Caux, C., Briere, F., Jouvenne, P., Peyron, E., Peyron, F., and Banchereau, J. (1996) Identification of human IgG autoantibodies specific for IL-10. *Clinical and Experimental Immunology*, **104**, 173–179.

46. Sorensen, P.S., Deisenhammer, F., Duda, R., Hohlfeld, R., Myhr, K.M., Palace, J., Polman, C., Pozzilli, C., and Ross, C.for the EFNS Task Force on Anti IFN-Beta Antibodies in Multiple Sclerosis (2005) Guidelines on use of anti-IFN-beta antibody measurements in multiple sclerosis: report of an EFNS Task Force on IFN-Beta Antibodies in Multiple Sclerosis. *European Journal of Neurology*, **12**, 817–827.

47. Goodin, D.S., Frohman, B., Hurwitz, P.W., O'Connor, W.O., Oger, J.J., Reder, A.T., and Stevens, J.C. (2007) Neutralizing antibodies to interferon beta: assessment of their clinical and radiographic impact: an evidence report of the Therapeutics and Technology Assessment Subcommittee of the American Academy of Neurology. *Neurology*, **68**, 977–984.

48. Bender, N., Helig, C., Droll, B., Wohlgemuth, J., Armbruster, F.P., and Helig, B. (2007) Immunogenicity, efficacy and adverse events of adalimumab in RA patients. *Rheumatology International*, **27**, 269–274.

49. Package Insert. HUMIRA (adalimumab). Abbott Laboratories. Available at http://www.fda.gov/Cder/foi/label/2002/adalabb123102LB.htm#clin.

50. Richards, S. (2002) Immunological considerations for enzyme replacement therapy in the treatment of lysosomal storage disorders. *Clinical and Applied Immunology Reviews*, **2**, 241–253.

51. Schellekens, H. (2002) Immunogenicity of therapeutic proteins: clinical implications and future prospects. *Clinical Therapeutics*, **24**, 1720–1739.

52. Parish, T., and Wilmalasena, R. (2005) Practical considerations in developing assays for immunogenicity testing of biotechnology products. *American Pharmaceutical Outsourcing*, **6**, 14–19.

████████ **CHAPTER 9**

Macromolecular Reference Standards for Biotherapeutic Pharmacokinetic Analysis[*]

MARIE T. ROCK

Midwest BioResearch, Skokie, IL, USA

STEPHEN KELLER

Facet Biotech, Redwood City, CA, USA

9.1 INTRODUCTION

9.1.1 Biopharmaceuticals and Biologics

Biopharmaceuticals (or "biotherapeutics") are generally produced through the application of recombinant DNA technology, where genetic manipulation of cells is required. The pharmaceutical agents produced this way are often either humanized monoclonal antibodies directed at targets involved in disease processes, or recombinant endogenous molecules used in replacement therapy. The intersection of monoclonal antibody and recombinant DNA technologies has resulted in a variety of novel therapies ranging from A to Z (Avastin® to Zenapax®), treating a broad spectrum of human diseases. The same is true of recombinant replacement therapeutics, with molecules like erythropoietin, insulin, and many others now serving unmet medical needs.

Biologics may be considered a class of therapeutics directly purified from an original biological source. This category would include blood products, vaccines, and some hormones. Insulin, a peptide hormone (51 amino acids), is an example of a biologic that has been commercially available since about 1923 [1]. With the advent of

[*]This chapter is dedicated to Dr. Michael Hirsch, the invisible, unsung hero of so many, many immunoassays that he developed for all of us as his clients. His ready wit, sensibility, creativity, infectious enthusiasm, and pure love of life are sorely missed. The immunoassay world is simply not the same without him.

Ligand-Binding Assays: Development, Validation, and Implementation in the Drug Development Arena. Edited by Masood N. Khan and John W.A. Findlay
Copyright © 2010 John Wiley & Sons, Inc.

recombinant DNA technology, insulin can now also be provided as a biotherapeutic. Insulin has a very interesting history [2], with multiple Nobel laureates associated with its discovery and innovations around its use. The Nobel Prize Committee in 1923 credited the practical extraction and discovery of insulin to a team at the University of Toronto, and awarded the Nobel Prize in Physiology/Medicine to Frederick Banting and J.J.R. Macleod. The patent for insulin was sold to the University of Toronto for one dollar. In the early 1930s, Eli Lilly made a breakthrough in the purification process that enabled the widespread sale of insulin for the treatment of diabetes. Of particular interest to the bioanalytical scientist, in 1977 the Nobel Committee recognized the innovative development of a radioimmunoassay for insulin by Rosalyn Yallow and Solomon Berson. This breakthrough opened up the cascade of immuno-based assays that continue to charm, beguile, and puzzle bioanalytical scientists as the analytical mainstay of protein bioanalysis.

Biopharmaceuticals and biologics, often grouped together as "macromolecular therapies," or just "macromolecules," differ in many ways from small-molecule drugs. The differences between these two general classes of therapeutics are summarized in Table 9.1. It is the very nature of these differences that necessitates different methods of bioanalysis as well as a dedicated look at both types of molecules as reference standards.

9.1.2 The Challenge

The quantitative analysis of macromolecules, particularly as applied to characterization of pharmacokinetics (PK), presents a broad scope of challenges. First and foremost, methods must be calibrated using an appropriate reference standard. A reference standard is generally defined as a drug substance, drug product, or biologic product that is well established and characterized for use as a calibrator or control for quantitative and qualitative analysis. Calibrators (or "standards") are dilutions of the reference standard, which when analyzed in a bioanalytical PK method are used to generate a standard curve (or "calibration curve") for interpolating unknown sample concentration values. The analytical procedure used to quantify macromolecules is generally an immunoassay that depends upon the affinity and specificity of the antibody reagents used. The antibody reagents are exquisitely sensitive to the conformational structure of the macromolecule being measured, and small changes

TABLE 9.1 Differences Between Small-Molecule and Macromolecule Therapeutics

Characteristics	Small Molecules	Macromolecules
Size	<1000 Da	>5000 Da
Synthesis	Chemically produced	Biologically produced
Structure	Small organic crystalline	Large complex tertiary/quaternary
Purity	Can be determined, nearly homogenous	Difficult to establish, can be heterogeneous
Impurities	Chemically characterized	Difficult to detect, process/host derived
Solubility	Varies	Usually hydrophilic
Instability	Chemical	Chemical, physical, and biological

in the three-dimensional configuration can have a profound impact on antibody binding, and therefore accurate quantitation. In fact, even subtle changes in the three-dimensional structure of the reference standard can alter standard curve characteristics, shift apparent assay sensitivity, and introduce assay bias. The affinity of antibody reagents for standards used during early-stage development (sometimes referred to as "development reference standards") versus reference standards produced at later development stages can differ, as transitions from small- to large-scale production occurs during the natural course of drug development. These changes are often related to the presence of higher levels of chemically or enzymatically degraded drug substance in large-scale batches that can lead to unexpected alterations of the standard curve. Furthermore, the matrix used to formulate the immunoassay calibrators can influence accuracy of methods since there may be unanticipated binding of matrix components to the drug, altering binding of immunoreagents and thus analytical recovery. These effects may be significant, as is often the case with calibrators prepared in biological matrices, or relatively less significant as when formulation changes introduce miniscule amounts of altered protein and thus influence binding characteristics of the standard.

The ideal PK immunoassay standard curve, which is nonlinear and heteroscedastic, is derived from solutions of well-characterized macromolecules added to a relatively nonreactive sample matrix. However, rarely does one encounter an ideal situation when describing bioanalytical methodology, thus developing and validating analytical methods for macromolecules, and analyzing samples from preclinical or clinical trials must include an evaluation of these variables and possibly many others. Careful consideration must be given to the topics described in this chapter to achieve the goal of accurate and reproducible quantification of biotherapeutics necessary for pharmacokinetic analysis.

One intent of this chapter is to describe the role of the United States Pharmacopeia (USP) in the generation and use of small-molecule reference standards to provide some historical and scientific context, and then discuss the features of non-USP macromolecular reference standards and the specific challenges related to their generation and use in ligand-binding assays (LBAs), including such topics as purity, stability, concentration determination, and interaction of reference standards with various matrices. These points are illustrated practically by the use of case studies that demonstrate the importance of a thorough understanding of these challenges, and thoughtful experimental design to avoid incorrect interpretation of experimental data.

A pure, stable, and well-characterized reference standard is a vital component of a validated PK assay. When accompanied by appropriate sample collection and storage procedures, such a validated assay is the only means to accurate quantitation of protein therapeutics in biological samples.

9.2 UNITED STATES PHARMACOPEIA

9.2.1 Mission

Founded in 1820, the United States Pharmacopeia is the official public standards-setting authority for all prescription and over-the-counter medicines, dietary supplements, and other health care products manufactured and sold in the United States [3]. Among other duties, the USP is tasked to standardize formulation of pharmaceutical agents. To accomplish this, the USP compiles and distributes reference standards or specifications for the drug(s) and information used to maintain and improve health care delivery. The Federal Food, Drug and Cosmetic Act of 1938 states that the quality principles established by the USP and National Formulary (NF) are enforceable by the FDA.

9.2.2 Organization and Process

The development of new reference standards for biologics and biotechnology is managed by the Division of Complex Activities Expert Committees. The process is predicated on establishing an initial set of expectations for testing and performance of the compound/protein. The "chapters" in the USP state what is expected with regard to purity, stability, and potency. Later in the development, an actual reference standard is provided and made available for use. This part of the process often takes several years to complete all the testing required.

To begin, members of industry or other interested groups collaborate with a USP scientific staff expert to draft a document (chapter in USP or monograph) to be published in the USP or NF. The USP Expert Committee reviews and approves the monograph or chapter for publication in the USP Pharamcopeial Forum (PF) as a proposal. After review and edit by the USP scientific staff liaison, the document is published in PF for public review. Public comments are received and processed by the liaison and forwarded to the Expert Committee. The Expert Committee provides review and submits a response to the liaison. If there are significant changes required, the revised document is republished in the PF for another round of review. If there are no additional revisions, the proposal is approved by the USP and the monograph or general chapter becomes accepted in the USP-NF.

Biologically derived therapies are more complex and developing standards of performance or providing reference standard proteins is much more involved than for chemically synthesized drugs. As a result, the process is more elaborate and less well defined. The Expert Committees involved for biologics include those for blood and blood products, vaccines and virology, cell and gene therapy; for genetically produced biotherapeutics; and for proteins, nucleic acids, and polysaccharides. Their mission is to write standards of performance and to identify and develop analytical reference standards to be used in testing of such biotherapeutics. The document describes the expectations for purity, quality, and strength/potency of the active ingredient. In addition, there are expectations outlined for identity testing, excipients, major impurities, and degradation products. The USP reference standards are used as a comparator during the analysis of the test article. The challenges in meeting the expectations for purity and activity are related to the complexity of the methods used and the inherent variability due to the biological source of the test article and some of the reagents used in the testing procedures.

The development and use of procedural reference standards can be helpful in managing the test variability. The procedural reference standards are provided as nonproduct-specific standards to qualify and validate the analytical methods and instruments used for the analysis of the product. Molecular weight markers used in electrophoresis, mixtures of amino acids for amino acid analysis of proteins and peptides, and cocktails of monosaccharides for glycoprotein analysis are examples of the more easily obtainable standard preparations. As one might imagine, given the complexities of producing and characterizing this class of therapeutic, developing a "standard" is a daunting challenge [4]. This is the task of the manufacturer, although the USP does assist with the process, and it needs to be completed prior to patent expiration, as described below.

9.2.3 Collaborative Testing

Once the drug is off patent, the USP becomes involved in collaboration with industry to produce the reference standard. The process used by the USP to develop and certify reference standards has been published [5]. To briefly summarize, the process begins with a collaboration of two departments within the USP, the Department of Standards Development and the Department of Monograph and Reference Standard Development, and the associated Expert Committees. The Department of Standards Development is responsible for the content of the USP-NF, which includes all the monographs and general chapters. If the Expert Committees decide a monograph or general chapter is required to demonstrate compliance, the next phase of the process occurs. The Department of Standards Development works with the Department of Monograph and Reference Standard Development scientists to provide the testing and characterization protocols that generally include testing to assess identification, purity, and content/ potency, for the drug application and stability.

Collaborative laboratory testing is essential, and may involve quite a few laboratories to assure reference standards are well characterized and fully suited for the purpose. Scientists from the Department of Monograph and Reference Standard Development oversee the testing process, review the data, and prepare the summary. Upon review by the Department of Standards Development and Expert Committees, the document is reviewed for approval by the USP Reference Standards Committee. The USP Reference Standards Committee must provide unanimous approval for acceptance; otherwise the process goes through another round of modification(s) until it can be adopted as an official reference standard. The process can take several years, and the complex nature of biomolecules presents a tough task for the National Institute of Standards and Technology (NIST) and for those intending to provide generically produced macromolecular drugs.

9.2.4 Generics (Biosimilars)

Prior to 1984, generic drug manufactures in the small-molecule sector were required to run clinical trials to demonstrate safety and efficacy. In 1984 when Congress enacted the Hatch–Waxman Act, two routes became available for the approval of generics, allowing the generic manufactures to rely on results from the original new drug applications. This seems a logical evolutionary step in generic drug development given the fact that small-molecule drugs are characterized by specific well-defined molecular structures and are produced using standardized synthetic chemistries. Following that logic, it is reasonable to rely heavily on analytical characterization data for an innovator small-molecule drug to demonstrate equivalence to a generic follow-on product, and allow relaxed requirements for additional nonclinical and clinical in-life studies [6].

However, at that time, the biotechnology industry was in its infancy, with Humulin (recombinant insulin) as the only approved recombinant protein available. It was recognized that the situation was quite different for macromolecular biotherapeutics that involve biologically based processes using living cells in difficult-to-control growth conditions and purification processes that were less easily standardized [7]. The difficulties for the originator to provide a true "reference standard" for use in the development of generic forms of the drug have been described [6,7]. Perhaps even more challenging is the task of the generic, or "follow-on," manufacturer in demonstrating bioequivalence to successfully get a generic (or biosimilar) form of the drug approved. In addition to classical demonstration of bioequivalence, further testing is necessary to assure the safety of the follow-on product. One major concern found in generic forms of macromolecules not shared with small molecules is the risk of altered immunogenicity of the generic compared to the original drug. Unwanted immunogenicity of biomolecules is most commonly a result of epitopes that are seen as foreign to their host. In addition to the unintended introduction of *de novo* epitopes arising from changes in the tertiary and quaternary structure of a follow-on biotherapeutic, immunogenicity can arise from small amounts of degraded or otherwise chemically or physically altered forms of the drug. These anomalous alterations are not easy to detect. In fact, small changes in the biotech manufacturing process can have profound consequences on the end product, yielding minute quantities of antigenic impurities that can go unnoticed in standard analytical characterization that may, unfortunately, result in occasional serious clinical sequelae [8]. The potential for an unwanted immune response to biotherapeutics, whether original products or follow-on generic/biosimilars, has driven regulatory agencies to require immunogenicity testing as part of any new license application [9,10]. This additional testing requires longer term clinical testing, involving repeat dosing and postdosing follow-up to facilitate drug "wash out," allowing optimized detection of anti-drug antibodies. Naturally, this will require a suite of complex, sensitive, and specific bioanalytical methods to be developed and validated to detect and evaluate any anti-drug antibody development. Since the development and characterization of these methods rely on highly specialized reagents that are not commercially available, are subject to constantly evolving industry standards and regulatory expectations for method performance (e.g., sensitivity), and will certainly vary significantly from company to company, the idea of conclusively demonstrating equivalence with respect to immunogenicity is simply impossible.

This additional equivalence testing requires significant resources and may limit the cost savings realized with macromolecular biosimilars/generics in comparison to those associated with the small-molecule generic drug industry. The economic advantage of small-molecule generics compared to the cost of obtaining approval to market follow-on biotechnology drugs is currently a hotly debated topic [6,7,11].

Whether discussing the equivalence, pharmacoeconomics, or the nonclinical/clinical development path for follow-on biotherapeutics, the importance of obtaining a well-characterized reference standard is crucial.

9.3 CHARACTERIZATION OF NON-USP REFERENCE STANDARDS

When discussing macromolecular reference standards in the context of pharmacokinetic analysis, one is typically referring to non-USP material derived at biopharmaceutical companies and used during the preapproval phase of drug development. There are a number of challenges with producing, characterizing, and using these reference standards. This section focuses on the proper characterization of reference standards. It is no exaggeration to state that without proper characterization of reference standards, particularly the assessment of purity, potency, concentration, and stability, accurate calibration of PK methods is not possible.

9.3.1 Purity

The FDA Code of Federal Regulations (21CFR Part 600.3) defines purity as it applies to reference standards as the relative freedom from extraneous matter in the finished product, whether or not harmful to the recipient or deleterious to the product. Purity includes but is not limited to relative freedom from residual moisture or other volatile and pyrogenic substances. The purity of a reference standard protein can be problematic to assess. As a guide for biologics in development, the USP guidelines [5] that are used for proteins where "standards" are available can be followed. The official USP reference standards include the following required testing: amino acid analysis, capillary electrophoresis, isoelectric focusing, peptide mapping, polyacrylamide gel electrophoresis, and protein determination [1]. A variety of additional purity analyses are commonly performed to ensure acceptably low levels of product (e.g., aggregates or degradation products) or process-derived (host cell protein/DNA, Protein A, etc.) impurities.

The most common sources of impurities are derived from the fermentation process and would include such factors as host cell protein or DNA, or components from cell culture growth media. In addition, endogenous retroviruses from hybridomas in monoclonal antibody production can also be present as impurities, all of which should be removed and tested for in the final product. [1]. These impurities can be present as lipopolysaccharides, oligonucleotides, and leachates from containers. The most common tests that are conducted for the reference standard and production batches are shown in Table 9.2.

As discussed in the section on biosimilars, a significant concern for biotherapeutics is the risk of an unwanted immune response to drug exposure resulting in serious safety sequelae. Among other origins, these anti-drug antibodies can result from trace amounts of impurities in the product that may represent denatured, aggregated, or fragmented proteins arising from the production process. In addition to these potentially immunogenic degradation product impurities, host cell proteins and

TABLE 9.2   Impurity Testing Methods Used for Macromolecule Therapeutics

Impurity Testing	
Protein Impurities	Nonprotein Impurities
Electrophoresis (SDS PAGE; isoelectric focusing)	Endotoxin testing
Dimensional electrophoresis	USP rabbit pyrogen test
Peptide mapping	Limulus amebocyte lysate
Multiantigen ELISA	Endogenous pyrogen assay
HPLC—size exclusion/ion exchange/reverse phase	

production enzymes used to cleave the product during a downstream processing step can cause an immune reaction in patients receiving the therapy. A summary of the tests for quality and identity is shown in Table 9.3. Testing for host cell proteins in drug product is mandated. However, the assays are difficult to develop and characterize, often suffer from a lack of specificity and sensitivity, and vitally depend on specialized reagents. Unfortunately, host cell proteins can occasionally be difficult to remove through the product purification process.

Detection and monitoring of host cell proteins is commonly conducted using SDS-PAGE, 2D electrophoresis, Western blot, and immunoassays. SDS-PAGE separates by molecular weight and has a sensitivity of approximately 100 pg/band. Greater separation, and therefore resolution, may be achieved when an additional dimension is added to the procedure; however 2D electrophoresis can still only detect approximately 100 pg/spot. Western blotting techniques add increased specificity, allowing demonstration of immunological similarity, but are less sensitive (0.1–1 ng/band). Immunoassays are the most commonly employed technique for monitoring host-cell-derived impurities in drug substance and drug products; however, these methods exquisitely depend on the specificity of the antibody reagents used. Immunoassay provides the greatest sensitivity (<0.1 ng/mL), and there are some commercially available generic ELISA methods that are configured to detect host cell proteins for a given recombinant expression system. Most drug companies generate host cell protein assays specific for the cell line(s) used to produce their products. However, assays do exist for generic host cell proteins for some of the more common cell lines in use. Not only can these be utilized for certain final product release assays,

TABLE 9.3   Testing Performed for Quality and Identity of Macromolecules

Tests for Quality	Tests for Identity
Color/appearance/clarity	Peptide mapping
	Amino acid analysis
Particulate analysis	SDS PAGE
pH determination	Capillary electrophoresis
Moisture content	HPLC
Host cell DNA	Western blot
Host cell protein	Immunoassay

but they can also be a valuable tool to monitor production processes to detect steps that introduce, or are especially effective at removing, host cell impurities. Immunoassays also offer the advantage of not requiring sample denaturation and solubilization needed in Western blot technology and provide relatively semiquantitative data, rather than the more subjective interpretation required in blotting technology. It is certainly true that host cell protein immunoassays, especially commercially available methods for common cell lines, have their limitations as well. Antibody reagents have varied affinity and specificity, and the generic calibrators used may have similar, but not identical, reactivity with the cocktail of host cell protein variants present in the unknown test samples. Therefore, the capacity to demonstrate true accuracy is compromised, and the data may show a bias. These assays can provide useful data, but some of the assay validation parameters may need wider acceptance criteria, and validation data certainly warrant more careful interpretation than for other immunoassays.

Aggregated protein can form at any stage of the production and manufacturing process. Aggregates are multimeric clusters of molecules typically linked together by covalent intermolecular disulfide bonds or by hydrophobic association. Aggregation can arise from drug formulation components, storage, and transportation conditions, or from product changes where oxidized or degraded forms of the molecule are unintentionally introduced. Since aggregated protein is large and may introduce novel epitopes, aggregates are well recognized for their immunogenic potential. The aggregation of proteins is favored at high concentrations, and intermolecular disulfide bond formation between cystinyl moieties occurs at alkaline pH under oxidizing conditions. Proteins naturally containing intramolecular disulfide bonds, such as antibodies, can undergo intermolecular disulfide bonding due to disulfide bond rearrangement at neutral or alkaline pH. Production batches of macromolecular biotherapeutics are routinely tested for percent aggregate composition. When present at unacceptable levels, these aggregates can often be removed by a variety of procedures, including size exclusion and ion-exchange chromatography, and filtration methods.

As mentioned above, there are many ways in which aggregated material can form during or after product formulation and final packaging. Triggers can include small amounts of detergent and/or excipients to stabilize the formulation, as well as a host of other causes. Unfortunately, aggregated protein can even form after the release testing of the packaged final product. It is not uncommon for aggregated material to demonstrate either enhanced or diminished potency as determined by the bioassay used for lot release and stability testing. In addition, aggregated material present in the assay calibrators can behave differently from nonaggregated protein, as illustrated in the following case study where a significant analytical bias was observed.

9.3.1.1 *Case Study: Reference Standard Compared with a Lyophilized Formulated Dose*   In this case study, calibrators for an immunoassay were prepared from a lyophilized formulated dosage material for a therapeutic protein, and compared with the corresponding liquid formulation reference standard. Spiked control samples were likewise prepared from both sources of material and run in the

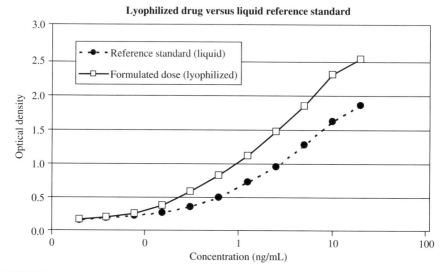

FIGURE 9.1 A comparison of two calibration curves, one prepared from the reference standard and another from the lyophilized formulated dose. The reference standard was provided as a frozen aqueous solution. Each was spiked into assay buffer and dilutions were made to provide the corresponding calibrators with the same concentrations.

method. Recoveries of control samples were then derived from both standard curves. The standard curves prepared from these two materials are shown in Fig. 9.1.

As the figure clearly shows, the dose responses for the two formulations were significantly discordant. An investigation revealed that the lyophilization process for the formulated drug, despite the fact that it included the addition of stabilizers, introduced aggregated protein that was estimated at 5% of the total mass. Of importance is the fact that the lyophilized product met the product release criteria by all physical and chromatographic analyses performed. It should be noted that the release criteria allowed the presence of a limited amount of aggregated protein up to 5%. However, using these materials interchangeably for calibrator preparation was certainly not advisable to avoid a significant bias. This bias is clearly seen when looking at the recovery data for controls, summarized in Table 9.4.

TABLE 9.4 Case Study: Analytical Recovery of Drug Spiked Controls Determined Using Calibration Curves Prepared from Nonlyophilized Versus Lyophilized Standards

Spike (μg/mL)	Nonlyophilized Standard		Lyophilized Standard	
	Nonlyo Recovery	Lyo Recovery	Nonlyo Recovery	Lyo Recovery
100	99.7	248.8	33.1	110.7
50	48.7	133.7	16.4	48.9
5	5.1	15.4	1.5	4.9

Using the reference protein to prepare calibrators resulted in an approximate threefold overestimation for samples prepared from the lyophilized drug. As would be expected, a similar degree of underestimation was seen when calibrators were prepared from the lyophilized material and used to test liquid solutions of reference material. Clearly, this example illustrates the fact that formulation or other manufacturing changes can affect relative immunoreactivity of protein biotherapeutics, presenting challenges for accurate quantitation. One would be advised to match materials for calibration with the test samples whenever possible, and certainly when insufficient characterization data exist to assure that materials are equivalent.

9.3.2 Potency

As with purity, the determination of biological potency (also referred to as biological activity) is included in the battery of testing done to release batches of drug, and can also be used as a component of stability testing. *Potency*, as defined in 21 CFR 600, refers to "the specific ability or capacity of the product, as indicated by appropriate laboratory tests or by adequately controlled clinical data obtained through the administration of the product in the manner intended, to effect a given result" [12]. To assess potency, 21 CFR 610.10 continues that "tests for potency shall consist of either *in vitro* or *in vivo* tests, or both, which have been specifically designed for each product so as to indicate its potency in a manner adequate to satisfy the interpretation of potency given by the definition in 21 CFR 600."

The potency of a therapeutic agent can be described as its ability to elicit a defined biological effect. The methods used to demonstrate this effect generally include animal-based models where a physiological end point is the readout or *in vitro* cell culture models using a biochemical marker as an indicator of activity. When *in vivo* or cell-based *in vitro* methods are not feasible, other biochemical and binding assays using antibodies and/or receptors as surrogates for pharmacological activity can suffice. Among these, perhaps the most commonly used potency paradigm is the *in vitro* cell culture model. These assays offer many advantages over other methods, including improved cost and feasibility compared to *in vivo* methods, a direct measure of biological activity with mechanistic relevance, and well-defined mathematical models for dose–response readout that can be applied to obtain semiquantitative information [13]. Initial potency specifications to release drug product can generally be expected to be within a 30% range of the reference lot.

This broader range in comparison to requirements for purity and content is a reflection of the fact that these are cell-based methods with greater variability and constitute the most challenging aspect of the drug-release test package. Typically, a cell line is identified or developed in the discovery phase of the drug development program and is modified and optimized for use as part of the release package. In the simplest model, the cells used to assess biological activity respond to the drug and yield a measurable response that is directly proportional to the biological activity or potency of the drug. The greater the concentration of the drug, the more intense the signal observed. The activity of the drug might be measured in the simplest model as an increase or decrease in cell count, where the cell proliferation or viability is directly impacted by the drug. In this case, the cells are either counted directly or exposed to reagents that respond to cellular activities (proliferation/death) and produce a measurable spectrophotometric, fluorimetric, or chemiluminescent signal.

In more complex or indirect potency models, the drug might act upon an external factor involved with signal transduction in the target cells to either stimulate or inhibit the production of a downstream marker of bioactivity. In these methods, the biomarker is used as a measure of the bioactivity of the drug. The biomarker can be any molecule that is produced or inhibited by the action of the drug upon the cells. When a biomarker is used to follow a cellular response to a drug, it may be necessary to measure the concentration of the biomarker in a complex matrix such as cell culture supernatant, which requires a relatively quantitative method to achieve required accuracy. The assays used for biomarkers are often ELISAs or other binding immunoassays where standard curves are required. Not surprisingly, those calibrators are subject to variations in batch-to-batch performance that can influence the results from the potency bioassay.

Potency assays are generally performed using a range of concentrations for the reference standard and for the test lot being evaluated. The dose–response curves are typically nonlinear and require careful optimization to achieve reproducible dose–response curve parameters. Such curves can be analyzed using models for parallelism (such as parallel line analysis) and the midpoint (EC50) computed to allow comparisons between test and reference materials [13]. This type of analysis is similar to but somewhat more rigorous than the evaluation of standard curve characteristics in assays for the determination of drug levels for the assessment of pharmacokinetics. The parallel line analysis approach has become more widely adopted since it allows the assessment of the response from test or reference material over a range of concentrations. In addition to potency, this can provide useful information related to formulated drug stability and purity.

In the development and validation of the bioassay method, the performance of the drug standard/reference lot is documented to rigorously define the reproducibility of the method and to establish the reference ranges that will be applied to the analysis of subsequent production lots of the drug. This can be challenging since it frequently takes some time to scale up and optimize the production procedures. During the early phase of development, and also later when new formulations may be introduced, seemingly small changes in production can have pronounced effects on the biological activity of the drug product. Moreover, the changes in biological activity may or may not be evident in any of the other required testing. The following three case studies illustrate how changes in manufacturing and improper calibration can impact the perceived potency of drug products.

9.3.2.1 Case Study: Changes in Potency Caused by Lot-to-Lot Differences in cAMP

In this example, THP-1 cells (a human leukemia cell line) were found to be responsive to a biotherapeutic agent in development. The biotherapeutic caused a stimulation of cAMP that accumulated in the cells exposed to drug and could be released after lysing the cells. Therefore, determination of cyclic adenosine monophosphate (cAMP) levels in THP-1 cell culture lysates was used as an indicator of potency for this biotherapeutic candidate. The procedure used to determine cAMP levels was validated using commercially available cAMP reagents and, during the development of the drug, the lot of this cAMP reagent changed. The assay was competitive with anti-cAMP antibody as a capture reagent, and a cAMP peroxidase conjugate used as a competitor for unlabeled cAMP in lysates. The procedure involved incubating the calibrators or unknowns in anti-cAMP antibody-coated wells along with the cAMP peroxidase conjugate. The cAMP in the test sample lysate competes for binding to the anti-cAMP antibody with the cAMP peroxidase conjugate. After incubation, the wells are aspirated and washed. The bound cAMP peroxidase conjugate is detected with the addition of TMB substrate (3,3',5,5' tetramethylbenzidine/ hydrogen peroxide) and produces the characteristic blue color amendable to optical density reading on a plate reader. The concentration of cAMP in the sample is inversely proportional to the signal.

During the course of sample testing, a new lot of commercially available cAMP was used to replace the existing, but depleted, lot. The change in the standard cAMP reagent resulted in a shift in the standard curve (data not shown). As a consequence, the determination of the concentrations in the unknowns was significantly biased (+20%), which led to inaccurate measurements of potency. This difficult lesson should serve as a cautionary note to bioanalysts relying on commercial reagents for their assays. Despite claims to the contrary, and no different than for critical assay reagents produced "in-house," it is not uncommon for significant lot-to-lot differences in these reagents to alter method accuracy and confound interpretation.

9.3.2.2 Case Study: ELISA and Cell-Based Bioassay Measurements of Potency During Manufacturing Process Development

A recombinant cytokine was being scaled up from bench size lots to small production runs to initiate IND-enabling safety studies [14]. The larger batches being released from the production scale-up facility were failing the cell-based bioassay. The bioassay used a dose-dependent proliferation curve, with the EC50 as the assay end point. The larger production batches did not meet acceptance criteria, with results falling below potency specifications. A companion immunoassay, which was a double-antibody sandwich assay configured with a monoclonal capture and an enzyme-tagged rabbit polyclonal detection reagent, also showed differences between the small- and large scale product batches. The differences in the ELISA assay were expressed as shifts in the EC50 values. In addition, when the new lots were tested as unknowns using the small-scale batch material as calibrators, results were approximately 30–40% lower than expected. When serial dilutions of each were compared, although the patterns were linear, they were not parallel. The combination of the cell-based potency data and ELISA results led to an investigation into possible denaturation of drug substance during the production process. To determine the point in the production process where the denaturation may be occurring, samples were taken at strategic points and tested in the ELISA procedure. This identified a mechanical pump used in the large-scale chromatography process that was producing shearing force and denaturing the protein. This was corrected by substituting the mechanical pump with a less-vigorous peristaltic pump.

9.3.2.3 Case Study: Improving Recombinant Calibrator Improves Robustness and Accuracy of Potency Assay

A biotherapeutic with a target in the coagulation cascade was being evaluated for efficacy in early Phase II clinical trials. A hematology assay, prothrombin time, which is a marker of the extrinsic coagulation pathway and generally used for the diagnosis of inborn errors of coagulation, vitamin K deficiencies, and for monitoring the effect of oral anticoagulation therapies [15], was selected to determine the potency of batches of the biotherapeutic. The assay uses thromboplastin as a substrate for the coagulation reaction, with thromboplastin derived from rabbit brain as the initial source of material for preparation of calibrators. The assay was validated and the results were correlated with the pharmacology models used during drug development. Overall, the method demonstrated between-run precision within 20%, which is considered quite reproducible for cell-based methods of potency. During the clinical trial, a new batch of the drug was produced, tested, and accepted for use in the continuing Phase II program. Prior to the introduction of the new batch into the randomized placebo-controlled trial, the candidate drug demonstrated superior efficacy compared to the standard of care control arm of the study. Once the new batch was put into use, the results were reversed, and the standard therapy was demonstrating greater efficacy. After several rounds of troubleshooting and investigation, the source of the discrepant clinical results was determined to be the bioactivity of the new drug batch. The data from the coagulation/ prothrombin time assay showed that the new batch, although it passed the release specification ($\pm 20\%$ of reference lot), was on the low side of that range. In addition, the calibrator for the assay (rabbit brain thromboplastin) was from a new lot, and was found to introduce an additional high bias in the potency result. When the low, but acceptable, potency result was combined with the high bias, it was estimated that the "true" potency of the new clinical lot was approximately 30% lower compared to the reference lot of drug. This more than accounted for the apparent loss in efficacy. When a recombinant human thromboplastin was substituted for the rabbit prothrombin to prepare assay calibrators and the new batch of drug was tested in the modified assay, a clear difference in bioactivity was observed. In fact, the new drug lot would have failed the potency criterion for lot release and would never have been introduced into the clinical trial. Ultimately, the introduction of a recombinant source of the thromboplastin substrate demonstrated greater consistency and provided for a more reliable and rugged method but the cost of this lesson to the company was significant.

9.3.3 Concentration Determination

Unlike the use of small, organically synthesized reference standards, proteins or biomolecules do not have qualities that enable the gravimetric determination of mass, so a reference standard solution cannot be simply prepared. The large size and fragile nature of the molecules preclude drying to constant weight. Current knowledge of the predicted molecular composition, based upon the amino acid sequence, may not take into account the addition of carbohydrates or other posttranslational modifications to the protein in the molecular mass. However, one approach to assigning a concentration to reference standards is the use of quantitative amino acid analysis. This approach is used on very pure protein reference standards when they become available, often in the later stages of development. Prior to the availability of such standards, other approaches are taken to estimate the concentration of protein reference standard solutions, as described below.

9.3.3.1 *Ultraviolet Absorption*

The ultraviolet absorption characteristics of the aromatic side chains of the primary amino acid sequence are often used to estimate an extinction coefficient for a protein. The extinction coefficient is calculated based upon the number of tyrosine, tryptophan, and phenylalanine (aromatic) residues in the protein. Phenylalanine has a relatively weaker absorptivity and may not be included in the calculations. One advantage of this approach is the fact that it is relatively nondisruptive, leaving protein conformation undisturbed. In addition, the same solution used for the concentration assessment can be removed from the cuvette and used for additional experiments. The measurement is based upon Beer's law:

$$\mathrm{OD}_{280} = E \times C \times L = H \times C \times L \div \mathrm{MW}$$

where OD_{280} is the optical density at 280 nm, E is the absorptivity (nm × mL/(mg × cm), C is the protein concentration in mg/mL, L is the light pathway (cm), H is the molar extinction coefficient, and MW is the molecular weight in g/mol.

The most common practice is to use an extinction coefficient of 1.0 when the purity and characteristics of the molecule are being determined. The sensitivity is typically in the range of 0.05–1.0 mg/mL, and one must be aware of the fact that impurities, particularly those that contain aromatic side chains, may lead to inaccuracies. Further interference that can skew results may be encountered with pigments, organic cofactors, and phenolic constituents of the solution. In addition, the extinction coefficient for a protein is pH dependent. On the whole, this approach is the most common one in use and although it can only be expected to yield an estimate of the true concentration, sometimes this is the best that can be done.

9.3.3.2 *Colorimetric Methods*

The concentration of protein solutions can also be determined using colorimetric methods that employ very pure bovine serum albumin (BSA) or bovine gamma globulin (BGG) as a calibrator. As with A280 methods, there are a number of challenges associated with accurate colorimetric protein determination. Notably, factors such as assay calibration, specificity, and sensitivity must be carefully considered. The bovine serum albumin or gamma globulin assay calibrators used are also proteins, and are likewise affected by the same issues as the unknown protein being measured. There is always going to be some amount of lot-to-lot variability linked to the source of the protein and isolation and downstream purification processes used. Not all colorimetric assays yield the same absorbance dose responses with BSA and BGG, which introduces another variable when interpreting results. A comparison of four commonly used colorimetric protein assays is shown in Table 9.5. These assays can simply be adapted to using the biotherapeutic reference standard for calibration when that is available.

TABLE 9.5 Comparison of Analytical Methods for the Determination of Total Protein Concentration

	Total Protein Assays			
Method	Biuret Reaction	Bicinchoninic Acid	Lowry	Bradford
Readout	540 nm	562 nm	750 nm	595 nm
Calibrators	BSA or BGG	BSA or BGG	BSA or BGG (~15%)	BSA or BGG (~30%)
Std curve	Linear	Linear	Nonlinear	Nonlinear
Specificity	Tripeptides or greater; Cu complexes with pep bonds	Tripeptides or greater; Cu complexes with pep bonds	Dipeptide or greater; Reacts with tyr, try, cys, his, asn, pro	MW ≥ 3K; Reacts with arg, lys, his
Interferents	Cu reducing or chelating agents; Free aa: cys, tyr, try	EDTA, sucrose, glucose, glycine; NH$_4$ sulfate; Na acetate and phosphate; Mercapto reducing agents; Free aa: tyr, cys, try	Detergents, K$^+$, free thiols; Cu chelating agents; Carbohydrates and N-acetyl derivatives	Low pH required: solubility issues; BSA and BGG stds 30% difference; Detergents; Chromogen stains cuvettes
Advantages	Surfactants do not interfere; All proteins behave similarly	Color stable for hours; Urea and detergents do not interfere	Relatively small difference in BSA and BGG calibration curves	Simple, compatible with most salts, solvents, buffers, thiols, chelating, and reducing agents

The Lowry assay [16] uses the reaction of cupric sulfate at alkaline pH in the presence of tartrate, producing a blue chromogen formed from four peptide bonds and one atom of copper. Addition of folin phenol reagent further enhances the color, with a maximum absorbance at 750 nm. The Lowry assay demonstrates the greatest sensitivity of the common protein concentration determination methods and varies only slightly when using the two common calibrators, BSA and BGG. Not surprisingly, this remains a very commonly used method.

The Biuret reaction [17] is based upon the coordination of at least three amino acids in a peptide, with Cu^{2+} under alkaline conditions, reducing it to Cu^{1+} and forming a blue/violet colored complex absorbing at 540 nm. In the bicinchoninic acid (BCA) assay, the Cu^{1+} complex is further reacted with bicinchoninic acid and a more elaborate complex is formed that has a greater absorptivity with a maximum at 562 nm [18]. Both chromogens demonstrate linearity in the 0–20 µg/mL range. In the expanded range to 2000 µg/mL, the method becomes nonlinear, with the observed curve introducing as much as 20% variation between the BSA and BGG calibrators.

Another assay, the Bradford assay, also known as the Coomassie dye binding method, was first described in 1976 [19]. In an acidic environment, proteins will bind to Coomassie dye and cause a shift from the reddish brown color (465 nm) to the blue dye–protein complex read at 595 nm. The development of the color is attributed to the presence of the basic amino acids arginine, lysine, and histidine. Van der Waals forces and hydrophobic interactions account for the dye binding and the number of Coomassie blue dye molecules bound is roughly proportional to the number of positive charges on the molecule. A protein molecular weight of about 3 kDA is required for successful color development. The Bradford assay dose–response is nonlinear and this method demonstrates the greatest difference in reactivity with BSA compared to BGG.

With so many choices, it is important to be aware of the advantages and limitations of these methods. The following case study illustrates the importance of appropriate protein concentration determination methodology.

9.3.3.3 Case Study: Quantification of In-Process Enzymes During Production

The use of absorption at 280 nm (A280) to perform concentration determination, as described above, is very common, but caution should be exercised when interpreting results. In this example, discordant concentration values were obtained when comparing A280 with an immunoassay specific for the enzyme used in a drug production process (data not shown). The protein production and purification process involved addition of a proteolytic enzyme followed by the removal of the enzymes using denaturants. Initially, A280 readings were routinely used to follow the presence of residual enzymes. Surprisingly, the apparent enzyme concentration did not diminish following the removal step. After some thoughtful consideration and more testing using an immunoassay specific for the enzyme, it became apparent that the A280 readings reflected the absorbance of the aromatic side chains of the amino acid residues and not necessarily intact protein. This highlights one of the shortcomings of determining protein concentration using this technique, namely, that A280 is a nonspecific technique, and thus no conclusions can be drawn regarding the purity of the protein solution being measured. It is important to keep in mind exactly what one is measuring when using A280 or any other method for protein quantification.

The concentration of large molecules may be expressed as mass units or activity units. There are challenges present in either approach. As discussed, mass unit determinations are difficult since the molecules are relatively large, complex, and fragile. Spectrophotometric approaches are at best a close approximation based upon the UV absorption of the aromatic moieties in the amino acid composition of the protein, and colorimetric assay results can vary depending on the unique chemical composition of the protein being measured relative to that used for calibration. On the other hand, activity units are assigned based upon a biological assay that responds in a dose-dependent manner to the protein. Such methods, by virtue of their biological nature, are semiquantitative and can be extremely sensitive to small conformational changes in the protein, not to mention the variability inherent in the biological assay itself. As an example, for therapeutic antibody drugs, slight alterations in protein conformation may be associated with significant changes in antibody affinity. The changes in antibody affinity may be observed in the binding curves that are used to calibrate assays and thereby may affect results, whether expressed in activity or mass units. It is always advisable to match as closely as possible the source of material for calibration with the antibody or other protein being measured, particularly in situations where the antibody has been shown to be susceptible to affinity-changing conformational alterations. Not doing so will likely lead to over- or underestimation of protein concentration.

9.3.4 Stability

The complexity and variety of biopharmaceutical recombinant products necessitate rigorous stability testing methods and schemes. The basic requirements and approaches for stability studies are outlined in ICH guidance documents [14] such as QA1 (R2), with the goal of "providing evidence on how the quality of a drug substance or drug product varies with time under the influence of a variety of environmental factors such as temperature, humidity, and light, and to establish a re-test period for the drug substance or a shelf life for the drug product and recommended storage conditions." Methods such as those described above to assess the purity of drug products (and considered "stability indicating") are used to test product samples subjected to accelerated or real-time storage conditions. A comparison is made to a reference standard stored under ideal conditions to finally determine the stability attributes of the product.

Drug substance/product stability may be separated into two categories, physical and chemical stability/instability. Physical instability is characterized by changes in secondary, tertiary, or quaternary structure of the drug resulting from processes such as denaturation, adsorption, aggregation, and precipitation. Excipients are often used to prevent aggregation, many of which are derived from animal sources such as bovine serum albumin. This raises additional safety-related purity concerns regarding potential infectious disease contaminants that are associated with the use of constituents from animals. Chemical instability of the protein biotherapeutic involves

TABLE 9.6 Macromolecular Reference Standards: Stability Challenges

Physical Instability	Chemical Instability
Denaturation	Cleavage
Adsorption	New bond formation
Aggregation	Deamidation
Stabilizers	Racemization
Precipitation	Proteolysis
Effects on biological activity	Effects on biological activity

changes to the primary structure and can result in the formation of a new chemical entity, making the development of a reference standard difficult. Chemical instability can occur as a result of cleavage and reformation of the peptide bonds, deamidation, proteolysis, racemization, and a variety of other chemical pathways. These unwanted alternate forms of the molecule often arise during the scaleup in manufacturing and may be more or less potent than the parent compound, and more or less stable. Table 9.6 summarizes the challenges in stability issues for macromolecules as standards.

Further, compounding the difficulty in generating an appropriate reference standard is the fact that this class of macromolecular therapeutics, even when free of process impurities and instability issues, contains significant structural heterogeneity. It is certainly conceivable that all the various heterogeneous forms existing in a final drug product may be biologically active, and that the overall biological activity of the product may actually increase or decrease over time as the balance of the various chemically modified forms tips toward the more or less potent constituents.

9.4 THE PK ASSAY

9.4.1 Preparation of Standard Curve

Once a well-characterized, pure reference standard of known concentration is available, one must be aware of the fact that the actual preparation of the assay calibrators can also influence the PK standard curve. The physical treatment and handling of concentrated protein solutions can be very challenging. Some reference standards require specific handling techniques to prevent aggregation or denaturation of the protein. The effects of vortexing can be disastrous as can the process used to thaw frozen reference standard or calibrator solutions. Details such as the dilution pattern that is used in spiking the calibration solutions can contribute to assay bias and between-laboratory discrepancies.

The pooled matrix used to formulate the calibrators can also significantly affect assay performance; thus, it is critical that sufficient volume of matrix pools that closely match the study sample matrix is available for use. Ideally, this would be a matrix pool from prestudy animals in safety studies or human subjects in clinical studies. The differences in patient-to-patient background effects can be detected in the assay selectivity and ruggedness experiments during method development. There are instances when it may be useful to add sucrose, immunoglobulins, or other components to the calibrator matrix and assay diluent to reduce nonspecific signal and enhance assay sensitivity. Finally, experiments should be performed to identify the minimum required dilution of matrix necessary to reduce signal background to acceptable levels, while maintaining adequate assay sensitivity to accommodate samples with low levels of drug. Lacking such information can result in unanticipated (and unwanted) surprises during study sample testing in which prestudy samples appear to contain drug, or where postdosing data appear to be inaccurate when using a baseline (prestudy sample) subtraction approach.

Calibrators are made by adding concentrated stock solutions of the purest form of drug available to the appropriate matrix, often serum or plasma matched to the species of test samples, or synthetic derivatives of either. These components may not be inert and one must always be on the lookout for drug binding or an extraction effect. This adsorption can also occur in preparing the assay controls. In preparing calibrators, one strategy is to prepare the highest concentration calibrator in 100% serum or plasma and aliquot for freezing. The standard curve is then prepared from serial dilutions of this high calibrator. On the other hand, controls may be made from individual spikes rather than serial dilutions of a single high concentration. If some of the drug product is lost to nonspecific binding to matrix components, incomplete recovery at low concentrations may be observed. The following case study illustrates the effect of seemingly insignificant matrix differences on standard curve performance.

9.4.1.1 Case Study: Effect of Anticoagulants on Standard Curve   In this example, a drug was found to be less soluble in K_3 EDTA plasma compared to Li heparin (lithium heparin), which may be related to the differences in pH of each anticoagulant type. The pH of lithium heparin is approximately 5.5, while the pH of K_3 EDTA can be above 8. Blood is readily collected in vacutainer tubes containing K_3 EDTA coated beads where the anticoagulation process occurs quickly. Lithium heparin plasma collection takes longer time and therefore is not always the first choice. In the assay of interest, a 50-fold dilution was used, leaving only 2% matrix present in the calibrators, samples, and controls. As is readily apparent in Fig. 9.2, a dramatic difference was observed in the performance of standard curves with Li heparin versus K_3 EDTA.

This effect was discovered during assay development when very basic experiments were conducted to determine background effects in potential matrices for safety studies. The significant differences in dose response for these curves would be expected to impact assay sensitivity. Equally important is the fact that, without further refinement of the method to reduce this matrix effect, accurate quantification of drug in-study samples can only be assured when samples are collected with the same anticoagulant in the matrix as that used to prepare the standard curve. Whenever possible, experiments to evaluate the effect of the matrix on the assay should be conducted before the in-life phase of the study begins.

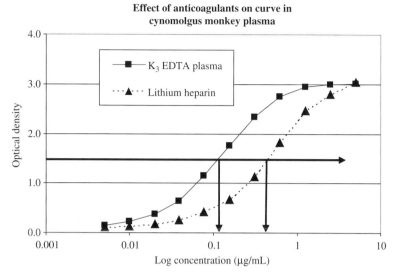

FIGURE 9.2   A comparison of two calibration curves in cynomolgus monkey plasma. One curve was prepared in K_3 EDTA plasma and the other in lithium heparin plasma. Each calibrator contained 2% of the corresponding matrix prepared from the same stock solution of drug, spiked directly into 100% plasma and then diluted 50-fold in assay buffer. The pH of the diluted calibrators was 7.4 for each matrix.

9.4.2 Critical Reagents

A well-characterized reference standard is of obvious importance to properly calibrating PK methods. Perhaps less well appreciated is the importance of well characterized, or at least well understood, critical reagents in PK methods. Critical reagents generally include such things as the entity coated onto a surface (e.g., an ELISA well or bead) and used to capture the drug from the sample matrix, the reagent used to detect the captured drug, any factors added to diluents to reduce the background or otherwise improve the performance of the assay, and the molecules necessary to generate a signal for detection. To reduce the chances of poor assay performance due to surprises during sample testing or, in other words, to ensure that methods perform optimally and as expected, the more one knows about the properties of these critical reagents, the better. The following case study illustrates this point.

9.4.2.1 *Case Study: The Effect of Amino Acid Substitutions on ELISA Reactivity*   This case study illustrates how manufacturing changes can impact biopharmaceutical drug product purity and a standard curve prepared from that drug and highlights the narrow specificity of monoclonal antibodies used for bioanalysis. Two monoclonal antibodies were used as capture reagents for each of the two ELISA methods for determining the quantitative blood levels of a biotherapeutic drug. One of the antibodies was specific for the N-terminus of the protein and the other for the C-terminus. The assays were otherwise identical. The combination of the two methods

enabled the assessment of total and intact protein concentrations in preclinical safety studies.

During the development of the drug (227 amino acids), the production method was modified to increase the yield and this resulted in the substitution of 27 leucine residues with norleucine, a seemingly small change. All of the analytical testing performed using typical methods to assess physical protein structure showed that the modified molecule was indistinguishable from the original configuration. In addition, the bioassay results showed equivalency between the original and modified drugs.

A bioequivalence study was conducted in nonhuman primates to assess *in vivo* equivalence for the two forms of the drug. In preparation for sample analysis, the assays were optimized and standard curves were prepared using each form of the protein in study matrix. In addition, spiked controls were serially diluted and each series was measured in the N-and C-terminus-specific assays. The results for the C-terminus assay were equivalent, as shown in Fig. 9.3, demonstrating acceptable dilutional linearity with either sample type. However, as one can see in Fig. 9.4, the N-terminus assay clearly does not equivalently recognize the two forms of the drug.

Acceptable accuracy and parallelism of the C-terminus assay are likely due to the C-terminal specificity of the capture antibody and the N-terminal location of the norleucine substitutions. Conversely, with the N-terminal specific assay, dramatic differences in recoveries were seen for the two forms of the drug, a direct consequence of these N-terminal modifications and differential binding of the immunoreagent directed at this region. Although each assay demonstrated good linearity upon

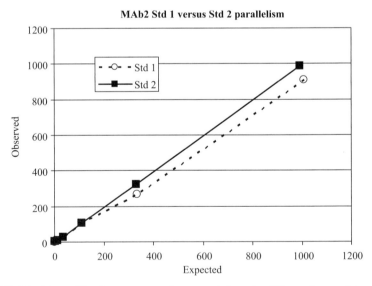

FIGURE 9.3 Two calibration curves, each prepared from the different forms of the protein. The MAb2 was used as the capture antibody and had specificity for the C-terminal of the protein. The similarity of the dilution pattern shows that the amino acid substitutions in the N-terminus did not alter the conformation of the C-terminus of the molecules, so that both were recognized by the capture C-terminal-specific antibody.

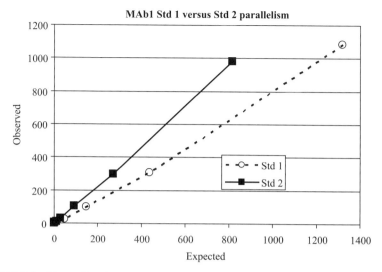

FIGURE 9.4 Two calibration curves, each prepared from the different forms of the protein. The MAb1 was used as the capture antibody and had specificity for the N-terminal of the protein. Although each set of serial dilutions demonstrated linearity, they were not parallel using the N-terminus-specific capture antibody.

dilution, significant nonparallelism was observed with the N-terminal assay when the concentration for either form of the protein was interpolated from a standard curve prepared from the other form. Interestingly, since bioactivity of the molecule is located in the C-terminal epitope(s), it was not surprising that both forms of the molecule performed equivalently in the lot release bioassay. In the end, it was determined that accurate quantification of these two distinct drug forms could only be achieved when calibrators and controls were prepared with matched forms of the drug. This case study highlights the importance of fully understanding the specificities of immunoreagents and matching materials to be tested with those used for calibration.

9.4.2.2 *Curve Fitting*   Finally, one cannot optimally quantify drugs in complex biological matrices or many other macromolecular analytes commonly tested in immunoassays, without a thorough understanding of dose–response relationships and curve fitting. This often underappreciated element of a validated method can ultimately be the key difference in achieving the necessary sensitivity of a method. Thus, the ideal PK bioanalytical scenario would include calibrators that have been carefully prepared from a well-characterized preparation of reference standard, run in an optimized and validated method by well-trained scientists, with the standard curve optimally modeled to interpolate unknown sample concentrations. It should also be understood that correct curve fitting does not start with the PK method. The characterization of the reference standard and release of production lots include a potency assay with the drug tested at multiple dilutions to create a dose–response curve. Often the readout of the potency assay will be a downstream biomarker that is

itself quantified by interpolation from a standard curve. Thus, we have layers of curve fitting that must be properly addressed by the time one is looking at PK assay dose–response data to avoid compounding inaccuracy. In fact, it is often advisable for bioanalytical and process scientists to swallow their pride and seek the counsel of statisticians with relevant expertise to assist with the evaluation of dose–response data and optimal curve-fitting strategies.

9.5 CONCLUSIONS

The use of reference standards for a variety of long-standing applications during all phases of a pharmaceutical product's life cycle—from drug development through the introduction of generic follow-on products—is well established, particularly for small-molecule drugs. Among these applications, bioanalytical scientists are especially interested in the role of reference standards to assess the pharmacokinetics of novel compounds, whether being developed for first-in-human studies or for label expansion of approved products. Biotherapeutic reference standards, in particular, present many challenges to bioanalysts, process scientists, and QC laboratory staff. This chapter presented some historical context, addressed some of these challenges, and offered some guidance with respect to this relatively new class of reference standard.

Establishing biotherapeutic drug product purity, potency, stability, and concentration is not as easy as one might believe, particularly if one's bioanalytical experience includes only small-molecule, chemically synthesized drugs. Despite this fact, it is vitally important to understand that whatever steps are necessary to generate the best possible reference standard need to be taken to achieve, among other things, accurate quantification of drug in PK samples from nonclinical and clinical studies. It is acknowledged that the "original reference standard," typically generated in-house early in the development cycle and subject to the same issues as drug product as it matures in a pipeline, is almost certain to change during the drug development process. As scale-up manufacturing/purification, formulation, storage, and other later-stage processes evolve, new reference standards will need to be assigned and characterized, as appropriate.

Likewise, to assess the pharmacokinetics of the drug product in its most evolved form, it stands to reason that one should use the most current reference standard available (or the drug lot used in the clinical study itself) to calibrate methods. Unlike some small-molecule drugs, biotherapeutics will typically never exist in the form of official USP reference standards except under certain circumstances as the compound comes off patent. For a USP reference standard to be accepted, many rounds of peer testing are typically required. The placement of assays in different labs to compare and qualify biologics in "round robin" testing in which identical samples are tested in multiple facilities—as is done with selected hormones, enzymes, and cytokines—is a daunting task, at least until the product becomes more widely produced and the methods are shown to be infallibly rugged. By virtue of the biological and heterogeneous nature of these molecules and the fact that the testing for potency (activity) is biologically based, the accuracy and precision familiar to the small molecule world, and possibly necessary for USP inclusion, are just not achievable. Finally, the product stability and stability testing represent another extremely difficult set of challenges. Thus, the task of creating and using appropriate reference material for establishing the pharmacokinetic properties of biotherapeutic entities falls on the shoulders of process and bioanalytical scientists at individual companies. It is hoped that some of the pitfalls and solutions highlighted in this chapter will help these scientists to work collaboratively to achieve the best reference standards possible in pursuit of the goal of ideal pharmacokinetic evaluation of biotherapeutics.

REFERENCES

1. Niazi, S.K. (2006) *Handbook of Biogeneric Therapeutic Proteins.* CRC Press, pp. 265–288.
2. Leahy J.L., and Cefalu W.T. (eds) (2002) *Insulin Therapy,* 1st Edition. Marcel Dekker, New York.
3. USP Reference Standards Catalog. United States Pharmacopeia, 12601 Twinbrook Parkway Rockville, MD 20852-1790, USA.
4. Bhattacharyya, I. (2004) The value of USP public standards for therapeutic products. *Pharmacological Research,* **21**, 1725–1731.
5. Williams, R.L. (2006) Project team 4, the 2000–2005 reference standards committee of the USP council of experts and its advisory panel and USP staff and consultant. *Journal of Pharmaceutical and Biomedical Analysis,* **40**, 3–15.
6. De Palma, A., and Thomas, P. (2006) A Wave Suspended: Follow-On Biologics. Pharma-Manufacturing.com.
7. Dudsinski, D.M., and Kesselheim, A. (2008) Scientific and legal viability of follow-on protein drugs. *New England Journal of Medicine,* **358**, 843–849.
8. Schonholzer, C., Keusch, G., Nigg, L., Robert, D., and Wauters, J.P. (2004) High prevalence in Switzerland of pure red-cell aplasia due to anti-erythropoietin antibodies in chronic dialysis patients: report of five cases. *Nephrology Dialysis Transplantation,* **19**, 2121–2125.
9. Guidance for Industry and Reviewers Nonclinical Safety Evaluation of Biotechnology-Derived Pharmaceuticals. U.S. Department of Health and Human Services, Food and Drug Administration, Center for Drug Evaluation and Research, August 2006.
10. Guideline on the Clinical Investigation of the Pharmacokinetics of Therapeutic Proteins. European Medicines Agency, Evaluation of Medicines for Human Use, July 2005.
11. Ben-Maimon, C.S., and Garnick, R. (2006) Biogenerics at the crossroads. *Nature Biotechnology,* **24**, 268.
12. Code of Federal Regulations, Title 21, Vol. 1, Biological Products, Section 600.3, Definitions, Edition 4-1-09.
13. Gottschalk, P.G., and Dunn, J.R. (2005) Measuring parallelism, linearity and relative potency in bioassay and immunoassay data. *Journal of Biopharmaceutical Statistics,* **15**, 437–463.
14. International Conference on Harmonisation of Technical Requirements for Registration of Pharmaceuticals for Human Use (1996).

15. Marlar, R.A., Cook, J., Johnston, M., Kitchen, S., Machlin, S., Shafer, D., and Worfolk, L. (2007). One-stage prothrombin time (pt) test and activated partial thromboplastin time (APTT) test. Approved Guideline, 2nd edition, Vol. 28(20), Clinical Laboratory Standards Institute, HA47-A2.

16. Lowry, O.H., Rosbrough, N.J., Farr, A.L., and Randall, R.J. (1951) Protein measurement with the Folin phenol reagent. *Journal of Biological Chemistry*, **193**, 265.

17. Stoscheck, C.M. (1990) Quantitation of protein. *Methods in Enzymology*, **182**, 50–69.

18. Wiechelman, K., Braun, R., and Fitzpatrick, J. (1988) Investigation of the bicinchoninic acid protein assay: identification of the groups responsible for color formation. *Analytical Biochemistry*, **175**, 231–237.

19. Bradford, R. (1976) A rapid and sensitive method for the quantitation of microgram quantities of protein utilizing the principle of protein–dye binding. *Analytical Biochemistry*, **72**, 248.

CHAPTER 10

Strategies for Successful Transfer of Ligand-Binding Assays for Successful Validation and Implementation in GXP Environment

WOLFGANG KLUMP

SAFC Pharma, Carlsbad, CA, USA

HOWARD HILL

Huntingdon Life Sciences, Alconbury, UK

10.1   INTRODUCTION

The globalization of pharmaceutical companies means that, within the same company, the "same" assay may be carried out at different sites, within the same country or in a different continent. Under these circumstances, it needs to be assured that the assay transferred to each of these sites continues to perform as originally developed and validated. In addition to within-company transfers, there is an increasing tendency to outsource methods to contract research organizations (CROs). The method is usually developed within the "innovator" company and subsequently transferred to the CRO. The reasons for using CROs vary with the philosophy of the company.

To be successful, it is essential that the CRO is capable of fulfilling the requirements of the innovator lab. To achieve this, compatibility of equipment, skills, and resources to set up and routinely run the assay, in addition to being capable of troubleshooting in a timely manner, are important attributes a CRO should have to execute such studies. Minimizing downtime caused by assay failure is critical and helps to build confidence in the contracting lab as well as maximizing profitability for the CRO. For GXP applications, use of GXP compliant systems, for example 21 CFR Part 11 compliant software, validated storage space, and appropriate sample handling, is required.

Ligand-Binding Assays: Development, Validation, and Implementation in the Drug Development Arena. Edited by Masood N. Khan and John W.A. Findlay
Copyright © 2010 John Wiley & Sons, Inc.

Ideally, electronic and computer-based data systems should be e-compatible with the innovator lab.

Contract labs must have efficient, cost-effective systems that allow the samples to be processed and the data reported in an efficient manner. While use of automated sample processing systems is commonplace, automated data processing and tabulation systems are only now becoming a reality.

As the number of CROs increases, the need for the innovator lab to develop an efficient objective selection process becomes essential. Such a process is best initiated by a request for information (RFI) that provides the contracting laboratory with basic information with respect to the capabilities of the CRO, and this is discussed in detail subsequently.

10.1.1 The Goals of Method Transfer

Before initiating any method transfer, the intended use of the method for testing must be well defined, and expectations should be made clear. Depending on the scenarios mentioned above, the method transfer and subsequent qualification or validation may be performed following different strategies and stringencies. The goal of a method transfer can be divided into different categories: (1) PK and immunogenicity methods to be run under GLP, as for GLP animal studies, or following GLP guidelines, as for clinical or certain animal studies, (2) biomarker methods that may or may not be run under GLP, depending on the quality of the method and intended application of the method, and (3) release, stability, or in-process methods that may be run in a cGMP environment. Different goals may require different approaches during the method transfer, for example, GLP applications based on validated assays versus biomarker testing based on minimally qualified methods.

10.1.2 Regulatory and Industry Guidance

Very little regulatory documentation directly relates to method transfer and usually where it is mentioned, it refers to cross-validation of the method between two laboratories. It is mentioned in the FDA's Bioanalytical Methods Validation Guidance [1] page 3 under Cross-Validation, "When sample analyses within a single study are conducted at more than one site or more than one laboratory, cross-validation with spiked matrix standards and subject samples should be conducted at each site or laboratory to establish inter-laboratory reliability." It is also mentioned in the Appendix of the same guidance that defines reproducibility as "the precision between two laboratories."

Cross-validation is discussed by Viswanathan et al. [2] in the report from the 2006 Crystal City III AAPS workshop/conference: "Cross-validation procedures and acceptance criteria need to remain flexible considering the various bioanalytical situations where it would be (may be) required. Specific cross-validation criteria should be established *a priori* in a standard operating procedure (SOP)."

The major contribution to establishing criteria for method transfer is to be found in the guide of International Society of Pharmaceutical Engineers (ISPE) [3]. While the analytical aspects of this guide relate to procedures used to measure active ingredients in pharmaceutical products, many of the principles enshrined within are applicable to the transfer of any analytical method. The guide defines the "Sending Unit" as the lab that is responsible for developing the methodology, that is, the innovator lab, while the "Receiving Unit," for example, CRO, is the one to which the method will be transferred. It also describes the responsibilities of the sending and receiving laboratories:

- The primary task of the sending lab is to create the transfer protocol, execute training, and assist in the analysis, while the receiving lab provides qualified instrumentation, personnel, and data collection and processing systems and executes the protocol.
- The sending and receiving labs are jointly responsible for issuing the final report relating to acceptability of the method transfer.
- Successful transfer is based on meeting pre-established acceptance criteria. It is essential that the available personnel and equipment used to establish the assay in the receiving lab are able to meet the criteria and are compatible with those of the sending labs.

Transfer of ligand-binding assays may occur in a number of different scenarios: (1) between labs within a company, (2) between labs of a study sponsor and a CRO, (3) between laboratories of different CROs, and (4) between more than two labs as part of larger projects. In the context of this chapter, the ISPE terminology will be used, although not exclusively, that is, the lab that initiates the method transfer is the "sending laboratory," while the lab to which the method is being transferred is the "receiving laboratory," but in some cases will be referred to as the "testing laboratory." The transfer between the laboratories can be further defined by the level of regulatory scrutiny that will be required for the planned testing tasks, for example, as part of GLP-compliant animal studies, clinical trials or non-GLP-compliant animal studies, as well as for product release or in-process testing.

The primary objective of this chapter is to highlight current industry best practices in effecting successful method transfers for those carrying out ligand-binding assays in biological matrices, usually plasma or serum. In most instances, the data generated support pharmacokinetic and/or pharmacodynamic evaluations as part of the drug development process. However, the procedures and processes are applicable to any GXP environment; only the "acceptance" criteria will vary.

10.2 ESTABLISHING SUCCESSFUL WORKING RELATIONSHIPS BETWEEN LABORATORIES

Successful method transfer requires a good match of skills, experience, and team dynamics between the sending and receiving laboratories. If contract research organizations are involved, the initial selection step of a suitable contractor requires an evaluation of these compatibilities. However, if the transfer occurs within an organization or as part of already existing partnerships, the match between labs may be predetermined. In this section, criteria will be discussed that are essential for developing a good working relationship necessary for the method transfer, validation, and sample testing processes.

10.2.1 Finding the Right Match

When identifying suitable testing labs, the main emphasis should be on the method application requirements, for example, sample analysis for preclinical or clinical studies, testing in conformance with GLP guidelines and, last but not least, the extent and philosophy of method validation between the laboratories. The selection of a compatible laboratory as the receiving laboratory is pivotal to the success of the method transfer process.

It is important that a rapport is established between the receiving and sending laboratories, with respect to processes, procedures, culture, and personnel. Geography may play an important role, since communication in real time may be compromised if laboratories are several time zones apart.

A further complicating factor is the nature of the work to be undertaken. Where studies may be small in number, the relationship may be purely transactional, that is, analyses are carried out and reported on an ongoing basis according to a predefined plan. At the other extreme, the receiving lab, for example, CRO, may be integrated into the sending laboratory's operational plan for the development of one or more "drugs." With increasing complexity and breadth of service, it may be necessary to have a focal point of contact at both labs that can effectively and efficiently coordinate these activities. In contrast, at the purely transactional level, the interaction may simply be between the laboratory analysts.

A broad range of experience and expertise in ligand-binding assays for PK, biomarker, and immunogenicity applications is mostly found in larger companies. However, it is important that CRO in-house expertise is based on the latest trends in the field, that is, do they have an expert within their ranks that is in close communication with other leaders in the field? Although the sending lab may provide this expertise, it is important to be able to rely on the in-house expertise of CROs to accomplish the most straightforward approach to moving projects to completion. Such expertise can be evaluated, in part, by the contribution of the receiving laboratory's expert to conferences, white papers, and other publications.

10.2.2 Instrumentation and Data Systems

Compatibility of instruments is one of the criteria to be assessed early on to assure that assays can be transferred more reliably. Incubators, plate washers, and plate readers (including analysis software) are critical in assuring comparable method performance between laboratories. Ideally, sending and receiving labs should run their methods on equivalent equipment. If not, assay conditions may have to be adapted and the assay transfer could become significantly more cumbersome, requiring additional supportive partial validation.

In addition, availability of data collection and analysis systems or laboratory information management systems (LIMS), with or without a data analysis package, at the receiving laboratory will determine how assay analysis and data transfer can be accomplished. There is a significant chance that data analysis, processing systems and LIMS are different between laboratories. In these cases, comparability of the results from the data analysis should be verified early on. It should be determined whether the calibration curve algorithm is the same in both labs. If they are different, it needs to be verified that the data analysis leads to comparable results. It is also important that the data can be transferred between labs in a compatible format, for example, to allow transfer to an SAS database.

10.2.3 Quality Processes

Most testing labs will already have detailed mechanisms in place for sample and data handling, which are GLP-compliant based on a network of SOPs covering all aspects of GLPs. It is still important, however, that audits are carried out by the sending laboratory before final selection of a testing lab is made, to ensure that the GLP implementation, required instrumentation, handling of samples, and data are acceptable.

It is essential to ensure that acquisition and analysis of raw data occur in a well-controlled environment. For GLP, as well as GMP applications, validation of the required software or, at a minimum, a gap analysis covering the software application should be in place.

10.2.4 Management

For good communication and efficient progress, a well-functioning management team possessing compatible quality and service philosophy, experience and industry expertise, and maturity (years in industry and company, turnover rate at company) at the testing laboratory is important. At each level, from director to principal investigator or supervisor to lab technician, experience and competence should be assessed, by reviewing resumes and/or interviewing personnel during visits or by telephone.

Sponsors should request alerts about personnel changes and obtain resumes for new personnel. This becomes more important when dealing with new staff in the CRO or testing lab to assure that high quality is maintained.

10.2.5 Selecting a Testing (Receiving) Laboratory

Identification of CROs and other testing laboratories will include one or more of the following paths: selection based on past experiences, recommendations by colleagues and consultants, follow-up on recent nonsolicited contacts, or Internet searches. Although the first three choices are limited, they can save time in selecting a laboratory. While the Internet may provide a large number of unknown companies from which to select, this selection process can be time-consuming.

To identify the most suitable laboratory, it is necessary to send a questionnaire that addresses all of the topics mentioned above. Questions should cover the following areas:

- Size of the company (total number of employees, size (employees and space) of animal facilities (if relevant), LC/MS and/or ligand-binding assay groups, experience of management and lab technicians, and separation (or not) of development and testing teams),
- Turnover/retention record,
- Number of assay transfers per year per assay type (PK, biomarker, immunogenicity, and ELISAs),
- Number of clients (how many big and/or small clients),
- Lab instrumentation and software for data collection and analysis,
- Status of software validation (21 CFR Part 11 compliance),
- QC and QA functions,
- Preferred modes of communication with clients,
- Success rate for assay transfers and testing failure rates,
- Timelines for assay transfers and assay validations,
- Training and training records for technicians and management,
- Good and bad experiences with clients and resolution processes used,
- Lead times to project start.

When the pool of CROs has been reduced to the most promising candidates, RFPs (requests for prices) should be sent out to obtain information on cost.

It is recommended to summarize accumulated data on spreadsheets to evaluate testing labs by experience, throughput, dedication, reliability, and cost. The least expensive CRO is not necessarily the one with the best fit for your project.

After narrowing down the candidates to a very few, it is prudent to conduct an audit visit to further evaluate the prime candidates. At these visits, the main goal is to identify any red flags that could jeopardize the project, covering scientific expertise to regulatory compliance. Audits are covered in a later section of this chapter. At this stage it is useful to discuss the projects in more detail, which may require establishment of confidentiality agreements (CDAs). Sufficient time must be allowed for CDAs to be put in place and audits to be conducted in advance of the planned work.

During the lab selection process, it is not unusual for the sending lab to interview lab and managerial staff at the receiving lab who are likely to be involved in the client project. Focus should be on evaluation of the experience and expertise of the staff, such as how they handle troubleshooting, and their understanding of regulatory intricacies, as well as learning about the company philosophy as it applies to method development, validation, and troubleshooting.

10.2.6 Set Up of Contracts and Other Supporting Documents

As stated before, expectations and scope of transfer projects should be clearly defined to ensure a clear path toward the end goal, a successful method transfer. This is best accomplished by employing contracts, defining scope cost and protocols or plans that cover the content of the projects in detail and by defining the individual experiments, the specific goals for each experiment, and the project as a whole. For method transfer, the plan or protocol content will be covered in Section 10.3. Contracts should be specific from the perspectives of cost, timelines, and expected process, which will ensure that the project has an objective frame of reference.

Protocols and contracts may be subject to revision when project scope and directions change. Both should be adjusted as needed, perhaps less formally for protocol or plan changes, which can be done via amendments, e-mail directives, memoranda, and other means of documentation. In most cases, contracts, as legal instruments, require amendments defining changes of scope and the anticipated impact on timelines, cost, and resources with approval by both parties.

In the case of method transfer, contracts should include specific milestones defining successful completion of parts as well as the whole project. As a minimum, the contract should contain the number of experiments and documentation requirements for the method transfer results. In addition, early definition of criteria for success and failure of experiments and responsibilities for repeating failed experiments, sets the stage for a smoother process throughout the project. The contract should also state, as part of the deliverables, the level of documentation of method protocols and content of the final report.

In the case that qualification is included in the method transfer, the contract should contain an agreed list of all analytical characteristics to be addressed. Specific criteria for success and failure of qualification experiments should be agreed upon and described in a protocol. Responsibility for the cost of experimental repeats that are caused by "suspicious"/aberrant/anomalous results should be clarified. The criteria for defining anomalous results and how they would trigger repeat analysis should be well documented.

Other scenarios that could trigger expansion of work scope are changes in reagent batches, sample volume, matrix, and sample containers. The entire process can be resolved by addressing as many of these issues as possible at the earliest stage, specifying criteria, and agreeing to an objective process.

10.2.7 Setting Up Teams for Method Transfer and Beyond

Once the frame of reference in terms of contracts and other agreements is finalized, it becomes important to ensure that lines of communication are established. For smaller studies where only one analyst may be involved, direct communication with the bench analyst may be expected, while for bigger projects with multiple analysts, a focal point for communication is essential. For larger projects, teams on either side should consist of the following:

- A project manager keeping track of project progress and providing meeting minutes and action items.
- A technical lead with good understanding of the method technology.

- The lab technician to provide information on the ongoing experiments (receiving lab) or feedback on method peculiarities (sending lab).
- Occasionally, members from IT (information technologies) may participate when discussing database and other software compatibilities, as well as to secure data transfer between labs.
- Depending on circumstances, senior team members may participate if decisions on work scope, timelines, and resources have to be made or other method-related issues arise.

Speed of communication is the essence of success, and solving problems quickly to mutual satisfaction is essential to prevent stalling of a project. Establishing weekly updates, be they by e-mail or tele/video conference, can expedite the process until a "natural" routine develops. There should be an agreement on how much latitude/flexibility/discretion the sending lab is prepared to "delegate" to the receiving lab. Generally, the longer the relationships, the greater the degree of delegation.

10.3 METHOD TRANSFER

The method transfer process can represent a full gamut of scenarios. Method transfers can be straightforward if the method is robust, fully validated, and being transferred between experienced labs. At the other end of the range, transfer may occur between inexperienced labs with a method that is neither robust nor fully characterized or validated. Here, we present a set of recommendations that should help streamline and simplify such transfers and increase their success rate.

The intended use of a method plays a decisive role in scrutiny of transfer. This will depend on whether the transferred method needs to be qualified for non-GXP use or eventually be validated for use in a GXP environment (e.g., for release testing of drug substance or product, testing in support of toxicology studies, or clinical trials). For example, to transfer a method successfully for clinical testing, the method needs to be robust and exhibit characteristics that can be easily validated. Any weakness that could impact validation should send the method back to development.

Due to their important impact on product release and study analysis, validation of ligand-binding assays has been highly scrutinized. A great effort put into providing guidance for method validation over the last decade has led to a series of publications and guidance papers. Although one FDA's guidance document exists [1], significant contributions, more recently, have been made by the Crystal City lll [2] report. While the FDA guidance document [1] is the prime document, other publications [4,5] based on workshops present some industry consensus of thoughts as well as how to interpret the FDA's prime document. In summary, these papers should be taken into account when assessing the process for a method transfer. If full validation of a method is required for its intended purpose, the most relevant validation characteristics that could be impacted by method transfer to another lab should be tested early on during this transfer. These include precision and accuracy, sensitivity, and, above all, the shape and reproducibility of the standard curve.

When transferring methods that will eventually require validation for GXP applications, relevant expertise on the side of the receiving lab is desirable. Such expertise can assure that relevant method parameters are acceptably addressed during method transfer. Publications and guidelines provide a good path toward validation; however, there is some flexibility in the FDA guidance, and discussions are ongoing to establish the best criteria for assessing method performance.

Method transfer is the first step toward the end goal, that is, being able to use this method for testing at the appropriate level. However, this step sets the tone for the whole process. It is important to consider the following when initiating method transfer between labs:

1. Clear understanding of the status of the method and its intended use.
2. Spelled out milestones and goals for the completion of the projects.
3. An effective communication mechanism set ahead of project start.

In the following sections, we will cover these and other areas that we consider relevant for an efficient and successful transfer process.

10.3.1 Expectations of the Receiving and Sending Laboratories

To set the stage for a successful method transfer project, the development status of the method as well as its intended use must be well defined. Both will have an impact on the scope of work to be accomplished and can impact timeline and resources significantly. As such, it is important to share data on performance of the method to assess the status of the method at the beginning of the process. The less developed the method, the less reliable the estimates on required resources and time frames. One mistake often made is to force a method through transfer and validation although it may not be as robust as required for its desired application. This can lead to failure either during validation or later during a testing phase, constituting a catastrophic scenario. Any loss of time resulting from further development of the method and subsequent revalidation could have been minimized if this had been addressed early on.

As part of the method transfer, training of operators can be crucial and hence options for this should be discussed early on. Such training could be triggered if the transfer of the method does not go smoothly. Depending on the situation, it may be desirable to initiate training of the operators at the start of the project. It is feasible that certain method steps are more sensitive to operator manipulation, like plate washing, sample treatment, and sample dilution steps.

It should also be taken into account that CROs base their lab work, qualification, validation, and documentation on their historically developed systems, which may differ from those of the sending lab. Here, a good early understanding of the capabilities of the receiving lab should be established, and their impact on the transfer process evaluated. For example, availability of raw data based on the LIMS used, software versions, limitations based on 21 CFR Part 11-compliant software used, delays in reporting data due to internal reviews, and compatibility issues of software to share raw data need to be addressed. The receiving lab may not have implemented the newest software versions of databases or analysis software, since each upgrade requires revalidation of the software.

The number of experiments and the required time frame need to be determined early on in the method transfer process. Since CROs serve many clients in parallel, it is important to understand the time and resource demands on both sides. It is also important to set expectations for communication of anticipated delays from either side. Frequency of project updates need to be agreed upon. The level of review by the sending lab should be aligned with the expertise of the receiving lab and may require compromises to allow efficient progress on the project. To cover all aspects of the project, it is best to document scope of work and expectations before initiating the transfer.

Availability and choice of instrumentation and how use of different equipment could affect assay performance need to be discussed. Definitions of experimental and storage conditions, reagent sources and quality, and lab personnel experiences should be discussed early on. This also applies to the process of assigning expiry dates, assessment of reagent stability, reagent handling, and shipping processes.

Method transfer to an internal quality control unit could also be challenging, facing the tendency to streamline, simplify, and generalize methods where possible. This could apply to choice of reagents, handling and storage of samples, cleaning procedures, and material resources. Before starting the transfer, there should be discussions on whether and for which steps or reagents alternatives may be considered. Any changes to the method at this time should be investigated as part of the method transfer, for example, including side-by-side comparison of the original method with the modified one. Even if a change appears to be minor, it could balloon into a large problem if it unexpectedly affects the method performance.

10.3.2 Setting Up a Transfer Protocol

A lot of effort is invested at the beginning of the project in defining the scope of work and expectations for transfer completion. This is best covered in a document defining the scope and goal of the method transfer, the regulatory standard to be applied (e.g., following GLP or not), experimental outline, acceptance criteria for assay performance, and transfer or development summary or report. It is useful to spend some time on such a protocol to reduce the risk of misunderstanding and to assure that expectations from both sides match.

These protocols should include a description of the assay, including, for example, range of standard curve, number and level of QCs, number of replicates for standards, controls and samples, dilution schemes, and source of matrix. Assessment of method characteristics, such as precision, accuracy, and selectivity, including number of assays to be run, number of QCs, and number of individual matrix samples and spikes with test agent and spiking level(s) should be addressed. This also includes the definition of cut point for immunogenicity assays and its calculation formula, source of anti-product antibodies (monoclonal, polyclonal, and derived from a specific species), and design of the confirmatory assay. For determining equivalence of methods, study design and choice(s) of statistical analysis should be specified in the transfer protocol.

In the case of commercial kits, comparison of kit and reagent lots should be addressed early on and, due to cost, the scope and goal of the transfer and development should be clearly defined. For example, use of additional or modified controls, modified standard curves, and sample treatment options (dilution scheme, assessment of minimal required dilution depending on matrix concentration) should be included.

The transfer protocol should be approved by both sides. If changes to the protocol or plan occur, they should be noted and be approved by both sides. For the purpose of the method transfer and development, such a protocol should be seen as a living document that should be used as guidance and not "set in stone." Any summary or report written afterward should address changes to the original protocol and reasons for such changes.

If method transfers between partners are happening frequently, the design of the protocol and follow-up report may follow a routine format and be relatively minimal. However, for a first transfer between parties, such protocols and reports will be valuable for evaluating the efficiency of the process and potential issues that may occur during method transfer and will help alleviate problems in future method transfer projects.

10.3.3 Experimental Design and Analysis

The design of the transfer experiments should be carried out with an understanding of how the data are going to be analyzed. The results generated need to be evaluated against set criteria, for example, standard curve performance, evaluation of variability, accuracy, or specificity. Consideration should also be given to what type of samples should be used for the comparison, that is, plain controls and spiked or incurred samples, and whether any of these samples should be blinded. Gilbert et al. [6] discuss strategies for performing cross-validation experiments using prepared biological samples of known concentration (spiked) and incurred samples from clinical trials. Similar schemes can be evaluated during method transfer. In many cases, controls are used to assess accuracy; however, blinded samples provide a higher level of scrutiny of the receiving lab's performance.

The use of incurred samples should be taken into consideration if they are likely to behave differently from spiked samples. Use of pooled, incurred samples eliminates spiking errors and minimizes the impact of spiking solvents and buffers that can cause differences in binding to endogenous proteins. If such interactions are considered likely, it should be demonstrated that the methods compare acceptably for both spiked controls and incurred samples.

Statistical evaluation should be considered, from its simplest form of assessment of the precision and accuracy to complex statistical analysis, as discussed by Kringle et al. [7]. Although Kringle's focus is on methods for analysis of pharmaceutical formulations, his application of statistics could be expanded to ligand-binding assays. He concludes that the acceptability of two methods should be evaluated using equivalence testing rather than difference testing. This approach determines "the amount of difference in true means between sites that would be considered 'analytically important' by the analyst." A similar approach has been discussed by Hartmann [8].

The recommended procedure involves the comparison of observed bias and precision with predefined acceptance limits. However, to better define the sources of variation, Kringle et al. [7] recommend the need to analyze on multiple days with different analysts and different equipment. Ideally, the process should take place in the sending and receiving lab at the same time to minimize temporal changes. These requirements are not always possible when carrying out pharmacokinetic assays. Therefore, pragmatic use of acceptance criteria may be necessary. In addition to those processes described above, the student t-test is widely used. It should, however, be used with caution. It carries the assumption that the variance of the two labs is similar, which is not always the case. The use of the point t-test is further confounded by the fact that a comparison of poorly run tests may pass, while highly precise results generated in either lab can reveal statistically significant differences that may be practically irrelevant. Therefore, statistical analysis requires rigorous review to assess its relevance, that is, that it is "fit for purpose."

If the data are not acceptable, it is essential that an investigation is carried out to determine the source of the difference, for example, which data are "wrong" and why. The SOPs to be used to carry out this investigation, whether those of the sending or receiving lab or a composite SOP, should be agreed upon during the "set-up" phase.

10.3.4 Transfer Issues

Law [9] defines some "typical" problems encountered with ligand-binding assays, such as loss of binding, shifted calibration curves, contamination issues, and changes in precision and limits of detection, but potential problems are by no means limited to these issues. For example, there may be subtle procedural changes that have been overlooked in the method documentation that are not performed consistently. There may be minimum or critical freeze–thaw and standing times for matrix/QC samples that allow equilibration to take place prior to analysis. This is particularly important if serum-binding proteins or receptors for the analyte are known or suspected. It can be anticipated that length of mixing or vortexing as well as the mixing equipment used can be influential. Although the same model of equipment may be available throughout the world, small differences in specification may cause problems in method transfer. Thus, differences in local voltage may mean a different specification motor is installed, resulting in arbitrary "speed"/mixing settings that are not comparable with shakers of the same make sold in different parts of the world. In some cases, the problem may be solved only after lengthy troubleshooting, including visits by the analyst from the sending lab to the receiving lab, and observing that the speed of rotation for the same setting was slower.

Preparation of control samples may lead to problems if the volume or the order or speed of addition is changed. This can be particularly important where addition of small volumes of spiking solvent can cause localized protein precipitation and localized adsorption and/or entrapment of the drug, resulting in lack of homogeneity.

Changes in lab temperature, even in air-conditioned labs, by up to 5°C, depending upon the time of day (or night) may have an impact on method performance. Use of the term "ambient temperature" is fraught with problems. We recommend that the receiving lab monitor lab temperature to determine whether temperature may contribute to method variability, or at least an understanding of the impact of temperature changes is determined at the development stage.

Similarly, environmental or seasonal changes may have an impact, where the routine use of local microenvironments during incubation steps has been found to be essential. In such cases, there may be a requirement for using incubators that are capable of maintaining constant "ambient" temperatures. Such anecdotal issues can be used to develop a checklist that can be used for future method evaluations and/or troubleshooting.

When issues arise with the performance of the method during the transfer, troubleshooting should be coordinated through both teams (sending and receiving labs). Troubleshooting guidelines are discussed subsequently.

10.4   MONITORING THE METHOD TRANSFER PROCESS

Monitoring the method transfer process is a necessity for both the sending and the receiving labs. The most important things to keep track of are the progress of the transfer process and the agreed-upon schedule. Depending on the experience of the sending and the receiving labs, the monitoring process could be more or less stringent. If this transfer is the first between the two labs, then the monitoring may include timely evaluation of transfer experiments, frequent communication via telephone or e-mail, in addition to the regularly occurring conference calls, and immediate troubleshooting if the transfer does not proceed as planned.

All of these activities should be defined and mechanisms established to allow the monitoring process to occur smoothly. Some of the details of the monitoring process may not be included in the transfer plan directly, but should be documented as part of meeting minutes or notes.

In the following sections, important steps in the monitoring process will be discussed in more detail, including evaluation of experiments and their data, impact of experiment failures on timelines, communication of changes in personnel and schedule on either side, and changes in the scope of the agreed-upon transfer work.

10.4.1   Evaluation of Experimental Data

The first experiments may be the most challenging during a method transfer. They can test the effectiveness of the established communication processes and can reveal immediate transfer problems. Data review by the sending lab will be crucial in identifying transfer problems early on. Reduced or increased signal strength, slope changes, and standard curve shifts can indicate suboptimal method performance.

Other warning signs are change or inconsistency in assay background or curve performance between assays.

Evaluation of experimental data can be done on raw data as well as analyzed data. For the transfer of raw data, it will be essential to have compatible software in both labs, which may require in many cases the same version numbers to be able to send back and forth experimental data. For example, a good comparison of data can be established if the standard (calibration) curves can be overlaid and differences in signal or shift of the curves can be visualized.

In addition, tabulated data from calibration curves, precision and accuracy data sets, selectivity experiments (spiking of matrices from individual sources), and baseline evaluations (for cut point analysis) will provide valuable information on method performance and should be compared with similar data sets from the sending lab.

Data analysis and review need to be well planned to minimize effect on the timeline. When discussing the monitoring strategies, it should be made clear that both labs have responsibility for timely communication back and forth to enable the project to go forward as scheduled.

Receiving labs with in-depth experience in the method to be transferred may propose to run the transfer relatively independently and communicate results on an as-needed basis, for example, weekly, or after a milestone has been reached.

To capture the whole path of a method transfer, all experiments, including failed experiments, as well as the troubleshooting experiments, should be included in a final report. If no final report is being provided, then meeting minutes or at least summaries of troubleshooting events should be generated to document essential findings, which eventually could have value in helping troubleshoot assay problems in the future.

10.4.2 Impact of Experimental Failures on the Method Transfer Timeline

Any experimental failures can be expected to have an impact on the method transfer schedule. Therefore, experimental failures should be communicated and addressed immediately. It should be expected that the receiving lab provides well-organized data or reasonable explanations for the failure(s) and provides scenarios for follow-up experiments to resolve the failure and rerun the experiment successfully. If the experimental failure requires troubleshooting, it is recommended to set up a trouble-shooting team that contains analysts, PIs, and project managers from both teams, who jointly develop troubleshooting strategies and review progress in an agreed-upon time frame. They also need to assess impact of the troubleshooting event on resource, timelines, and cost.

10.4.3 Changes in Personnel and Schedule

Both the sending as well as the receiving lab should communicate changes in personnel that could impact the transfer project. This should also include changes in control of QA, QC, and higher level positions with direct effect on the transfer team of the receiving lab. Depending on the circumstances, new personnel may join a conference call to acquaint the teams with their roles with respect to the ongoing project(s).

Changes in schedule can be caused by many different circumstances, for example, changes in priority by either party, personnel changes, illness, and assay failures and required troubleshooting efforts. Any changes in schedule should be decided upon by the joint transfer teams, and a new schedule should be agreed upon by both parties. Any loss in transfer time may require reassessment of the effort to be spent on the project and changes to the scope of the transfer.

10.4.4   Changes in Scope

A significant change in scope for a transfer project may occur when the initial method transfer fails and either training of personnel at the receiving lab is required or additional method development needs to be initiated. Any additional experiments represent a change in work scope, and should be clearly spelled out and added to the method transfer plan.

10.5   AUDITING CROs

In general, there are several stages in the relationship where the client may want to inspect a CRO, these are,

- Preagreement facility audit or due diligence to determine if the lab is fit for purpose. This is usually carried out by the sending lab's QA unit, although sometimes they may be accompanied by the relevant lab scientist.
- Project-specific inspection carried out when there is an ongoing relationship. The facility audit has usually been carried out previously, so the objective of this is to ensure the current project is within the capabilities of the operation.
- Poststudy inspection is where the sending lab wants to satisfy itself as to the integrity of data with respect to data trails, decisions made regarding choice of data reported for repeat analysis, and to investigate any unusual observations.

The emphasis in these inspections is on ensuring that the receiving lab complies with the appropriate GXP, if required, and is scientifically qualified and experienced to conduct the work requested using appropriately qualified and trained staff.

These inspections usually follow a standard format that is well documented and is similar in all regulated laboratories. The emphasis is on ensuring that there are well-controlled processes and that these are adhered to during the study. One of the major areas of concern is instrumentation, with focus on essential maintenance and routine calibration. The depth of the inspection can vary ranging from the extensive to the basic. Thus, for maintenance, it may only be necessary to ensure that maintenance was carried out at prescribed intervals (as covered in relevant SOPs) and was authorized and confirmed by the lab's representative at the time. At the other extreme, auditors may require evidence of the "engineer's" competence, for example, access to training records and/or confirmation that his/her employer is a member of a relevant recognized quality system, for example, ISO.

There are almost as many interpretations of regulatory requirements as there are different levels of inspection. Sending labs may have their own preferred options that may or may not be easy for the receiving lab to implement. Where the sending lab's QA unit has deemed the receiving labs to be in compliance, it is usually better to let the receiving lab adhere to their idiosyncratic practices to minimize errors. Where these practices are not GXP compliant, obviously, changes must be made before any work can commence.

10.5.1 Sample Transport and Integrity and Data Systems

Most receiving labs will have a prescribed format as to how samples should be transported consistent with IATA (International Air Transport Association) rules. The essential part of this requires the packer to be trained to IATA standards. The documentation from the receiving lab should define package type and required amount of dry ice to sample ratio (based on the expected duration of transport).

Labeling to identify destination address and, where appropriate, customs agents at the destination airport is required. If samples are of animal origin, specifically those covered by CITES (Convention on International Trade in Endangered Species), it is essential that clearance is obtained from both the sending and receiving countries' relevant authorities. Without this, delays will ensue and more than likely samples will be compromised.

It is pivotal to ensure that the receiving site has facilities and trained personnel capable of handling samples out of normal business hours, that is, particularly weekends. They should know how, where, and under what conditions the samples should be stored before they can be individually logged in.

The sample accession/logging in process should be secure, that is, there should be no possibility that samples received from outside "labs" will be left at the wrong temperature for extended periods of time. The sample identity should be unique and trackable. The storage facilities must be qualified and fully documented, that is, temperature probes are monitored continuously and calibrated against internationally accepted standards.

Data systems compatibility is an essential component of this process. This is especially important when sharing data between labs. The receiving lab should be able to format the data in a manner acceptable to the sending lab's "data" systems. This can range from identifying each sample with a unique single "number" to one that requires the inputting of multiple lines of demographic data. While the receiving lab might be able to commit to the complexity of inputting multiple demographics, the implications of multiple entries could be immense, for example, increased chances of input errors requiring additional auditing cycles. The ideal scenario is to assign a unique identifier with the demographics early on in the process so that the demographics follow the identifier wherever the sample goes.

LIMS and/or other data processing systems should be validated and be in compliance with 21 CFR Part 11. If not, a gap analysis should be carried out to understand any limitations. Compliant systems only exist if they are fully validated by the user.

In addition, for full compliance, the analysts should be fully trained in the use of the data system and processing procedures, and their training records should reflect this. Their status on the organogram should be appropriate for the actions and responsibilities they will have for this study.

10.5.2 Project-Specific Inspection

Project-specific inspections are usually carried out by the "relevant" scientists from the sending lab and are usually a follow-up to the general facilities audit that precedes the implementation of a specific project. A growing, but not yet dominant, trend is for the sending lab representative to "interview" the scientists at the receiving lab—in informal discussion. The objective is to identify a "compatible" study director as well as analysts on a personal basis. In addition, it is essential to identify the study director's competencies with respect to the specific project in terms of their CV and training records.

10.5.3 Poststudy Inspection

The main rationale for a poststudy inspection is to confirm that the study was carried out to GXP and to the agreed plan, including all set criteria and specifications. The depth of this inspection can vary, ranging from confirmation of audit trail (sample integrity to final results) to evaluation of "exceptions," that is, what decisions were made when repeat analyses were carried out, what triggered the repeat, were there appropriate SOPs, and were they followed. If there were exceptions not covered by SOPs, were decisions made objectively and consistently? How much decision making was automated, for example, if repeat analyses were carried out, was a decision tree used, and if so, was this automated or manually applied? If automated computerized systems are used, any manual intervention should arouse suspicion. In such a case, the level of auditing should be raised.

10.6 METHOD TROUBLESHOOTING

A method breakdown can happen any time, often when least expected. In most cases, a method failure is indicated by "unexpected" results. However, it may also happen that method breakdown occurs gradually, and identifying such an assay failure is not trivial. Therefore, it may take several assay runs before a method failure becomes obvious. In such a case, it is important to identify method failure early on, to prevent excessive reanalysis of test samples or significant repeats of experiments that are part of method transfer or validation.

When assay results are deemed anomalous, an investigation should be initiated. In many cases, troubleshooting will be required to get the method back on track.

An important aspect of the investigation and the troubleshooting process is documentation. All activities, starting with initiation of the troubleshooting process and ending with a summary of the outcome of the investigation, should be thoroughly documented. This allows reviewers, not familiar with the method failure event, to understand what the failure was and how it was investigated and what the outcome of the investigation was. This will also be of value for resolution of future assay and method issues since they may be related to this earlier investigation.

Method failures can, of course, occur at any stage in the progression from transfer to validation to sample testing. Therefore, the troubleshooting process discussed in this chapter applies to any of these stages.

10.6.1 Identification of Method Failures and Trending of Assay Performance

Method failures may be easily identified if significant changes in the regular assay performance occur, for example, changes in plate background or changes in standard signals. Such failures may require an investigation after just one failed assay. Method failures could be more difficult to identify and describe if there is a gradual shift in performance, for example, if controls fail at an increased frequency or if variability in the assay is increased to an unacceptable degree. In such cases, method failure may become obvious only after several assays have been run.

For early identification of method failures, trending of assay performance markers can help tremendously. Besides monitoring control values and variability between replicates, following other criteria, for example, assay background, standard signal levels and percent recoveries for lower and upper limits of quantification, and standard curve parameters (e.g., for four-parameter fit calculations), allows evaluation of the method performance over time. Trending should be established early on and include transfer, qualification, validation, and testing runs. This becomes especially important if assays are run over several years using the same method, for example, for product release or clinical trials. Trending should be done by the testing labs, but may also be conducted by the sending lab, for example, if several testing labs are contributing to the data set.

10.6.2 Steps in the Investigation and Troubleshooting Process

Formal initiation of a failure investigation should be based on a well-controlled process defined by SOP or company guidelines. This requires documentation using worksheets or forms to be completed manually or electronically using LIMS or electronic lab notebooks. These forms should contain a section for description of the occurred failure and a preliminary action plan.

The first step in the investigation and troubleshooting process is the formal description of the observed assay failure, which serves as the justification for the investigation. Building on the failure description, a proposal for proceeding through the investigation should be generated. It can be expected that this initial plan will likely change due to findings during the investigation. Therefore, the investigation process should include reassessment of potential root causes after each experiment. Ideally, each experiment should be justified by the outcome of experiments performed before, and each experiment should be followed up with a conclusion that will move the investigation process forward. The investigation will be closed after the root cause has been identified. In general, a root cause may be identified and confirmed by a sequence of 5–10 experiments. However, in some cases, a root cause may not be identified although the method performs well again. Either way, the closure of the investigation should follow a predefined process. The investigation should be summarized, the root cause (if identified) described, and recommendations for preventing reoccurrence of the same failure provided. To finalize the investigation, teams from both labs should give approval to this document.

The first part of the investigation should evaluate the most obvious causes, for example, documented operator mistakes, erroneous dilution calculations, use of wrong reagents, the omission of a method step, or selection of wrong wavelengths for measurement. If no obvious errors can be identified, all information about the failed assays, as well as bracketing well-performing assays, should be assembled and listed. This list can then be used to identify whether a compromised reagent or method step could have been the cause for assay failure. Of course, assay performance could also be affected by unsuspecting changes in assay steps, for example, incubations, reagent and matrix mixing, pipetting, and dilution schemes. This information should help in identifying root causes and contribute to the design of experiments to solve the method failure at hand.

At the conclusion of the investigation, a summary report should be prepared that contains the experimental strategy and data. Such a report may be reviewed by QA at the validation and especially at the GLP testing stage and QA's approval may be part of the investigation process. For investigations during validation or testing, procedures should be in place to guide the troubleshooting process. It is appropriate that recommendations for modifications of methods or changes in training should be reviewed and approved by QA.

Troubleshooting taking place during method transfer will require less oversight by QA. However, any changes from the original method should be documented. If the method is to be run in parallel at different labs, any proposed changes should be cleared with the other labs involved to ensure that these changes can be implemented at the other labs and that the changes do not interfere with the already established performance of the method.

10.6.3 Developing Hypotheses and Designing Troubleshooting Experiments

Hypotheses to explain method failures will be based on available facts. Therefore, it is of advantage to gather as much information as possible about the failed assays, as well as assays that performed well, to narrow down potential causes for the failures. Creating tables containing, for example, information on all reagents and buffers (and their lot numbers), disposables, assay conditions for each step, operators, and instruments, is a first step in identifying potential culprits. Based on the nature of the failure, deductions can be made with respect to the cause of the failure, for example, if controls fail, signals change (high or low), variability increases, or standard curves shift. Increased control failure could indicate instability; signal changes could point at changes in enzyme activity or substrate. If variability increases, coating, washing, or pipetting steps could have contributed. Standard shifts may be caused by changes in the critical assay reagents.

Depending on the hypothesis, experiments are designed to either confirm or eliminate causes from the working list. If assay conditions, reagents, or reagent lots are changed, it is important to run the original conditions as well as the original reagents in parallel to be able to see differences. Therefore, only one condition or reagent at a time should be changed to be able to assign any observed changes in results to a specific condition or reagent change. This may require more experiments or larger experiment sizes. Having several operators to help in the troubleshooting could move the process along. In some cases, it may be useful to run experiments in parallel in both labs. The quality of the evaluation will be enhanced if both labs participate in the analysis. Both labs should provide new designs for experiments, and they should be finalized via conference calls or other communication paths.

Troubleshooting plans should have clear timelines to keep the project moving forward at full speed. Early agreement has to be in place on how to keep the project on track and how the communication during the troubleshooting phase should be structured. Results need to be reviewed in a timely manner and between conference calls and transfer of raw data together with data tables should be the first priority for the receiving lab. Clearly, a quick response to the data packages by the sending lab is also essential to move resolution of the issue forward.

After identification of a root cause, it is important to determine whether any assay runs besides the obvious failures may be affected. Depending on the investigation outcome, validity of these assays should be reassessed and the outcome documented well.

10.6.4 Corrective Action

The result of the investigation should be the identification of a root cause and a proposal for the elimination of this root cause in future testing. This could include change of storage conditions and reagent or sample handling (to increase stability), changes or clarifications to certain method steps (pipetting, dilutions, and mixing), tightening of incubation conditions (time and temperature by using incubators), choice of materials (selection and screening of reagent lots, e.g., antibodies, BSA, Tween, and microtiter plates), and precoating of boats and tips.

In case of operator mistakes or instrument failures, changes in the method may or may not be required to prevent future assay failures. In many cases, retraining may be the best solution.

If the root cause is not identifiable, the outcome of the troubleshooting may just include recommendations for minimizing this failure by adding certain precautions or additional training, for example, training in pipetting and generation of dilutions in a more reproducible way, or clarifying mixing steps by adding more detailed information on mixing conditions.

10.7 SECRETS OF SUCCESSFUL METHOD TRANSFER

One of the major contributors to success is for the sending and receiving laboratories to develop a rapport—understanding one another's strengths and weaknesses. This can only be achieved in an honest, open relationship where there is mutual respect between the groups, along with a "can-do" approach. A good relationship can be enhanced by direct face-to-face meetings, either during an audit or at conferences, and should be encouraged.

The method transfer project should be embedded in a functional network of documents governing the process, from contract to protocols to final report. In combination with a well-defined communication process ensuring timely follow-up and effective monitoring, the path toward successful completion of a transfer project should be set. It is important to cover expectations and requirements from both labs early on, including intended use of the method, status of the method at time of transfer, equipment requirements, capabilities, personnel, and training. This also includes clearly defined goals, milestones, and acceptance criteria that help guide the project along to completion.

There are also apparently minor, but important, things to keep in mind that can help keep the transfer process moving smoothly:

- Never assume processes in other labs will be the same as in your lab, and never be afraid to ask what may appear to be simplistic questions.
- Communicate concerns that could influence timelines or quality of a project early on, for example, clear expectations on availability, shipments, and quality of reagents.
- Account for vacations and other leaves, and assure that there is a backup plan to keep the project moving.
- Be aware of obstacles that can slow down progress, for example, incompatibilities of materials, equipment, and software, which may require method adjustments and make the data review cumbersome.
- Account for reviewing time in other departments on either side, for example, quality checking of data and QA review of SOPs, protocols, and reports, as well as legal and financial departments addressing contract and cost issues.

When things go awry, for example, failures occurring during method transfer, apply enough resources to the project to allow efficient and timely troubleshooting. Consider early on in the project whether sending an analyst for training and helping in troubleshooting may eventually be more time-saving and cost-effective than a long and protracted investigation.

As part of the process of method transfer and troubleshooting methods, the production of some form of checklist or *aide-memoire* of historical issues should be developed to ensure history is not repeated. Problem-solving and method-development "tricks" should not rely on the memory of the senior analysts but should be recorded for posterity.

ACKNOWLEDGMENTS

The authors acknowledge the input and experiences of colleagues past and present who have been involved as part of receiving or sending lab teams.

REFERENCES

1. Food and Drug Administration (2001) *Guidance for Industry: Bioanalytical Method Validation.* U.S. Department of Health and Human Services, Food and Drug Administration, Center for Drug Evaluation and Research, Rockville, MD.

2. Viswanathan, C.T., Bansal, S., Booth, B., DeStefano, A.J., Rose, M.J., Sailstad, J., Shah, V. P., Skelly, J.P., Swann, P.G., and Weiner, R. (2007) Workshop/conference report— quantitative bioanalytical methods validation and implementation: best practices for chromatographic and ligand binding assays. *The AAPS Journal*, **9**, E30–E42.

3. International Society of Pharmaceutical Engineers *Good Practice Guide: Technology Transfer*, 2003.

4. Miller, K.J., Bowsher, R.R., Celniker, A., Gibbons, J, Gupta, S., Lee, J.W., Swanson, S.J., Smith, W.C., Weiner, R.S., Crommelin, D.J.A., Das, I., DeSilva, B.S., Dillard, R. F., Geier, M., Gunn, H., Kahn, M.N., Knuth, D.W., Kunitani, M., Nordblum, G.D., Paulussen, R.J.A., Sailstad, J.M., Tacey, R.L, and Watson, A., (2001) Workshop on bioanalytical methods validation for macromolecules: summary report. *Pharmaceutical Research*, **18**, 1373–1383.

5. DeSilva, B., Smith, W., Weiner, R., Kelley, M., Smolec, J., Lee, B., Kahn, M., Tacey, R., Hill, H., and Celniker, A., (2003) Recommendations for the bioanalytical method validation of ligand binding assays to support pharmacokinetic assessments of macromolecules. *Pharmaceutical Research*, **20**, 1885–1900.

6. Gilbert, G. T., Barinov-Colligon, I., and Mikisic, J.R., (1995) Cross-validation of bioanalytical methods between laboratories. *Journal of Pharmaceutical and Biomedical Chromatography*, **13**, 385–394.

7. Kringle, R., Khan-Malek, R., Snikeris, F., Munden, P., Agut, C., and Bauer, M.A., (2001) Unified approach for the design and analysis of transfer studies for analytical methods. *Drug Information Journal*, **35**, 1271–1288.

8. Hartmann, C., Smeyers-Verbeke, J., Penninckx, W., Heyden, Y.V., Vankeerberghen, P., and Massart, D.L., (1995) Reappraisal of hypothesis testing for method validation: detection of systematic error by comparing the means of two methods or two laboratories. *Analytical Chemistry*, **67**, 4491–4499.

9. Law, B. (ed.) (1996) *Immunoassay: A Practical Guide*. Taylor & Francis, London.

CHAPTER 11

Application of Automation in Ligand-Binding Assays

CHRIS MORROW

Genentech, South San Francisco, CA, USA

11.1 INTRODUCTION

Laboratories that run ligand-binding assays in support of clinical and nonclinical studies face ever-increasing pressure to analyze more samples with fewer resources in less time. Data quality and regulatory compliance requirements can limit a laboratory's ability to increase process efficiency. In this arena, laboratory automation is a tool that has the potential to greatly reduce the time and effort required to analyze samples [1]. Automation can also increase data quality and regulatory compliance and reduce repetitive strain injuries and exposure to hazardous materials. For this reason, many laboratories have begun implementing automated systems to run ligand-binding assays. Due to the high barriers to entry into automation (particularly, cost and regulatory compliances) and the relative lack of turnkey solutions, there is a wide variance in how these systems are implemented. This chapter elucidates some basic strategies for approaching ligand-binding assay automation as well as discussing specific systems. In the end, each laboratory must itself implement automated systems as per its specific needs; what follows in this chapter may serve as a useful starting point.

Laboratory automation can produce real gains in efficiency and throughput. If not done well, it also has the potential of wasting large sums of money and distracting a laboratory from its core mission. Laboratory automation is nothing more than a tool; if it is implemented properly to solve the right problem, the benefits can be substantial. If it is not implemented in the right way or if it is applied to the wrong problem, there may be no benefit at all. Therefore, laboratory automation should be viewed as one of

Ligand-Binding Assays: Development, Validation, and Implementation in the Drug Development Arena. Edited by Masood N. Khan and John W.A. Findlay
Copyright © 2010 John Wiley & Sons, Inc.

the many tools available to a laboratory. As with any tool, it must be carefully chosen to solve a specific problem. Once a clear problem has been identified, it is important to follow an organized and methodical approach to successfully implement an automation project.

The focus of this chapter is on automating ligand-binding assays in support of clinical and nonclinical studies. This chapter will not specifically address laboratory software systems or LIMS, although many of the tools for implementing laboratory automation can be applied to these systems as well.

11.1.1 Why Regulated Ligand-Binding Automation is Unique

Good laboratory practice (GLP) ligand-binding automation has several unique characteristics. The first is regulatory compliance. Automation projects are complex by their very nature; by adding GLP [2] and 21 CFR Part 11 [3] requirements and the need for validation, the projects become orders of magnitude more complex [4]. The resources required for configuration and validation can significantly increase the cost of a system. The second factor that makes this type of automation unique is the diverse skill sets required to successfully implement an automated system. Required skills include knowledge of assays and lab processes, familiarity with computer programming, liquid handling, technical writing, understanding of 21 CFR Part 11 and GLP regulations, computer system validation, and project management. Above all, laboratory automation requires creativity to envision a system and overcome the inevitable obstacles that arise in the course of implementation. The third factor that makes GLP automation unique is the relative lack of turnkey solutions. There are many vendors offering automated systems for clinical labs (e.g., in a hospital setting) and for high-throughput screening applications, but few that specifically target GLP ligand-binding assays. The result of this is that the laboratory must play a much greater role in implementing systems that were originally designed for research or clinical environments. Finally, GLP automation is unique in that it includes a wide range of processes and procedures to ensure regulatory compliance. It is not sufficient to simply get a system to work properly; processes must be put in place for troubleshooting, end user training, problem reporting, securing data storage, and change control. Therefore, when we speak of automated GLP "systems," we mean much more than just hardware and software.

11.1.2 An Example of What Can Go Wrong

Before beginning the discussion of how to implement an automation project, it is helpful to first look at an example of what can go wrong. This example is all too familiar: A laboratory manager decides to increase the use of automation tools. A scientist is asked to automate LBAs. After meeting with several vendors, a system is chosen and purchased with only a vague idea of how it will actually function. The system is very expensive and the vendor seems very responsive, so everyone assumes that they are on the right track. The system is installed in the lab and a couple of lab personnel (whose education, experience, and aptitude are in biochemistry, not in automation) are assigned to get the system working. The vendor starts configuring the system and some issues start to surface. Perhaps it can only run four plates per run, or it cannot save data files in a format compatible with the lab's LIMS. The lab goes back and purchases additional peripherals or software and the vendor gets back to work. After a few weeks or months, the vendor turns the system over to the users. Several problems appear: the vendor only programmed the system to process one assay, and no one really knows how to program another assay protocol. What is worse is that the results of the automated assay do not match the manual assay. After several months of frustration, management starts to wonder why they are not seeing returns on their investment. The vendor is called back who explains that the commitment was fulfilled and the system does everything it was supposed to. At this point, a small project team is formed to work through the issues. At every turn, they find unanticipated problems: their assays are not sufficiently standardized for one automation process, or they see that carryover is affecting their assay, or they find that computer programming skills are required to make the system do what they want. Soon, other lab personnel start wondering why they bought such an expensive piece of junk. After many more months of work, the team finally gets the system up and running, often after major process reengineering and scaling back to the original system requirements. At this point, the validation group is brought in to validate the system. They immediately find that the system does not meet some key 21 CFR Part 11 requirements. The team goes back to the drawing board and reconfigures the system, or pays the vendor even more money to create a custom application that meets regulatory requirements. Once this is completed, the team realizes that they need to create processes for calibration, assay incorporation, and training for users and administrators. This delays the project another 3 months. The system finally goes live several years after it was purchased. The team is justifiably proud of their accomplishments, but they soon discover another problem: no one wants to use the system. Other scientists in the lab have serious doubts about the ability of the system to generate good data or have heard so many bad things about the system that they would not touch it. At this point, the system is either left idle in the corner of the lab or the team attempts to create a strategy to prove the system's worth. The net result is a system that cost much more than originally budgeted, required much more resources than planned, does not function as originally intended, and is underutilized.

Although this is obviously an extreme example, every company has encountered at least one of these obstacles and many first automation projects end up running into many of these roadblocks. The root causes of the above problems can be summarized as follows:

- Failure to create detailed requirements prior to purchase
- Insufficient thought given to standardizing lab processes
- Insufficient skills of project team
- Failure to manage the expectations of end users
- Insufficient attention to processes for the use and maintenance of the system
- Failure to apply project management principles

11.2 IMPLEMENTING AUTOMATED SYSTEMS

11.2.1 Phases of an Automation Project

To avoid these problems, an automation project must be planned and executed in an orderly manner. A GLP automation project can be broken down into the following general phases:

1. Defining a problem statement
2. Forming a project team
3. Requirements
4. System selection and purchase
5. Setup and configuration
6. Complying with 21 CFR Part 11
7. System qualification
8. Documentation
9. Validation
10. System rollout
11. Ongoing maintenance

Each phase will be discussed in further detail below.

11.2.1.1 Defining a Problem Statement The first step in successfully implementing an automation project is to clearly define the problem that needs to be solved. Automation can solve a number of different problems. Each laboratory must ask itself which specific problems it wants to solve. The best place to start is in thinking about the needs of the laboratory. Is there a need to analyze more samples with fewer people or to shorten sample turnaround time? Is there a need to increase the consistency of an assay or process? Is there a need to reduce exposure to hazardous materials or to minimize operator fatigue or repetitive motion injuries? Is there a need to reduce the cost per sample? Is there a need for a process to run overnight or over the weekend?

The answers to these and other questions determine the approach that will be taken at every subsequent stage of the project, so it is critical that sufficient attention is given to this step [5,6]. For a first automation project, it is recommended to choose one or two primary goals. Once the system is successfully implemented, work can begin on the others. If a laboratory already has a solid track record with automation, then it may be appropriate to set a loftier goal.

Most laboratory managers will have an intuitive sense of which problems need attention. Nevertheless, it is a good idea to solicit feedback from other members of the laboratory, if for no other reason than to give people at all levels in the organization a common understanding of what is needed. It is recommended to document this problem statement so that it will be clear in the future what the goal is. Note that at this point it is not necessarily an automation project—it is only a problem statement. In the

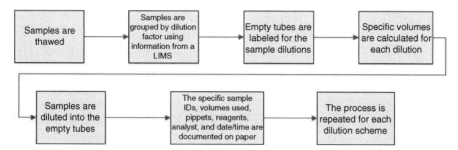

FIGURE 11.1   As-is workflow example diagram for manual sample dilution.

process of refining the problem statement, a laboratory may come to the conclusion that a nonautomation solution would be a better option.

Once a high-level problem statement has been identified, the next step is to analyze the problem in more detail. A good way to do this is to create an as-is workflow showing the various steps before, during, and after a particular process (see Fig. 11.1). This does not have to be complicated; the goal is simply to describe who does what, when and how data flow through the process. Once this as-is workflow is created, key individuals should review it. The laboratory should think about the problem statement in the context of the workflow. Which steps are absolutely required and which steps are not? Which steps are holdovers from an outdated system or process? Which specific steps are problematic? Look for bottlenecks in the process—if a bottleneck was removed, would it have any meaningful impact on the overall process, or would it simply move the bottleneck to the next step in the process? This process of documenting the workflow often leads to insights about a particular problem. It may become clear, for example, that the sample dilution step is the primary bottleneck—an automated assay system that can run more plates may have no effect on overall sample throughput.

Next consider various solutions to the problem. Is there a simple process change that would help to solve the problem? Are there multiple bottlenecks that must be removed? Are the benefits of solving a particular problem worth the cost? Now that the problem is better understood, is this still the problem that requires the most attention? Finally, is this a problem that automation could solve? If the answer to the last question is yes, then an automation project can begin with a well-defined goal.

11.2.1.2 *Forming a Project Team*   The next step in implementing an automation project is to form a project team. Depending on the size and scope of the project as well as the laboratory's resources, the project team could consist of as few as one person to as many as five or six. The key requirements are that the team has sufficient skills and sufficient time to implement the project. The core skills for an automation project are as follows:

- *Project Manager*   Someone to manage the project, create timelines, project documents, and project communication.
- *Technical Resource*   Someone familiar (or at least having aptitude) with software and hardware systems.

- *User Representative*   Someone with detailed knowledge of the process or assay to be automated as well as the business needs of the laboratory.
- *QA Representative*   Someone who can judge the GLP and 21 CFR Part 11 compliance of the automated process.
- *Validation Representative*   Someone who can execute the validation phase of the project.
- *Project Team Members*   One or more people who can do the hands-on work of the project—programming and configuring the system, testing the system, ordering supplies, training users, configuring the lab space, and others.
- *Technical Writing Resource*   Someone to write system documents such as user manuals, administrator manuals, configuration documents, SOPs, and training courses.
- *Project Owner or Sponsor*   Someone who approves various project deliverables and ensures that sufficient resources are dedicated to the project.

It is rare (and perhaps undesirable) to have eight different people fulfilling these various roles. The key point is to ensure that the project team possesses all of these skills. It is also often unnecessary to bring all of these skills to play at the same time. For example, the validation resource needs to play only a minor role until the system has been purchased and is partially operational. The other key element is that the team has sufficient time to dedicate to the project. It is a common mistake to underestimate the resources required for a GLP automation project. It is strongly recommended to have at least some of the resources completely dedicated to the project. Having team members who devote only a fraction of their time to the project and who have other competing priorities often leads to delays. Once the project team is formed, it is suggested to create a project charter with the roles and responsibilities of each team member. The project charter should be updated as the project progresses.

The project manager is key to the successful completion of an automation project. This role is, therefore, worth discussing in detail. The project manager should manage the project like any other complex technical project. The project manager should set up regular meetings with agendas, minutes, and detailed activities assigned to each team member with due dates. The project manager should also create a detailed project plan/timeline for the implementation phase of the project. The timeline should list high-level activities for each stage of the project along with the expected duration of each activity. The project manager should plan the order of execution of the activities and thereby link the activities to a comprehensive timeline. This allows the project manager to determine the critical path for the project that shows the timeline critical activities as the project progresses. Specific activities are listed later in the chapter for sample dilutors and assay robots.

It is also important to anticipate roles and responsibilities once the system goes live. Most systems require an administrator role to take care of activities such as creating new user accounts, programming new protocols, and performing maintenance and troubleshooting. It is also a good idea to have a management representative or system owner to oversee the high-level operation and use of the system. This management representative or system owner is responsible for ensuring that the system is maintained in a compliant state as well as for problem-reporting and change-control activities. This ensures that control of the system is maintained and the system is ready for FDA audit at all times. The other obvious role is that of the end users of the system. Some thought should be given to how many users will use the system on a day-to-day basis and how much training they require. If a laboratory will employ a small group of expert users, then less effort needs to go into user manuals and training. On the other hand, if a system will be used by a large number of nontechnical users, then considerable effort needs to go into making the system simple to operate.

11.2.1.3 *Defining the Requirements*   Although the natural tendency is to quickly purchase a shiny new robot and start playing with it, this is not advised. Now that the problem has been defined, it is necessary to start sketching out requirements for a solution. It is helpful at this point to get a general idea of what systems are out there and how they work, but the temptation of having a vendor do all the work should be avoided. Vendors rarely have the time or interest to understand all of the details of a particular process. This puts a considerable burden on the laboratory to understand exactly how a potential system might function. If this step is skipped however, the system is unlikely to meet the intended objectives without further modification. Another way of stating the situation is as follows: the laboratory will have to define every detail of how a system functions, one way or another. If this is done before purchase, the system will work with no modifications and the vendor will be very helpful. If this is done after purchase, the system may require additional hardware or software and the vendor may not be as motivated to help.

It can be difficult to define the specifics of a process that is only conceptual at this point, but there are several tools that can be applied. The first is to take the "as-is" workflow mentioned above and modify it to a "to-be" workflow (see Fig. 11.2). The workflow captures the relevant steps in a new automated process. Again, the focus is on who does what when and how data flow through the system. Keep it to an appropriate level of detail—a complicated workflow quickly becomes worthless if it is too difficult to read.

Next a "use case" can be created for each step in the workflow. Use cases [7] were originally developed as a tool for software development, but they can have considerable utility defining processes for off-the-shelf systems. In this context, the use case is

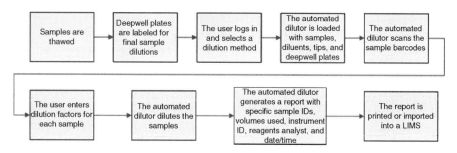

FIGURE 11.2   To-be workflow example for an automated sample dilutor.

basically a written description of the workflow that captures additional detail. The goal is to document more detail about the system and in the process raise questions that may otherwise have been overlooked. Use cases can have a number of different sections, but for an off-the-shelf system it is sufficient to have the following sections: title, description, basic course of events, alternative paths, exception paths, specifications, requirements, and questions.

An automated dilutor may have a workflow step for login and protocol selection. An example use case for this step is shown in Table 11.1.

The example in Table 11.1 shows how the process of creating the use case raised a number of relevant questions about the system. This may seem like a lot of work for an off-the-shelf system, but the questions raised by this use case are exactly the issues that delay automation projects. While there are other, less formal ways of getting at this information that may work fine, the key point is to spend some time thinking about what is required of the system and to document the process. If insufficient thought is given to what is required, there is no guarantee the system will meet the laboratory's requirements.

While defining an automated solution, some thought should be given to a related topic: standardization. Automating diverse, nonstandardized processes is a futile endeavor. If a laboratory has 10 different ways of running ELISA assays, for example, it will have a very difficult time automating all of them. Process standardization should, therefore, be seen as a critical prerequisite to automation. The standardization effort may run into two difficulties. The first is resistance to change. Some scientists will invariably feel that their particular way of running or developing an assay is preferable to others. They may perceive standardization as a process of "dumbing down" their work. It is important to anticipate these objections and work toward getting the people who develop and run assays to accept a certain level of process standardization. This is often best accomplished by laboratory management communicating a clear rationale behind the decision to automate. The second difficulty in standardization is the large number of nonstandard methods in use when the automation project is initiated. Converting existing assay methods to a more automation-friendly format may require considerable testing and revalidation. This effort may be worthwhile for some laboratories and prohibitive for others. If existing assay methods will not be standardized, then the full potential of the automated system may not be reached for several years until older assays fall out of use.

11.2.1.4 System Selection and Purchase

Once a detailed system used process has been documented, it is easy to create system selection requirements. These requirements define every function of the system that is absolutely required. It is also recommended to define a list of "nice-to-haves" that would improve the system, but are not absolutely required. These lists are basically a checklist of functions that can be completed for the various systems under consideration. This checklist could be sent out to various vendors as a Request For Proposal (RFP) or filled out in face-to-face meetings. Regardless, it is important to ensure that the vendor understands the questions and the laboratory understands the answers. See Table 11.2 for a list of categories for selection requirements.

TABLE 11.1   An Example Use Case

Title	Login and Select a Dilution Protocol	Requirements
Description	This use case describes the process of login to the automated dilutor selecting a dilution protocol	
Basic course of events	1. User logs in to software, initializes the system, and selects a protocol 2. The system asks for the following information: (a) How many samples will be diluted? (b) What are the sample dilution factors? (c) How many diluents will be used? 3. The user enters the relevant information 4. The system displays a deck layout that shows where to place samples, labware, tips, and diluent	System allows user to select multiple protocols System will ask user for the following: Number of samples Dilution factors Number of diluents The system will prompt the user to place labware in the correct location
Alternative paths	5. The user may select a protocol that does not scan sample barcodes and does not allow different dilution factors for each sample. In this case, all that the system asks for is the number of samples to be diluted	The system will support simple protocols that do not require user input
Exception paths	6. The system displays an error message if the number of samples to run exceeds the system's capacity 7. The system displays an error message if an invalid dilution factor is entered	System will check for and display input errors
Specifications	1. The system will dilute both clinical samples 2. The system will be able to dilute 100 samples in one run 3. The system will be capable of diluting samples to the following dilution factors: $1/10, 1/20, 1/50, 1/100, 1/1000, 1/10000, 1/100000$ 4. The system will be able to use either one or two diluents	
Questions	• What is the initialization process and how long does it take? • How many different protocols are required? • Should the user enter the number of samples, or should the system know this from scanning the sample barcodes? • How will the user enter the dilution factors—one by one, from an electronic file, or from some other system? • How will the system know when to switch from one diluent to the next?	

TABLE 11.2   Categories of Selection Requirements for Automated Systems

Category of Selection Requirement	Examples of Specific Questions or Requirements
Security	• Does the system allow multiple security roles? • Are protocols secure from routine user modification? • Are configuration settings secure from routine user modification?
Data integrity/Part 11	• Can data or reports generated by the system be modified? • Are audit trails available to capture changes to raw data, protocols, and configuration settings?
Performance	• How many plates or samples can be processed using the attached protocol? • Can the system use two different diluents? • Can the system process 100 samples per run? • Can the system dilute from both 3–5 mL round-bottom tubes and 1.5 mL centrifuge tubes? • Can the system be programmed to dilute samples to the following dilution factors: 1/10,1/20,1/50,1/100,1/1000,1/10000,1/100000? • How long will a run of 100 samples last? • Can the system detect insufficient sample or reagent volume? • Can the system detect sample clots?
Reporting	• Can the system generate a report of actual sample IDs, dilution factors, and sample locations? Is the report format configurable?
Service and support	• What is your service/maintenance policy? • What types of service plans are available? • What is your guaranteed turnaround time on service calls? • How many service technicians do you have in this area?
Vendor information	• How long have you been in business? • How many systems do you currently have in the field? • What is the financial state of your company?
Experience with GLP systems	• Has your company implemented a similar system in a GLP environment? • Do you have an internal QA group that is familiar with GLP and Part 11 regulations?
Error recovery	• Can the system notify the user of an error—how? • What options are available to recover after an error?

Specific questions/requirements should be generated in the process of creating use cases.

Once selection requirements have been created, the next step is to search for systems that meet the laboratory's needs. It is common for a few different vendors to offer systems for LBA automation. It is important to remember that by the time the system is validated, considerable time and effort will have been spent implementing the system—the last thing a laboratory wants is to find that the vendor is going out of business or has only one service technician covering the entire country. A common mistake is to select the technologically most impressive system while ignoring "softer" requirements such as vendor history and maintenance. It is recommended to ask each vendor how long they have been in business, who owns them, how big they are, whether they are financially sound, how they offer maintenance and support, and how many of their systems have been implemented or validated for a similar process. Some vendors may be able to arrange a visit to one of their customers who has a similar system. It is also recommended to ask others in industry about their experience with a particular vendor. In addition, some QA or validation groups may require a vendor audit or questionnaire that can give additional insight into the quality of a vendor.

Once a system has been chosen for purchase, the next step is to create detailed purchase requirements. These requirements are critical to getting a system that will function as intended. No matter how much effort the laboratory has spent in evaluating specific systems and vendors, there will always be details that were overlooked. Some of these details could have a significant negative impact on the final system. For this reason, the purchase requirements put the burden on the vendor to double check the proposed system and to make every effort to get the system running. These purchase requirements are similar to the selection requirements, but are specific to the system that will be purchased. They may also contain specific requirements for protocols that the vendor will program. The purchase requirements should be attached to the purchase order with specific consequences if the requirements are not met. For example, some vendors will agree to a 100% refund if the system does not meet all of the purchase requirements. In addition, it is recommended to specify payment terms where the last payment will be contingent on the system meeting the purchase requirements.

11.2.1.5 *System Setup and Configuration*   Setting up and configuring a new system can be a daunting task due to the sheer number of issues that must be overcome. Even if the vendor did the majority of the programming and configuration, there is quite a bit of work to be done in actually understanding how the system works, creating detailed configuration settings, optimizing performance, and confirming the system operates as expected (before the start of validation). Therefore, setup and configuration can be divided into three distinct phases: learning the system, programming, and configuration.

One of the major challenges in working with a new automation system is learning how to program, operate, and maintain the system. Even if the vendor did the initial programming, the automation team must become experts in the programming, use, and maintenance of the system. In fact, it is difficult to successfully implement a system until the automation team knows the system as well or better than the vendor. With this in mind, it is never too early to start learning about the system. When the system is first installed, it is recommended to participate in the process as much as possible. Assign some team members to watch everything the vendor does and ask questions. The service or application engineer who is installing the system is an invaluable resource for information about the system (especially details that the salesman did not mention). Once the system is installed, the vendor will generally give a brief training course on how to use the system.

Depending on the complexity of the system, the quality of the vendor training, and the experience of the automation team, some laboratories may be comfortable working with the system right away. More commonly, people may be a little intimidated by the prospect of damaging a brand new, quarter-of-a-million-dollar system. The best way past this is for the project manager to assess the team's comfort with the system and start assigning simple tasks to get familiar with the system. With an automated sample dilutor, for example, the team could start with the simple assignment of creating a protocol to transfer liquid from one location to another. The complexity of the tasks should be gradually increased until the team has a good grasp of how the system works. This could take from several weeks to several months depending on the complexity of the system and the skill set of the automation team. It is important to write down everything the team learns about the system since it is easy to forget details later in the project. This documentation will serve as the basis for SOPs, user manual, and administrator manuals later in the project.

Once the team is up to speed on how the system works, they can begin programming and configuring the system. These two activities are closely related, but distinct. Configuration can be defined as the specific settings required for correct operation that are not expected to change in the normal use of the system. Examples of this could be liquid class settings, e-mail error notifications, or audit trail settings. Programming can be defined as the process of creating new protocols that may change periodically as new assays or dilution protocols are added. Drawing a distinction between the two allows a clear differentiation between activities that require validation change control (configuration) and those that do not (programming). Some systems will have very little configuration and very detailed protocols. Other systems will have extensive configuration, but very simple protocols. The dividing line between programming and configuration will also depend on the needs of the laboratory. For example, if a laboratory has a need to add new liquid classes on a regular basis, then it may not make sense to consider these to be configuration.

The goal of the configuration stage is to understand every setting in the system and know how each one should be set. This should result in a configuration document that defines all settings required for the correct operation of the system. This document is an invaluable resource for the installation qualification stage of validation and also for maintaining the system in a compliant and operational state. If the computer hard drive were to fail, it is critical that the system can be restored. Frequent software backups are a key part of this, but it is also necessary to have the configuration documented separately. For systems with hundreds or thousands of configuration items, it can be difficult to understand the exact function of every setting. Many of them may apply to functionality that is not being used. In these cases, a setting should be chosen and documented. The validation of the system will prove the system (and therefore the configuration) works. All that is required is that the configuration is not changed from the validated state without change control.

Programming should take place in parallel with creating the configuration settings since the two activities inform each other. Again, the vendor training and documentation are important resources, but trial and error is the primary tool for programming. The project manager should organize the programming and configuration activities into well-defined categories and should ensure that the team makes steady progress. Specific programming and configuration activities are listed later in this chapter for automated dilutors and assay robots.

11.2.1.6 *Complying with 21 CFR Part 11*   One of the challenges in implementing GLP automation is complying with 21 CFR Part 11 regulations. This is difficult due to the sheer amount of electronic information required to operate an automated system and also varying interpretations of Part 11 itself. It is important to start thinking about Part 11 before the purchase of a system since the purchase order may need to include specific Part 11 requirements or a commitment from a vendor to improve the compliance of their software. Each laboratory's QA group should be the main guide in regulatory issues such as this, but what follows are some practical ways of organizing an approach to Part 11. The major automation vendors now understand the basic concepts of Part 11 and their software usually includes some "Part 11 friendly" features, but few systems have technical controls to meet every aspect of Part 11. This means the customer must carefully assess each system's Part 11 compliance and implement technical or procedural controls wherever required.

The usual first step to assessing a system's Part 11 compliance is to ask, "What electronic records are created, used, or maintained by this system?" The answer to this question depends on the definition of "electronic records." This is where things can get messy. There are many types of electronic data associated with an automated system, many of which are not organized into distinct "records." In addition, there are several different categories of data, ranging from original study records (an Optical Density data file from an assay robot) to settings that describe mundane physical characteristics (the coordinates of the top left corner of a plate sitting on an instrument). Obviously, these different types of data are associated with different risk profiles. If an Optical Density data file were incorrect, study data would be compromised; if a labware definition were incorrect, the system would not be able to dilute samples (an undesirable result, but an operational concern, not a compliance one).

With this in mind, it is useful to think about the different types of electronic "data" in a system. The following questions provide a good starting point:

> Is the data considered to be an original study observation? Is the data used to show the compliance of a certain process? What would happen if a setting was inadvertently changed? Would study data be impacted? Would someone be able to detect the change? How many people should have access to change this setting? How often will the setting need to change?

After going through these and other questions for the various types of electronic information associated with a system, it should be possible to categorize electronic data and settings into one of the categories listed in Table 11.3.

TABLE 11.3 General Categories of Electronic Information Associated with an Automated System

Electronic Setting or Data	Security	Audit Trail	Signature
Raw data file, including run information (user name, date, protocol used, etc.)	No one should have access to change these files	No one has access to change these files. Utilize network server or document management systems for audit trail if needed	Required when a run is being set up
Configuration settings	Users should not have access to change these settings. System administrators may have access, but should only change them as part of change control	Software should generate audit trail records for these settings. They are also documented in the configuration document	Software should prompt for a signature. Configuration document revisions require signature
Protocols	Users should not have access to modify protocols. System administrators have access to modify protocols	Software should generate audit trail records for protocols, but will not capture user requests. Augment with a paper protocol request form	Software should prompt for a signature. A second QC signature may need to be recorded in a paper log
Liquid classes (except calibration factors)	Users should not have access to modify these settings. System administrators may have access, but should only modify them as part of change control. Calibration factors may need to change in response to wear or maintenance and should, therefore, not be considered to be configuration	Software should generate audit trail records for liquid classes. They are also documented in the configuration document that is under change control	Software should prompt for a signature. Configuration document revisions require signature
"Maintenance settings" such as robot position coordinates that may change on a regular basis	Users should not have access to modify these settings. System administrators have access to modify them	Software should generate audit trail records for these settings. Changes should also be described in equipment log books	Software should prompt for a signature
Metadata reports showing incubation times or actual sample dilutions	No one should have access to change these files	These files are audit trails in and of themselves that can be associated with an assay run	Required when a run is being set up

11.2.1.7 System Qualification Proving that data generated by automated systems are acceptable can be a difficult task. There are a number of potential ways that automated assays can differ from manual assays and each one of these can have an unexpected effect on the data. Furthermore, proving that an automated system produces acceptable data for a handful of assays does not necessarily mean that it will produce acceptable data for all assays. Therefore, system testing should be seen as consisting of two main components: system qualification, an in-depth, proof-of-concept test that shows the system is capable of producing acceptable data for a variety of common conditions (e.g., pipetting both serum and buffer), and assay-specific validation test to confirm that the system generates acceptable data for specific assay methods [4]. Operationally, it is preferred to do more qualification testing and less assay-specific validation testing since it allows new assays to be automated quickly.

Regardless of how the testing is done, it is important to start thinking about system qualification and method validation before selecting a system. The general principle is to make an automated system as similar as possible to the manual processes it replaces to eliminate as many sources of bias as possible. The first way of doing this is to design it into an automated system. If disposable pipette tips are used for manual dilutions, they should be used for automated dilutions as well. If a certain type of plate washer is used for manual assays, the same type should be used on an assay robot. The second way of making manual and automated processes more similar is to modify the manual processes. This may sound backward, but it can save quite a bit of effort in the long run. If an assay robot requires reagents to be prepared at the start of the run and left at room temperature until use, then the same thing should be done with manual assays. The goal is to get to the point where the only difference between a manual and automated assay run is that one uses a robot arm to move the plates around and pipette, and the other uses a human arm. This allows minimal assay-specific testing and the rapid incorporation of new protocols. The importance of this step should not be underestimated. Similarly, every effort should be made to make automated sample dilution as similar as possible to manual sample dilution. This is not as straightforward as it is for assay robots due to the number of complex adjustments a human makes while pipetting, but the principle still applies.

System testing can also be complicated by the variety of comparison methods that can be used and the amount of data required. It is important to establish clear criteria based on the intended use of the system. It is recommended to establish a validated, manual method as a "gold standard" that the automated system will be compared to. Due to the inherent variability of LBAs, care must be taken in designing testing methodologies that either minimize variability or are statistically powered to overcome it. In addition, care must be taken to avoid characterizing an automated method more than a manual method. A data set of 200 values from an automated method may very well look different from a data set of 20 values from a manual method, though no fault of the automated system. A biostatistician is an invaluable resource in designing comparison methods. More specific recommendations are discussed later in this chapter for automated dilutors and assay robots.

11.2.1.8 Documentation Good documentation is critical to a GLP automation project. It helps to organize the team's approach, ensures that standardized processes

TABLE 11.4   List of Project Documents for an Automated System

Document	Description
Project charter	Describes the overall goal of the project, scope, deliverables, resources, roles and responsibilities, risks to the project and how they will be mitigated, and due date
Project timeline	Describes the high-level tasks of the project, the expected and actual duration of each task, dependencies between the tasks, the expected completion date as well as the critical path
Meeting agenda/ minutes	Documents the agenda and minutes for project meetings. A good place to capture discussions and decisions
Detailed activity list	Detailed list of activities assigned to each team member each week
Project notes	Document that describes everything that is known or learned about the system during the setup and configuration stage of the project
Lab notebook	Documents experiments performed during the setup and configuration of the system. For example, several experiments may be performed to determine the optimal sample mixing practices (e.g., number of mix cycles, mix volume, aspirate/dispense speeds)

are followed for system use and administration, centralizes the team members' combined knowledge, and ensures the continued functioning of the system in spite of personnel changes. It is recommended to utilize the vendor manuals as much as possible, but they are often too general to describe a laboratory's specific use of a system. There are three general types of documents: project documents used to manage the initial setup of the system, validation documents, and system documents that guide the use and administration of the system itself. Tables 11.4 and 11.5 list the various project and system documents required for a GLP automation project.

TABLE 11.5   List of System Documents for an Automated System

Document	Description
Configuration document	Documents all hardware/software settings required for the correct operation of the system that are not expected to change. This could include operating system security settings, liquid class information such as aspirate/dispense speeds, e-mail settings for error notification, pipetting or scheduling software settings, and others
System administrator manual	Describes the detailed processes for system administration including user account creation and management, programming and testing new protocols, crash recovery, troubleshooting, maintenance, and calibration
User manual	Describes the detailed process users must follow to use the system
SOP	Describes the system at a high level, roles and responsibilities, and associated processes such as training, maintenance, problem reporting, and change control. It is often easier to put the details in other documents to keep the SOP from becoming too long
Training course	Describes the specific topics and steps of the training process

Validation documents are not listed since most companies have well-defined processes in place for computer system validation.

11.2.1.9 Validation   The validation phase of the project proves that the system meets user requirements and complies with GLP and 21 CFR Part 11 regulations. Each laboratory should have detailed procedures for computer system validation, so only high-level considerations will be discussed here.

The most important point about validation is also the most obvious: the system should work flawlessly prior to the start of validation. Given the pressure to get these systems up and running as soon as possible, there is a real temptation to start validation before configuration and programming is complete or to rely on validation testing to prove that the system functions as intended. This is a mistake. Given the complexity of these systems and associated processes for maintenance, training, and calibration, it is critical that the function of the system is proven before validation starts. Therefore, it is recommended that the validation resource only play a minor role in the project until the system has passed initial qualification testing.

One important distinction between automated laboratory systems and computer systems (with no automation hardware) is that automated laboratory systems perform physical processes. These physical processes have different levels of risk associated with them and can be observed, measured, and calibrated. Computer system validation procedures were originally instituted to control "black box" software applications that could not be observed, measured, or calibrated. Therefore, if a LIMS "crashes," it usually requires validated problem reporting and change control to diagnose and fix the problem. If a robot arm crashes by colliding with a plate washer on an assay system, it generally does not. The point is that it is necessary to separate physical processes from solely software processes and employ appropriate controls to each category. This is not to say that physical processes should not be validated, only that it is necessary to define which system functions or parameters can change without validation and which ones require change control. As an example, consider a specific labware on an automated dilutor. The user requirements for such a system may specify that the system is capable of diluting into 2.2 mL deepwell plates, and the validation would prove this. A month after the system goes live, however, the labware definition may need to be adjusted in response to system wear or a physical crash. This adjustment is a physical process that can only be verified visually by a system administrator and should therefore not require revalidation. This concept can be difficult for QA or validation groups that have not worked with automated laboratory systems before, but it is important to allow for ongoing maintenance.

11.2.1.10 System Rollout   Once a system has completed validation testing, it needs to be rolled out to end users. It is important to start planning for this early on in the project since the users' perceptions of the system can make or break an automation project. Obviously, the most important factor for the successful rollout of a system is to ensure that the system meets the needs of the users. This is why it is so critical to get key users involved in defining system requirements early on. A second factor that is critical is the expectations of the end users. If these are not carefully managed, users can feel distinctly let down by a system when it goes live. This is especially true if the system was oversold by the automation team. It is important to remember that resistance to change, even positive change, is a universal trait. It is also important to remember that no matter how thorough the automation team was in implementing the system, there will be inevitable minor oversights that make the system a little less efficient or more difficult to use. For these reasons, it is important to carefully communicate the benefits and drawbacks of the system leading up to the go-live date. Users will form their own opinions soon enough. They will be much more accepting of a system that exceeds their expectations compared to one that falls short. It is also important to remind users that the transition period may feel uncomfortable and that processes and procedures may need to be adjusted before the system reaches its full potential.

It is also important to respond to real or perceived problems with a new system quickly and decisively. This will give the users confidence in the automation team and the system, and will reinforce the lines of communication about the system. Rather than relying on rumors from coworkers, users will naturally look to the automation team for information.

11.2.1.11 *Ongoing Maintenance*

Once a system has been rolled out and is in use, it must be maintained in good working order and in a compliant state. This is likely to be the first time a laboratory has experience using the system on a day-to-day basis for an extended period of time. For this reason, it is not uncommon to uncover problems or issues that did not surface before. This should be expected and additional resources should be devoted to deal with the inevitable issues that arise. Software bugs may be found, requiring a patch or updated version of the software. Maintenance deficiencies may be found that lead to changes in the frequency or type of routine maintenance. It is also common to learn what types of problems are most common and how they can be avoided. For these reasons, System Administrator Manuals, User Manuals, SOPs, and training procedures may need to be updated within a few months of a system going live.

11.2.1.12 *Key Points*

In summary, the following key points should be followed for a successful automation project:

- Have a clear and well-defined problem statement.
- Have the right people working on the project and ensure they have sufficient time to devote to the project.
- Know exactly how the system will function before purchase.
- The system must work perfectly prior to the start of validation.
- Standardize laboratory processes before an automated system is implemented.
- Document everything that is known about the system.
- Spend time creating detailed processes for system use, training, maintenance, programming, troubleshooting, problem reporting, and change control.
- Carefully manage the expectations of the end user group.

11.3 SPECIFIC LIGAND-BINDING ASSAY AUTOMATION SYSTEMS

11.3.1 Introduction

There are a number of different ways in which automated systems can be deployed in support of LBAs, ranging from the use of stand-alone, semiautomated workstations to complex integrated systems that perform both sample dilution and assay steps. In addition, a lab can opt for strictly off-the-shelf systems or custom integrated systems. The approach that is right for a particular laboratory depends on the lab's needs (throughput, cost per sample, etc.), budget, experience with automation, number of end users, and time horizon. Systems can be placed into one of the four general categories based on the degree of automation: stand-alone workstations, off-the-shelf combined dilution and assay systems, off-the-shelf independent dilution and assay systems, and custom integrated systems.

11.3.2 Stand-Alone Workstations

These are small, relatively simple (and inexpensive) instruments that have one or two dedicated functions such as 96-channel pipetting or reagent dispensing. Examples of the former include Velocity 11 Bravo, Tecan Aquarius, Caliper Sciclone, or Tomtec Quadra Tower. Examples of the latter include Biotek uFill, PerkinElmer Flexdrop, or Thermo Multidrop. These systems may or may not come with a plate stacker, and may or may not be controlled by an external computer. In general, these systems are easy to implement and require minimal setup and validation. In terms of impact, these systems have the potential more than double the number of plates that can be processed by a single analyst. However, they do not allow walk-away use.

11.3.3 Off-the-Shelf Combined Dilution and Assay Systems

A number of vendors offer systems that can dilute samples and run an ELISA on the same system. Examples include Tecan EVO, Beckman FX, Hamilton STAR, and PerkinElmer Janus. They are comprised of a single workstation with an 8 or 12 tip pipetting arm, a robotic plate-gripping arm, and various peripherals such as plate washers and plate readers. These types of systems are often a first foray into auto-mation, but they do have two drawbacks: throughput and complexity. The throughput problem comes from the fact that, if the system is diluting samples, it cannot run an assay and vice versa. In addition, there is usually insufficient deck space for both, an 8-channel and a 96-channel pipetting arm, plate washer, plate reader, samples, tips, diluent, and other labware needed for higher throughput. These factors typically limit throughput to less than 8 plates (320 samples) per day. There are ways of getting around this throughput problem such as integrating more than one system, but this adds complexity and limits the ability to independently upgrade either the sample dilution or assay functions. The second potential problem with combined systems is complex-ity. Not only do these systems require extensive liquid handling setup and testing, but they also require scheduling software to process the assay steps. These combined systems will not be discussed in further detail, but the sections that follow on automated dilutors and assay robots should cover most implementation details.

11.3.4 Off-the-Shelf Independent Dilution and Assay Systems

The next step up in cost and throughput is independent sample dilutors and assay robots. Sample dilutors are dedicated workstations that dilute samples from tubes to 96-well labware such as deepwell plates. Examples include Tecan EVO, Beckman FX, Hamilton STAR, and PerkinElmer Janus. These are the same instruments listed above but are configured differently. Since they are dedicated solely to sample dilution, they do not require 96-channel pipetting arms, plate washers, plate readers, or incubators. This allows them more space to hold samples, diluents, and pipette tips, resulting in increased throughput. These types of systems are less complicated than the combined systems since they do not require scheduling software and can generally dilute ~700 samples per day. Off-the-shelf assay systems are often built from the same systems as the sample dilutors, but are configured with 96-channel pipettors (with no 8 or 12 tip arm), plate readers, plate washers, and incubators. These systems are loaded with diluted samples in 96-well format and run the assay from the blocking or sample addition step to reading the assay plates. These systems are less complicated than the combined systems since their liquid handling is fairly straightforward. They can generally run 30 plates per day (~1100 samples).

11.3.5 Custom Integrated Systems

The final category of automation is comprised of large custom integrated system such as those from Velocity 11, CRS, Beckman, Tecan, Thermo, or Caliper. These larger systems are usually configured around a robot arm that moves the plate between the various peripherals. This category is very heterogeneous since no two custom systems are the same, but they generally have the potential for higher throughput as well as integrating separate sample dilutors and assay functions. Potential drawbacks of these systems are complexity and the potential for software bugs with custom software.

11.3.6 Recommendation

Given these four categories of system, which one is preferred? As mentioned before, it depends on the need of each laboratory, but here are some general recommendations:

- Start with stand-alone workstations. These systems will give experience with automation tools and processes and significant productivity gains without spending hundreds of thousands of dollars. They will also get a laboratory to start thinking about support systems such as user training and calibration.
- Next, add an independent sample dilutor or two. This is likely the major bottleneck in sample analysis since the stand-alone workstations increased assay capacity. Automated sample dilutors are discussed in more detail below.

- Once sample dilution has been automated, add an assay robot to further increase throughput and to allow overnight operation. Assay robots are discussed in more detail below.
- As throughput needs increase, add additional independent sample dilutors and assay robots. If needed, evaluate customized systems that may offer higher throughput, but be mindful of the difficulty in validating custom software in a GLP environment.

One important consideration is the decision to go with popular off-the-shelf systems from well-established vendors, similar systems from smaller vendors, or custom systems. It is important to keep in mind some of the vendor selection criteria mentioned earlier in the chapter: vendor support, vendor stability, and experience working with GLP customers. Smaller vendors or custom software are not necessarily bad, but they can have more software bugs since they have fewer customers using the software and reporting problems. Given the need for validation and change control, the system with the fewest problems is often the best investment.

11.4 AUTOMATED SAMPLE DILUTORS

11.4.1 Introduction

Sample dilution is one of the most labor-intensive tasks in running an LBA. Add standard curve and quality control dilution (which these systems can easily do) [8], and it becomes over half the effort to run an assay. Depending on the specific practices of a laboratory, samples can be diluted in duplicate, triplicate, at four serial dilutions, at eight serial dilutions, with one or more sample diluents, at different dilutions for each sample, and from different size tubes (e.g., clinical versus nonclinical). Similarly, standard curve and control dilutions can be performed in a variety of ways. For these reasons, it can be challenging to implement an automated dilutor to meet all of these requirements.

As mentioned in the previous section, sample dilutors are generally 8–12 tip (although some vendors now offer 16 tip versions) pipetting instruments. The channels are able to move to different "spans" to allow each tip to enter either sample tubes or individual wells of 96-channel labware. Traditionally, these instruments could be configured for fixed or disposable tips and used a liquid-filled line connected to a syringe that acts as the pipetting piston (Some vendors are now offering air displacement systems that skip the liquid system). These instruments are comprised of a pipetting arm that can move to various points on the system deck. Various carriers sit on the deck and hold different types of labware such as sample tubes, deepwell plates, pipette tips, and reagent reservoirs. Most vendors now offer a dizzying array of peripherals from robot arms to 96-channel pipetting arms, to plate washers, plate readers, shakers, and barcode scanners. These systems are, therefore, highly configurable to each specific application. The software that controls these instruments generally consists of user-definable protocols that control the pipetting arm and "liquid classes" that determine the exact specifications of how the instrument pipets. A typical protocol flexible enough to dilute each sample to an independent dilution factor may consist of hundreds of instruction lines and involve several thousand settings for factors like submerge depth, liquid level detection sensitivity, blowout volume, variable lookup, and others. Needless to say, these systems can be quite complex.

11.4.2 Needs Assessment

Before purchasing a sample dilutor, it is necessary to first define requirements. The previous sections covered the use of workflows and use cases to help define an automated process. This section gives more specific information for defining automated sample dilutor requirements. Depending on how standardized the current sample, standard, and control dilution process is, a laboratory may or may not have a "tight" set of requirements. Since no automated system can ever meet 100% of a laboratory's needs, it is suggested to focus on the first 80%. Users should be asked how they currently dilute samples. The following questions should cover the basics:

- What are the minimum and maximum dilution factors needed?
- How many replicates are diluted? Is each replicate an independent dilution from the source?
- Are samples serially diluted? If so, what serial dilution factors are used?
- How many serial dilutions could there be?
- How many diluents are used? At what dilution should the system switch from one diluent to the next?
- What is the final sample volume desired?
- What are the accuracy and precision requirements?
- With what size and shape tubes will samples come in?
- Are the samples barcoded?
- Should the system be able to dilute each sample to a different dilution factor in the same run?
- How are samples positioned in the plate? How are replicates positioned in the plate?
- What is the ideal number of samples to dilute in a single run?
- Are any of these requirements expected to change in the next 5 years? If so, how?

A spreadsheet can be created with the answers to the above questions. Using the 80% criteria, requirements should be categorized as in-scope or out-of-scope. In addition, it is important to look for opportunities for standardization. A finalized list of requirements should be created, reviewed, and approved by end users and laboratory management. The above process can be repeated for standard curve and control dilution if these steps are to be automated.

11.4.3 Programming and Logic

Even though each company will have a unique set of dilution requirements, there are some general practices that encompass most needs. The simplest way to use an automated dilutor is to create a separate protocol for each dilution method, with each sample undergoing the same dilution process. For example, there may be one "1/10" dilution protocol that dilutes all samples to a 1/10 dilution. All the instruments need to know is how many samples to dilute in each dilution run (and maybe the sample barcode ID if the instrument is used to scan the samples). The benefit of this approach is that the programming is relatively straightforward. It is also straight-forward to document the actual dilutions performed since it is the same for all samples in a dilution run. The drawback of this approach is that samples must be segregated by dilution factor before they are run. If samples for a particular study undergo three different dilutions depending on the dose and sample time points, then it is necessary to perform three different dilution runs for the different groups of samples.

A more advanced approach is to create a more complex protocol that can dilute each sample to an independent dilution factor. This eliminates the segregation of samples by dilution factor, but adds considerable complexity. The dilutor needs to know the specific dilution factor for each sample in a run, which requires that this information be imported into the protocol for each run from an electronic file. In addition, it is no longer obvious how each sample was diluted. This means that some sort of audit trail report must be created to report the dilution factor for each sample. Most popular automated dilutors have this capability, but it often requires custom programming by the vendor. This approach has the potential for the greatest efficiency, so it is worth further discussion.

As mentioned before, automated dilutors can be implemented in a wide variety of ways. The best way to figure out a dilution method is to prototype the process manually. This can be done by clearing some lab bench space and laying out some empty sample tubes. Next, labware can be added—that samples will be diluted into—usually deepwell plates or a rack of 96-well tubes. This labware defines the starting and ending points for the dilution run. The next step is to determine how each sample can be diluted. Samples could be diluted straight into the final labware, but this limits the dilution factors available since it is not possible to do much more than a 1/200 dilution in this labware. For this reason, some sort of intermediate dilution is often required. The intermediate dilutions can be performed in 5 mL tubes or deepwell plates. Using the requirements gathered above, a detailed set of instructions to perform the dilution run should be created. It will look something like this for samples diluted in duplicate:

1. Pick up 1 mL tips and add 300–990 µL of diluent to the first intermediate locations.
2. Add 300–990 µL of diluent to the second intermediate locations.
3. Add 300–990 µL of diluent to the third intermediate locations.
4. Get new 200 µL tips and aspirate 10–100 µL of sample and dispense into the first intermediate locations.

5. Get new 1 mL tips and mix the first intermediate dilutions three times with 600 μL.

6. Get new 200 μL tips and aspirate 10–100 μL of the first intermediate and dispense into the second intermediate locations.

7. Get new 1 mL tips and mix the second intermediate dilutions three times with 600 μL.

8. Get new 200 μL tips and aspirate 10–100 μL of the second intermediate and dispense into the third intermediate locations.

9. Get new 1 mL tips and mix the third intermediate dilutions three times with 600 μL.

10. Get new 1 mL tips and transfer 160 μL of the first, second, or third intermediate dilutions to the final locations.

The next step is to test the instructions by performing a mock dilution with dye manually. Once this works, steps can be added for adding a second diluent or for serial dilution—whatever a particular dilution method requires. This process should be continued until the protocol meets all of the user requirements. For example, it may be necessary to add steps for scanning sample barcodes, querying the user for the number of diluents, or the final dilution volume desired.

Once the dilution method is final, it is necessary to start thinking about how many samples, deepwell plates, and pipette tips are required for the method. It is important that the system have space for these materials. If it does not, a larger capacity system may be required or it may be necessary to lower the number of samples that can be diluted in a single run. This process will ensure that the laboratory understands exactly what the system will do. Once the dilution protocol is finalized, it can be attached to the purchase order to ensure that the system will meet these requirements. The vendor can also be asked to do the actual programming of the protocol, which can save quite a bit of time and effort. This approach will work for any potential dilution protocol, including standard curve and control dilution. The key point is to figure out exactly what the instrument should do to execute the protocol.

The following general guidelines may give a starting point for designing a protocol:

- The system should use only disposable tips for sample aspiration/dispense. Fixed tips can be problematic for carryover. This is not an insurmountable problem, but requires extensive assay-specific testing [9–11]. Furthermore, disposable tips are used for manual diluting, so they should also be used for automated diluting.

- The minimum aspiration volume should be set to 10 μL—it is fairly easy to get good accuracy and precision at this volume.

- The maximum total volume for any dilution should be 3 mL. Most systems have large disposable tips with a volume of 1 mL. It is fairly easy to mix a 3 mL sample with a 1 mL pipette tip.

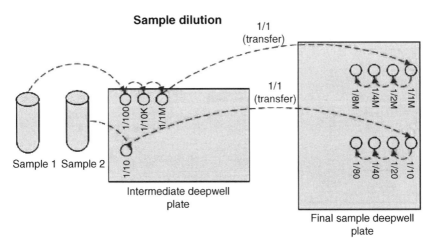

FIGURE 11.3 A flexible and efficient way of performing automated dilutions. Only 2 samples are shown, but one final deepwell plate can accommodate 18 samples diluted to 4 serial dilutions.

- Each sample may have a different dilution factor, but has the same number of replicates or serial dilutions. This is a good compromise between flexibility and complexity.

Figure 11.3 shows a diagram of a flexible and efficient dilution method that can handle a wide range of requirements. The basic approach is to use deepwell plates for intermediate dilutions. Each sample undergoes one to three intermediate dilutions depending on the total dilution factor required. Once the intermediate dilutions are performed, the sample is transferred into a final location where serial dilutions are performed (if needed). Figure 11.4 shows a Multiprobe II deck layout for this protocol.

Data flows for this type of protocol can be complex, but there are techniques that help to simplify the protocol. One of the most commonly used is the worklist. A worklist is a file containing specific information for the automated dilutor on how to dilute the samples (see Fig. 11.5). Worklists can contain a variety of information, but the simplest ones for automated dilutors contain the sample IDs and specific volumes of diluent and sample to pipette into each well or tube. They may also include specific well maps that guide the dilutor where to dilute each sample. The benefit of using worklists is that the protocol does not require complicated logic to calculate specific volumes for each sample. The worklist is usually created by an external application. For example, an Excel macro could be used to capture sample IDs and dilution factors, and then include this information into a worklist that can be imported into a sample dilutor protocol. Some laboratories have created applications that query a LIMS for the sample IDs and dilution factors and automatically generate the worklist [8].

A related approach is to use lookup files to store information about the protocol. A lookup file is similar to a worklist, but does not contain information about particular

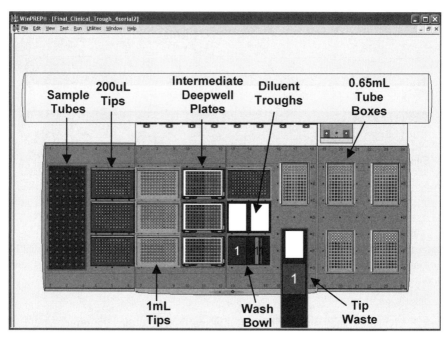

FIGURE 11.4 A Multiprobe II deck layout for the above dilution method.

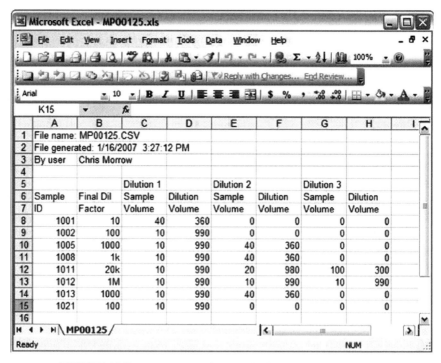

FIGURE 11.5 An example of a worklist for an automated dilutor.

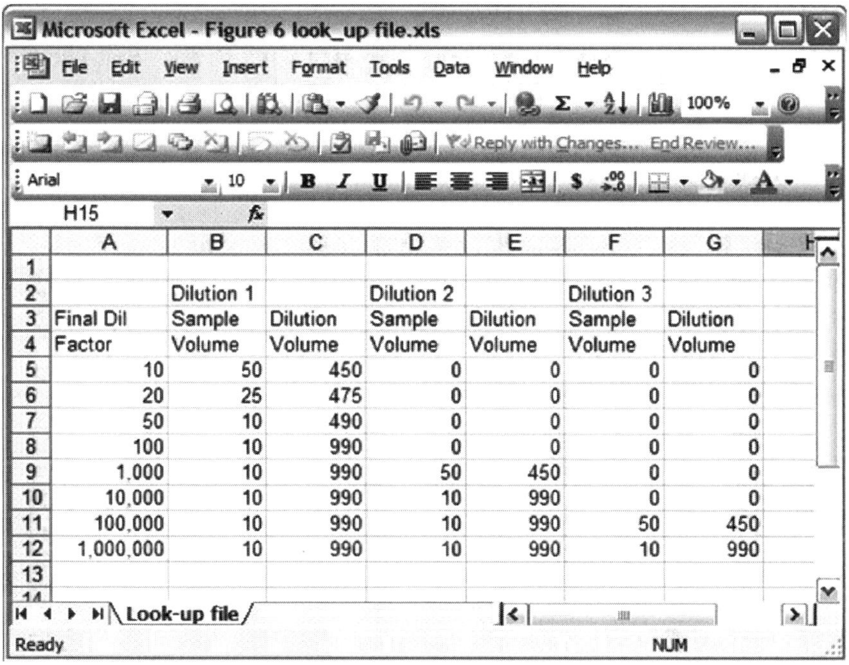

Final Dil Factor	Dilution 1 Sample Volume	Dilution Volume	Dilution 2 Sample Volume	Dilution Volume	Dilution 3 Sample Volume	Dilution Volume
10	50	450	0	0	0	0
20	25	475	0	0	0	0
50	10	490	0	0	0	0
100	10	990	0	0	0	0
1,000	10	990	50	450	0	0
10,000	10	990	10	990	0	0
100,000	10	990	10	990	50	450
1,000,000	10	990	10	990	10	990

FIGURE 11.6 Example of a simple lookup file for an automated dilutor.

samples. The sample-specific information (ID, dilution factor) is stored in a separate file that is imported into the dilutor protocol. The dilutor then looks up information in the lookup files based on keywords or specific columns of information. Figure 11.6 is an example of such a file. The dilutor can be programmed to look up specific volumes for each dilution factor. For example, if the dilutor imports a file that shows a 1/10 dilution factor for a particular sample, it looks up "10"in the lookup file and know to use 50 μL of sample and 450 μL of diluent. The benefit of this approach is that no external application is required to generate a worklist. A user can create a simple Excel file containing a column for sample ID and another column for dilution factor that is imported into each dilution run. Data can still be extracted from a LIMS by an external application, but the application is much simpler since it does not need to calculate specific volumes to use. It is also easy to add new dilution factors without modifying the actual protocol. Lookup files can contain other types of information such as well maps.

Protocols that accept electronic inputs such as the sample dilution factor or number of diluents present one additional complication: knowing what the instrument actually did. Just as a manual dilution process requires documentation of the various parameters used in the dilution, so does an automated dilutor. This information may be captured in an audit trail, but it is generally necessary to store this information with the assay documentation where it can easily be cross-checked against the parameters in a LIMS. This creates a requirement for the automated dilutor to generate a report of sample IDs, actual dilutions performed, number of diluents used, user name, date/time of dilution run, and others. A worklist may contain much of this information with one critical difference: the worklist tells the automated dilutor what it is supposed to do. This does not necessarily correspond to what was actually done. Some samples may have had insufficient volume to dilute, others may have had clots, and others may have encountered some kind of error. For this reason, it is important to know exactly what the automated dilutor actually did. Different automated dilutors have different capabilities in this regard but some may require customization to generate a concise report. Requirements should be generated for the reports and attached to the purchase order. It may be necessary to pay the vendor extra to get this functionality.

11.4.4   Liquid Handling

Liquid handling is a complicated subject due to the sheer number of options available. Most dilutors have extensive sets of settings organized into liquid classes (see Fig. 11.7.) Liquid classes allow the definition of specific pipetting techniques for different types of liquids.

It is important to try to simplify the liquid classes as much as possible. It is preferred to use only one or two liquid classes. Some laboratories try to create a separate liquid class for each liquid that will be pipetted (serum, diluent, etc.). This is a nice idea in principle, but what liquid class should be used for an intermediate dilution that is 50% serum and 50% diluent? A simpler approach is to adjust the settings in a single liquid class so that both serum and diluent can be pipetted accurately. With a little trial and error, this approach seems to work for many biological matrices. Of course, the data should be the guide.

If a system uses multidispensing (aspirating once and dispensing multiple times), then it may be necessary to create a liquid class specifically for this type of pipetting. It is often necessary to perform tip-wetting, predispense, or postdispense steps to ensure that equal volumes are dispensed in each dispense step.

The actual process of defining a liquid class can be laborious given the amount of data required. Vendors can recommend basic settings, but the lab will have to prove that a particular class works acceptably. This can best be done utilizing a gravimetric scale that is offered with some automated dilutors, or with dye if no gravimetric option is available [12]. It is important to carefully observe the instrument performing the pipetting steps during the liquid class definition since settings like "submerge before aspirate depth" or "liquid tracking" can best be set by watching the interaction of the pipette tip and the liquid surface.

11.4.5   Liquid Level Detection

Most automated dilutors have capacitance liquid level detection. The conductive pipette tips sense a change in capacitance when they come in contact with a liquid. This feature is critical for these instruments since excess sample may be transferred if the tip submerges too far into the sample. On the other hand, if the liquid level detection setting is too sensitive, the pipette tips may touch the wall of the sample tube and

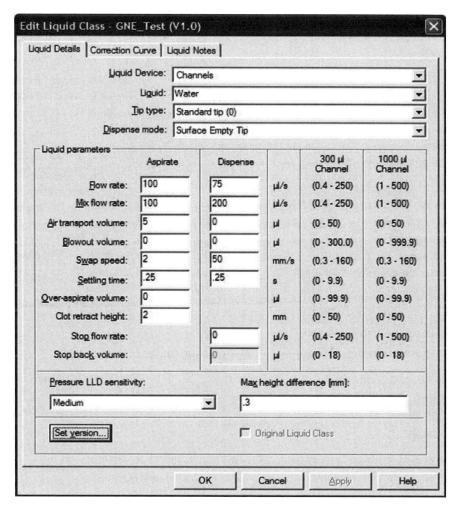

FIGURE 11.7   An example of a liquid class from a Hamilton STAR.

mistakenly aspirate air. Getting this setting right can be a challenging balancing act. If it is insufficiently sensitive, the system may not detect smaller sample volumes, if it is too sensitive, the system may occasionally aspirate air. To reduce the likelihood that the pipette tips will touch the sides of the sample tube, every effort should be made to ensure that all samples are held perfectly vertical. Many systems come with spring-loaded sample racks that do a good job of this.

Since the liquid level detection settings are critical to the proper aspiration of samples, this should be tested extensively. It is important to create a reliable testing method with the volumes, liquid types, and sample tubes that will be used in the actual protocol. It may also be necessary to perform this testing with mock sample labels since thick labels can affect the position of the sample tubes. This experiment should be repeated with a large number of mock samples on different days to confirm the system aspirates all samples correctly.

11.4.6 System Qualification

System qualification proves that the system generates acceptable accuracy and precision as defined in the user requirements. This testing should not be performed using dye or gravimetric methods since these do not accurately reflect the full complexity of a dilution run. Due to the variability of LBAs, designing a testing protocol and acceptability criteria can be challenging. Wherever possible, it is recommended to eliminate as many sources of variability as possible. One approach that works well is to create spike samples for each matrix that will be tested and for several different assays. The same samples should be diluted manually and on the automated dilutor at the same time. The diluted spike samples from the manual and automated methods should then be assayed on the same assay plate to minimize interassay variability. The experiment should be repeated on several different days with different people performing the manual dilutions. It is important to allow some variability in the results. A requirement that states that *all* samples must be within 10% of manually diluted samples, for example, may be difficult to meet. A biostatistician is invaluable for designing this type of testing protocol.

11.4.7 Project Activities for an Automated Dilutor

There are a number of other issues to deal with while implementing an automated dilutor. Table 11.6 shows a high-level list of project activities for implementing an automated dilutor.

TABLE 11.6   High-Level Project Activities for an Automated Dilutor

• Define selection requirements	• Liquid level detection
• Evaluate systems	• Clot detection
• Define purchase requirements	• Mixing
• Purchase	• Error notification
• Prepare lab space	• Error recovery
• Install system	• Calibration procedures
• System acceptance testing	• Maintenance procedures
• Learn system	• SOP
• Data flow	• User manual
• Programming and logic	• Administrator manual
• Configuration	• User and administrator training course
• Security (application, workstation, network folder)	• System qualification
• Account creation and management	• Protocol request, testing, and approval process
• 21 CFR Part 11 compliance	• New assay incorporation process
• Reporting	• Validation
• Liquid classes	• System rollout

11.5 ASSAY ROBOTS

11.5.1 Introduction

Assay robots can automate the laborious process of running an LBA: washing, adding diluted samples and reagents, adding substrate and stop solution, incubating, and reading the plates. As with automated dilutors, assay robots can be implemented in a number of ways depending on the needs of the laboratory. One laboratory may require coincubation of samples and conjugate, others may require fluorometric or luminescent plate readers; others may require 37°C incubation or plate lids.

As mentioned previously, assay robots can be built from off-the-shelf systems or can be custom-made by integrating a number of different peripherals. These systems generally have a robot arm to move plates, tips, and diluted sample boxes, storage hotels or a storage carousel, a plate washer, a 96-channel pipettor, some type of regent dispenser, shakers/incubators, and plate readers [13]. Depending on the system, it may be possible to use the 96-channel dispenser to add both samples and reagents to the assay plates. This simplifies the system and eliminates the need for priming steps. The software that controls these systems must include drivers for each peripheral and some type of scheduler that can determine the order of steps for the various plates the system is processing. Liquid handling is usually straightforward on these systems since they only transfer samples and reagents into the assay plates.

11.5.2 Needs Assessment

As with automated dilutors, the best place to start in implementing an assay robot is with the needs of the laboratory. A similar process should be followed to define the most important 80% of requirements by talking to end users. The following questions should provide a good start:

- What sample and reagent volumes are required?
- How many and what type of wash steps are required?
- What type of labware will be used?
- What are the minimum and maximum incubation times required?
- Are there any coincubations?
- What type of plate readers are required?
- What temperatures are required for incubations? Are two different temperatures required for the same assay?
- Is plate shaking required for incubation steps?
- How many plates will be processed in a single run?
- How will reagents be added—from troughs on the 96-channel dispenser, or from dedicated reagent dispensers?
- What data file format is required?
- Will any light-sensitive reagents be used on the system?
- Are plate lids required?

Again, a spreadsheet can be created with the answers to the above questions. Using the 80% criteria, requirements should be categorized as in-scope or out-of-scope. Look for opportunities for standardization. A finalized list of selection requirements should be created, reviewed, and approved by end users and laboratory management.

The next step is to talk to vendors to learn more about how specific systems function. Use cases can be refined with specific system functions in mind. The use cases should address the following questions:

- What information should be included in the data file (user name, comments, assay procedure, date/time, unique plate number)?
- How will the user enter the above information?
- Where should data files be saved? How will they be controlled?
- How will protocols be requested, programmed, tested, and approved?
- How will the system notify the user of errors (e-mail, pager)?
- Can the system be recovered in the event of a crash?
- What steps are required to set up and initialize the system prior to run?
- What steps are required to clean up after a run?
- How will the user know the exact incubation times for each plate?
- How many plates can be run at once, and how long will each run take?
- What is the dead volume for samples and reagents?

As the laboratory works through the use cases and the above questions to define selection requirement, it should get a good idea of which systems may best meet the requirements. It is recommended at this point to perform some proof-of-concept testing to determine whether the automated assay will produce acceptable results. There is no way to prove this definitively until the system is purchased and installed, but it is possible to test specific parameters such as:

- Reagent handling and stability. Can the reagents sit on the system at room temperature for the required amount of time?
- Can the assay be run without the use of plate sealers? If not, can it be run with plate lids instead?

11.5.3 System Components and Layout

Once selection requirements have been created and a laboratory begins to meet with vendors to discuss specific systems, some thought must be given to the peripherals used (pipettors, washer, readers, incubators, etc.). This will depend on the specific requirements of the laboratory, but some general principles should be followed. The first of these is simplicity. If at all possible, it is best to select the simplest possible configuration. Each peripheral has electric motors, encoders, and other mechanical components, all of which will fail eventually. The fewer moving parts a system has, the better. Using a 96-channel pipettor to add reagents as well as samples eliminates

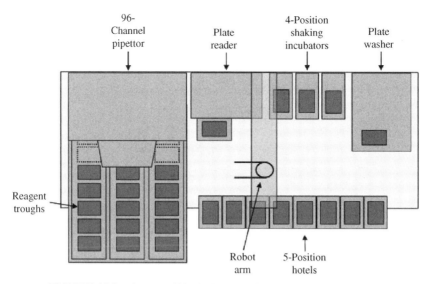

FIGURE 11.8   One possible deck layout for a Tecan ELISA station.

the need for separate reagent dispensers, thereby lowering the complexity, cost, and maintenance/calibration effort. The second principle is speed. Peripherals that can execute their operation quickly will allow more flexibility in the schedule and may allow more plates to be processed at once.

Once the peripherals have been selected, a deck layout should be created showing where each peripheral will be located. The vendor will usually be able to offer suggestions, but the laboratory should also give some thought to this. The peripherals should be located in a logical arrangement that minimizes the duration of robot arm movements. Some thought should also be given to the labware orientation. It is much better to have a system function solely in portrait or landscape orientation. If the robot arm must regrip a plate from landscape to portrait *en route* from the washer to the incubator, for example, it can take quite a bit of time and therefore have a negative impact on scheduling. Figure 11.8 shows a deck layout for a Tecan ELISA station.

11.5.4 Scheduling

The scheduling of operations for each plate in a run can be a difficult factor to measure before purchase. The algorithms these systems use to schedule an assay are quite complex with the result that schedulers often behave in an unpredictable, nonlinear manner. It is important to understand scheduling since it determines how many plates can be run in a single batch and how each plate is processed. The schedule depends on the time it takes for the system to execute each operation, the specific assay process, and the number of plates being processed. Small changes to any of the three can have undesirable results. Most vendors can simulate a schedule for a particular system, assay process, and number of plates. The schedule is viewed as a Gantt chart with the vertical axis being the plate number and the horizontal axis time. Individual equipment

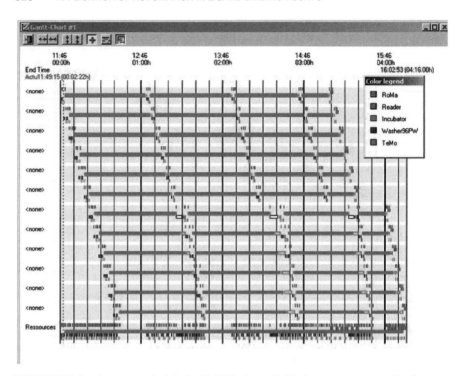

FIGURE 11.9 An assay schedule in FACTS where all 12 plates are processed in the same batch. Each row is a separate plate that undergoes three incubation steps.

operations for each plate are often shown as colored blocks. It is important to review this schedule carefully to ensure that the system functions as expected. If the schedule is not acceptable, more or faster peripherals may be required to get the desired result. Figure 11.9 shows an assay schedule created by the Tecan FACTS software for an EVO assay system. This schedule shows a consistent process where all plates are processed in one "batch." Figure 11.10 shows a schedule for another assay with different incubation times. Note that the last two plates are processed more than 3 h after the first plate. This is an unacceptably long time for samples and reagents to be sitting at room temperature on the system. This illustrates the point that the throughput of these systems can be limited more by the scheduling than the physical capacity of the system. The best way of avoiding scheduling problems is to specify exactly how many plates can be processed for a particular assay procedure and what the total run time will be. This requirement should be included in the purchase requirements with a money-back guarantee if the system does not meet the requirement.

11.5.5 Configuration

There can be a substantial amount of configuration for an assay robot due to the number of equipment drivers and scheduling settings. It may take quite a bit of trial and error to optimize and document these settings, but once this is done the actual programming of assay protocols is usually straightforward.

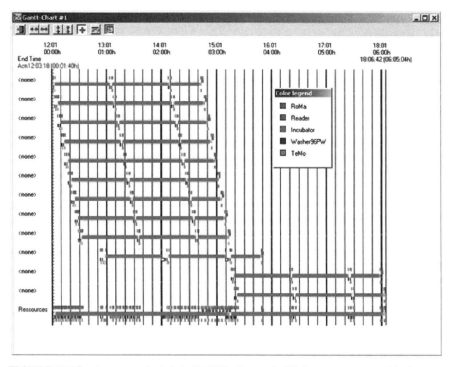

FIGURE 11.10   An assay schedule in FACTS where only 10 plates are processed in the same batch.

11.5.6 Reporting

Due to the dynamic nature of the scheduling software, it is often difficult to know exactly how long each plate was incubated. Since this is generally called out very specifically in the assay SOP, it is necessary for the system to generate a report of actual incubation times for each plate. Care must be taken in defining exactly what constitutes incubation. The time in the incubator may underestimate the actual amount of time a reagent was in a plate due to robot arm movements and delays in the start of the wash step. Again, several assay schedules must be carefully evaluated to determine how a specific system functions. Most vendors can create an incubation time report, but it may require customization to get a report of the required information (user name, run number, assay procedure, etc.) in a readable format. Figure 11.11 shows an example of such a report.

11.5.7 System Qualification

As mentioned in a previous section, one of the goals in implementing an assay robot is to make the manual and automated methods as similar as possible. If this is done successfully, then system qualification becomes a fairly simple proposition. As with automated dilutors, it is recommended to compare to a validated manual

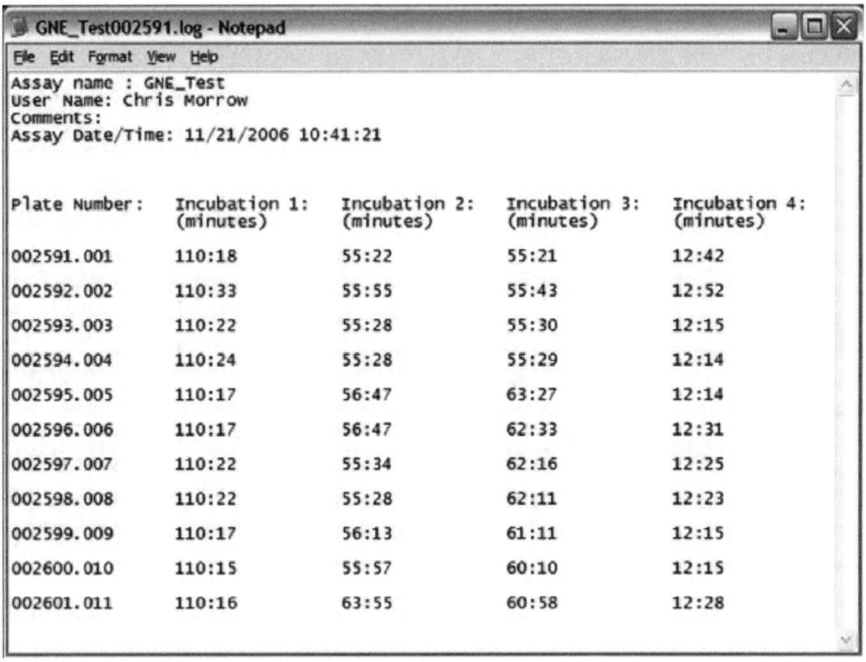

GNE_Test002591.log - Notepad				
File Edit Format View Help				

```
Assay name : GNE_Test
User Name: Chris Morrow
Comments:
Assay Date/Time: 11/21/2006 10:41:21
```

Plate Number:	Incubation 1: (minutes)	Incubation 2: (minutes)	Incubation 3: (minutes)	Incubation 4: (minutes)
002591.001	110:18	55:22	55:21	12:42
002592.002	110:33	55:55	55:43	12:52
002593.003	110:22	55:28	55:30	12:15
002594.004	110:24	55:28	55:29	12:14
002595.005	110:17	56:47	63:27	12:14
002596.006	110:17	56:47	62:33	12:31
002597.007	110:22	55:34	62:16	12:25
002598.008	110:22	55:28	62:11	12:23
002599.009	110:17	56:13	61:11	12:15
002600.010	110:15	55:57	60:10	12:15
002601.011	110:16	63:55	60:58	12:28

FIGURE 11.11   An incubation time report from an assay robot.

method. Again, this can be done by creating spike samples that will fall at different points in the standard curve. The spike samples should be run using the same preparation of standard curve, controls, and reagents on both methods at the same time. This should be repeated on different days with different analysts performing the manual method. This should also be repeated with different assay methods. A biostatistician should be consulted on the amount of data required and specific comparison criteria. As with automated dilutors, the comparison criteria should leave some room for the failure of one or two comparison runs through assay variability or analyst error.

If the automated assay method is sufficiently different from the manual method, then the differences between the two methods must be carefully examined to determine the best testing approach. This may result in the need to partially revalidate each assay on the automated system. Once this is done, a decision must be made about whether both the methods can be used to generate data for the same subject/study/ project. This involves quite a lot of work and serves as an example of why standardizing the manual and automated methods is so important.

11.5.8   Project Activities for an Assay Robot

Table 11.7 shows a high-level list of project activities for implementing an assay robot.

TABLE 11.7   High-Level Project Activities for an Assay Robot

• Define selection requirements	• 21 CFR Part 11 compliance
• Evaluate systems	• Reporting
• Define purchase requirements	• Error notification
• Purchase	• Error recovery
• Prepare lab space	• Calibration procedures
• Install system	• Maintenance procedures
• System acceptance testing	• SOP
• Learn system	• User manual
• Data flow	• Administrator manual
• Data file format	• User and administrator training course
• Programming and logic	• System qualification
• Configuration	• Protocol request, testing, and approval
• Scheduling	process
• Security (application, workstation,	• New assay incorporation process
network)	• Validation
• Account creation and management	• System rollout

11.6 INTEGRATION: TYING IT ALL TOGETHER

Automated sample dilutors and assay robots can independently have a beneficial impact on a laboratory's efficiency and throughput. Further improvements can come from integration of the two types of systems and a LIMS. There are many ways of accomplishing this, based on the needs of an individual laboratory; however, two general approaches are described:

1. Using a LIMS to direct the operation of automated systems
2. Using automated systems to direct the operation of a LIMS

The first approach is based on the fact that the LIMS contains information such as sample ID, run number, sample location, and sample dilution factor. This information can be extracted from the LIMS and used to create worklists for automated dilutors (see Fig. 11.12). This eliminates the need for an analyst to re-enter this information into the dilutor, thereby increasing efficiency and reducing transcription errors. Implementing this requires the creation of a custom application that can query the LIMS and translate the information into a worklist that can be read by the automated dilutor.

One potential drawback with this approach is that the automated dilutor may not dilute the samples exactly as instructed by the LIMS. There could be samples with insufficient volume, clots, errors, and others. For this reason, a manual QC step must ensure that the actual sample dilution information is reflected in the LIMS. If a particular sample was not diluted, then it must be deactivated or removed from the run in the LIMS.

The second approach overcomes this issue by starting with a report from the automated dilutor showing how samples were actually diluted. This report is then

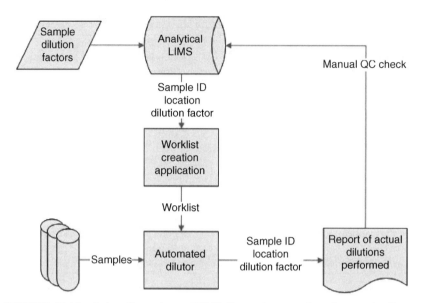

FIGURE 11.12 A data flow where a LIMS directs the operation of a sample dilutor.

imported into the LIMS, instructing the LIMS to create runs, with the specified samples, dilution factors, and sample positions (see Fig. 11.13). This approach does not require a manual QC step to ensure that the automated dilutor and LIMS information matches. It also saves time by automating the run creation step in the LIMS. Unfortunately, not all LIMS support automatic run creation.

Assay robots can also be integrated with the LIMS or sample dilutors. They could be physically integrated by implementing a system to transfer diluted samples from the automated dilutor to the assay robot. The cost/benefit of this approach should be carefully evaluated since the manual transfer of diluted samples from an automated dilutor to an assay robot is generally not a time-consuming step. Integrating data of the three systems may make more sense. The data flow for this type of integration will generally be more straightforward since the raw assay data can only flow from the assay robot to the LIMS.

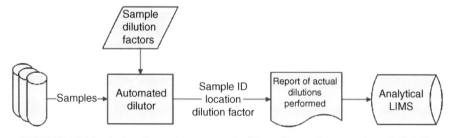

FIGURE 11.13 A data flow where a sample dilutor directs the operation of a LIMS.

11.7 FUTURE DIRECTIONS IN LIGAND-BINDING ASSAY AUTOMATION

The field of laboratory automation is developing at a rapid pace. Much of this progress is driven by high-throughput screening technology such as 1536-well plates and nanoliter pipetting [14]. It is unlikely that these technologies will have any immediate impact on the field of GLP ligand-binding assays, but it is likely that they will continue to have a trickle-down effect. One example of this is 384-well assays. 384-Well processing has been quite common in screening application for a number of years. Most vendors now offer 384-well capability with systems that can be used for LBA automation. Most GLP laboratories have not yet made the move to 384, but it may become common in the future. As with all automation initiatives, the move to 384-well assays should be carefully evaluated. Potential drawbacks include LIMS compatibility and the difficulty in running 384-well assays manually. There can be real throughput gains by moving to 384, but samples will still need to be diluted in the 96-well format (at least in the near term). Regardless, there is no doubt that ligand-binding assay automation technology will continue to evolve. Automated systems will continue to get faster, more flexible, and more reliable. Due to the small market size of GLP ligand-binding assay automation, it is unlikely that vendors will offer off-the-shelf, turnkey systems specifically targeted to GLP LBAs any time soon. For this reason, laboratories will need to continue to develop the capabilities to identify and implement the right solution to meet their specific needs.

11.8 CONCLUSION

In summary, ligand-binding assay automation has the potential of producing significant gains in throughput and efficiency. Along with these gains, however, comes the need to fully appreciate the skills and efforts required to implement robust and compliant solutions. For this reason, GLP LBA automation cannot be a half-hearted endeavor. Laboratories must view automation as a unique competency that must be fostered. If they do this, they have the potential to continually improve the quality of their data and the efficiency with which they produce it.

ACKNOWLEDGMENTS

The author would like to thank many people for their contribution to the knowledge and ideas presented in this chapter, namely, Patricia Siguenza, Director of the BioAnalytical Assays Department at Genentech; The BioAnalytical Assays Automation Team (Oliver Arceno, Scott Phillips, Ben Ordonia, Melissa Cheu, Gabrielle Hatami, Elena Lee-Villamizar, Ihsan Nijem, and Marco Palencia); and Ashwin Datt, Director of the Genentech Nonclinical Operations Department at Genentech.

REFERENCES

1. Gurevitch, D. (2004) Economic justification of laboratory automation. *Journal of Laboratory Automation*, **9**, 33–43.
2. Code of Federal Regulations (2006) Title 21, Part 58, Good Laboratory Practice for Nonclinical Laboratory Studies.
3. Code of Federal Regulations (2006) Title 21, Food and Drugs, Part 11. Electronic Records; Electronic Signatures; Final Rule.
4. Webster, G., Kott, L., and Maloney, T. (2005) Considerations when implementing automated methods into GxP laboratories. *Journal of Laboratory Automation*, **10**, 182–191.
5. Yates, I. (2006) Lab automation: implementing a successful system to support drug discovery. *Innovations in Pharmaceutical Technology*, **20**, 30–34.
6. Koppal, T. (2007) To automate or not to automate? *Drug Discovery and Development*, **11**, 10–14.
7. Cockburn, A. (2002) Use cases, ten years later. *Software Testing and Quality Engineering Magazine (STQE)*, **4**, 37–40.
8. Gu, H., Unger, S., and Deng, Y. (2006) Automated Tecan programming for bioanalytical sample preparation with EZTecan. *Assay and Drug Development Technologies*, **4**, 721–733.
9. Gu, H., and Deng, Y. (2007) Dilution effect in multichannel liquid-handling system equipped with fixed tips: problems and solutions for bioanalytical sample preparation. *Journal of Laboratory Automation*, **12**, 355–362.
10. Fregeau, C., Yensen, C., Elliott, J., and Fourney, R. (2007) Optimized configuration of fixed-tip robot liquid-handling stations for the elimination of biological sample cross-contamination. *Journal of Laboratory Automation*, **12**, 339–354.
11. Ouyang, Z., Federer, S., Porter, G., Kaufmann, C., and Jemal, M. (2008) Strategies to maintain sample integrity using a liquid-filled automated liquid-handling system with fixed pipetting tips. *Journal of Laboratory Automation*, **13**, 24–32.
12. Xie, I., Wang, M., Carpenter, R., and Wu, H. (2004) Automated calibration of Tecan genesis liquid handling workstation utilizing an online balance and density meter. *Assay and Drug Development Technologies*, **2**, 71–80.
13. Schneider, I., Stoll, P., Haller, D., and Thurow, K. (2007) Establishment of a flexible platform for an automated brain-derived neurotrophic factor: ELISA. *Journal of Laboratory Automation*, **12**, 219–229.
14. Ramachandran, C. (2006) Advances of laboratory automation for drug discovery. *Drug Discovery World*, 2006, Spring, 49–55.

CHAPTER 12

Documentation and Regulatory Compliance*

CT. VISWANATHAN and JACQUELINE A. O'SHAUGHNESSY

U.S. Food and Drug Administration, Silver Spring, MD, USA

12.1 REGULATORY PERSPECTIVES IN THE DOCUMENTATION OF BIOANALYTICAL DATA AND REPORTS

12.1.1 Introduction

Documentation of the events in an experiment and recording of the data as they are being collected are significant components in any good laboratory practice. In this regard, source records that document study events and the actual conditions of laboratory analysis are critical for verifying data integrity. Regulatory inspections use source records in various ways for the following purposes and to address the related questions:

- To evaluate method reliability; is the method accurate and precise?
- To re-create study conduct; were samples processed in accordance with the established method?
- To determine if the reported data are reliable for use in regulatory decisions; what was the impact on the accuracy of the reported results if the method was not followed?

---

*The views expressed in this chapter are those of the authors and do not reflect an official policy of the U.S. Food and Drug Administration (FDA). No official endorsement by the FDA is intended or should be inferred.

Ligand-Binding Assays: Development, Validation, and Implementation in the Drug Development Arena. Edited by Masood N. Khan and John W.A. Findlay
Copyright © 2010 John Wiley & Sons, Inc.

327

It is very likely that incomplete or missing records would prevent the verification of data integrity. Source records should be complete to facilitate an understanding of actual study conduct for critical phases of method development, method validation, and subject sample analysis. The records should confirm whether the testing was conducted in an appropriate manner, with well-designed and optimally controlled experiments. The documentation of actual laboratory events should demonstrate that the quantitative measures are suitable to achieve the objectives of the clinical or nonclinical protocol. The records should confirm that the reported results accurately reflect the actual concentration of the analyte in the biological matrix. It should be noted that the failure to adequately document critical details of study conduct has resulted in rejection of bioanalytical data for regulatory purposes.

Although complete and contemporaneous documentation of study events is critical from a regulatory perspective, it should not be viewed solely as a regulatory requirement. It is also essential to the bioanalytical laboratory in its effort to demonstrate that a method is reliable and can produce high-quality data. Furthermore, comprehensive recording of study events can assist the bioanalytical laboratory in troubleshooting efforts, when unexpected problems occur during routine sample analysis.

Our inspectional experience with the FDA and review of cases for regulatory submissions involve bioanalytical methods for both small and large molecules. We have conducted many audits of the bioanalytical portions of *in vivo* bioequivalence studies. In addition, our experience includes bioanalytical sample analysis for Phase 1 pharmacokinetic (PK) studies, population PK studies, and the toxicokinetic portions of nonclinical safety studies. Although our experience with bioanalytical methods for macromolecules is less extensive than for chromatographic assays for small molecules, the following discussion of documentation expectations is made without reference to a particular methodology. However, it is noted that methodology differences between small and large molecules might necessitate the documentation of distinct attributes of study conduct. Notwithstanding the specific methodology, it is the responsibility of the bioanalytical laboratory to make this determination and confirm that all aspects critical to study conduct are recorded and maintained in the study file. Furthermore, it should be recognized that documentation beyond the areas raised in this chapter might be warranted in specific circumstances.

12.1.2   Chapter Objectives

The purpose of this chapter is to address documentation issues related to method development, validation, and routine sample analysis from a regulatory perspective. The issues will cover both source records and reporting expectations, with the goal of obtaining a sufficient level of documentation to allow an after-the-fact reconstruction of study events. Appropriate documentation is needed for regulatory agencies, sponsors, and bioanalytical laboratories alike to demonstrate that the bioanalytical method and resulting data are reliable and can be used for regulatory review decisions.

The documentation approaches discussed in this chapter are based on an inspectional perspective. It is recognized that this point of view does not necessarily reflect other equally acceptable approaches utilized by bioanalytical laboratories. Although this detail-orientated approach might seem mundane, complete and contemporaneous documentation of all laboratory events and decisions is necessary to permit study reconstruction. In addition to the considerations presented in this chapter, FDA's 2001 guidance document regarding bioanalytical method validation [1] and the conference report regarding the May 2006 American Association of Pharmaceutical Scientists (AAPS)/FDA Crystal City workshop on best practices for chromatographic and ligand-binding assays [2] are useful references that discuss expected documentation practices. Reference is also made to a 2007 publication that discusses documentation considerations in the context of key elements for macromolecule bioanalytical method validation [3].

12.1.3 Responsibility for Documentation

The expectation for complete and thorough documentation applies to any laboratory conducting bioanalytical testing for regulatory purposes. Sponsor, contract, and academic laboratories alike should adhere to good documentation practices. In addition to laboratory analysts, good documentation practices should be carried out by supervisors, report writers, and others assigned by the management of the testing laboratory.

The involvement of a well-qualified quality assurance unit (QAU) to assure the integrity of the study data through inspections and audits is desirable. In fact, QAU oversight is required by FDA's Good Laboratory Practice (GLP) regulations (21 Code of Federal Regulations (CFR) Part 58) for nonclinical laboratory studies.[1] Although other program areas do not have this specific regulatory requirement, it stands to reason that all studies for regulatory submission can benefit from the involvement of an effective QAU that is independent of the individuals engaged in the direction and conduct of the study. Nonetheless, regardless of QAU involvement, bioanalytical laboratories are responsible for assuring the integrity of the data they collect. Furthermore, sponsors have an overall responsibility for all of the data they provide in their regulatory submission.

Beyond the need for individual bioanalytical laboratories to document adequately and report completely the results of bioanalytical analyses, it should be noted that sponsors submitting data to FDA have additional reporting responsibilities in their regulatory submissions. For example, sponsors should submit summary information regarding the various bioanalytical methods and validation reports used across the studies that support a new drug application. A table that details, in chronological sequence, the general attributes of the methods will enable a quick comparison of any differences. FDA's 2001 guidance regarding bioanalytical method validation [1] provides recommendations regarding the type of summary information that sponsors should provide.

[1]Nonclinical laboratory studies are *in vivo* or *in vitro* experiments in which test articles are studied prospectively under laboratory conditions to determine their safety [21 CFR 58.3(d)]. The International Conference on Harmonisation of Technical Requirements for Registration of Pharmaceuticals for Human Use (ICH) Guideline regarding toxicokinetic assessments (ICH S3A) states that bioanalytical analyses for GLP studies should be conducted in accordance with GLP requirements [4].

12.2 RECOMMENDATIONS FOR DEVELOPMENT, VALIDATION, IMPLEMENTATION, AND REPORTING PHASES

12.2.1 Method Development

In general, documentation related to the development of a bioanalytical method is seldom the focus of regulatory oversight. That being said, it is clear that method development activities provide critical information regarding the various processing procedures, reagents, matrices, instrumental conditions, and others considered to arrive at an optimized assay. In this context, comprehensive documentation that details the progression of a method is clearly useful to the bioanalytical laboratory and can prevent wasteful use of resources; for example, there is less value in repeating failed development activities or retesting reagents already deemed inappropriate for the method. The preparation of a report based on method development activities should be considered a useful supplement to the source records and can facilitate a quick, straightforward understanding of how the method arrived at its initial form for validation testing.

In 2003, a publication authored by the AAPS Ligand Binding Assay Bioanalytical Focus Group subcommittee [5] described that method development activities for macromolecules include assessments of critical assay reagent selection, the standard curve model selection, specificity of the reagents, sample preparation, and preliminary precision, accuracy, and stability, to name a few. The results of these assessments, and the preliminary evaluation of method robustness, should provide the bioanalytical laboratory sufficient information to prepare a written description of the assay procedure that should be approved by the responsible parties (e.g., bioanalytical investigator and management) prior to validation testing. The procedure should minimally describe the stepwise handling and processing of samples, the necessary reagents, the anticipated calibration range and standard curve model, and conditions of instrumental analysis.

12.2.2 Validation Protocols

Since the goal of validation is obvious (i.e., to verify whether a bioanalytical method is accurate, precise, and reliable for its intended use), a written description of the planned testing will facilitate an upfront assessment of whether the appropriate experiments have been considered and can be carried out in a scientifically sound manner. With regard to basic validation tenets, FDA's guidance document on bioanalytical methods validation is a useful reference [1]. In a nutshell, the guidance describes the various aspects of validation that should evaluate all variables (e.g., environmental, matrix, material, and procedural) with the potential to impact the estimation of the analyte in the study samples, starting from the time of sample collection through the end of analysis. Additional clarifications regarding validation testing that are intended to enhance data quality are discussed in the AAPS/FDA conference report on best practices for chromatographic and ligand-binding assays [2]. References focused wholly on bioanalytical method validation for macromolecules also discuss considerations and recommendations on issues such as assay reagent and matrix selection, nonlinear calibration models, and parallelism, to name a few [3,5–7].

For all validation testing, the issues to be evaluated and the design of the experiments should be recorded in advance of the testing. Such upfront preparation provides the bioanalytical laboratory the opportunity to evaluate whether the planned testing addresses all issues affecting assay reliability and sample integrity. This preparation and the resources spent are well justified, generally leading to a robust data bank that enables a more meaningful reconstruction of events, especially when questions arise later regarding the various aspects of the assay. Because the validation experiments for demonstrating accuracy, precision, and stability are typically similar across bioanalytical methods, a general protocol or standard operating procedure (SOP) is recommended for defining validation experiments common across methods. However, it is recognized that individual methods might require specialized validation experiments to address specific processing and analyte concerns. In these situations, the laboratory should clearly define the basis for and conditions of the additional validation testing. In this regard, a validation protocol specific to the bioanalytical method with reference to the general validation SOP might be appropriate for specially designed experiments.

In cases where an approved bioanalytical method is changed subsequent to validation testing, the changes must be documented and their impact addressed, with additional validation experiments as necessary. Thus, changes in matrix (e.g., plasma to urine, and rat to mouse), use of a different assay format, alteration of the relevant concentration range, and selectivity issues resulting from concomitantly administered medications are examples of modifications that would trigger additional validation testing [1]. A description of the testing conducted to demonstrate the performance of the revised method should be included as an amendment to the validation protocol. Beyond procedural modifications, changes in critical reagents, such as capture or detection antibodies (i.e., the use of a different batch/lot), should be evaluated to assure that the assay conditions remain optimal. The acceptability of batch-to-batch variability for the purpose of quantitative measures needs to be evaluated and considered part of method validation.

12.2.3 Assay Kits

In addition to methods developed in-house, it is recognized that commercially available ligand-binding assays (generally designed for use in clinical settings) are sometimes considered suitable for measuring analyte concentration in pharmacokinetic studies. Although kit manufacturers provide some validation data in the package insert, it is the responsibility of the bioanalytical laboratory to demonstrate the reliability of the assay under the specific operating conditions and equipment in the laboratory where sample analysis occurs.

Although the manufacturer's validation data and package insert generally convey the suitability of the kit to detect the analyte, the site-specific validation (and particularly the specificity of the assay) should assess acceptability of the kit for the protocol objectives (e.g., suitability of the assay for quantitative measurements) under the actual conditions of use. In-house validation of a commercial kit is expected even when the kit instructions are followed without modification. This is similar to in-house validation of a published method or a method transferred from a sponsor's laboratory. Any changes to the manufacturer's procedures must also be validated.

12.2.4 Validation Reports

The basis for determining whether a method suits its intended purpose rests, in part, with the data obtained during prestudy validation. In this regard, a comprehensive method validation report is an essential component for demonstrating the suitability of the method. The report should provide a complete and accurate description of the validation experiments conducted and the results obtained. A comprehensive report should discuss the general attributes of the bioanalytical method, the firm's standardized procedures for validating methods, specialized validation considerations, and the acceptance criteria used to establish the reliability of the method. It should clearly demonstrate that the method is suitable for routine sample analysis. Of course, problems encountered during validation should be reported and the impact of those problems on the integrity of the validation results addressed. Validation reports should be signed and dated by the responsible bioanalytical investigator.

Although not an exhaustive list, a validation report should include a description of the bioanalytical method, the reference standard and critical reagents, the calibration standards and validation samples, the validation experiments, SOPs, and the validation testing results. Table 12.1 provides additional details for the suggested content of the validation report.

In cases where the matrix for calibration standards and quality controls (QCs) differs from the subject study samples, the use of a different matrix should be justified. Issues related to the use of a different matrix should be investigated during validation testing and described in the validation report.

Appending the bioanalytical method and validation testing protocols/SOPs to the validation report provides the basis for evaluating the experimental design of individual validation tests in conjunction with the method's processing procedures. For example, it is useful to understand whether validation experiments covered all allowable variations in sample processing, as described in the approved method. In cases where specialized experimental designs are necessary, a brief description of the testing in conjunction with the protocol/SOP allows an assessment of the approach and the impact of the experimental design on the interpretation of the data.

Beyond the narrative description of the validation data, actual testing results are routinely presented in tables specific to each validation experiment. Validation batches should be identified by batch name (run ID), the date of sample processing, and the date

TABLE 12.1 Bioanalytical Method Validation Reports: Recommended Contents

Report Contents	Additional Details
Bioanalytical method	• Description of sample processing and instrumental analysis • Calibration range, regression type, and weighting factor (as applicable) • Computerized systems used • Bioanalytical method protocol/SOP as report appendix
Reference standard and critical reagents	• Source, purity, stability, and other pertinent characteristics • Lot number • Stock solutions (concentration, solvent, storage conditions)
Calibration standards and validation samples	• Date of preparation and storage conditions • Matrix type and source • Calibration range • Concentrations of calibration standards (including anchor points, as applicable) • Concentrations of validation samples • Regression model for calculating concentration results
Validation experiments	• Description of testing • Disposition of samples during testing (e.g., storage location/temperature) • Identify protocol/SOP for validation testing – Include as report appendix (as deemed necessary)
Standard operating procedures	• Brief description of critical SOPs (e.g., acceptance criteria for validation results) – Include as report appendix (as deemed necessary) • SOP deviations and their impact on the integrity of the validation results

Results	• Discussion of method specificity and selectivity, matrix selection, and potential interference issues
	• For chromatographic methods, representative chromatograms
	• Unexpected results
	  – Identify affected validation batches
	  – Describe any subsequent investigation
	  – Describe the impact of the unexpected results on the integrity of the validation experiments
	• Tabular presentation of data

of analysis. Result tables should include, but are not limited to, the following examples:

- All batches initiated during validation testing and their status (e.g., accepted, rejected, and other)
- Within- and between-batch accuracy and precision, calculation of total error (as applicable)
- Back-calculated concentration of calibration standards
- Standard curve parameters
- Stability determinations (bench-top, freeze/thaw, long-term, post-preparative, reference standard stock solutions, reagents)
- Batch size anticipated during routine study use
- Recovery (as applicable)
- Dilutional linearity (as applicable)
- Parallelism (if study samples available)
- Matrix effects (as applicable)

Data reported from accepted runs must include the results of all validation samples. Exclusion of individual data points from accepted runs because the results exceed the predefined acceptance limit is not acceptable. Along these lines, complete reporting of validation experiments includes a discussion of failed experiments, in conjunction with an explanation for rejecting the data. When experiments are rejected, the basis for the rejection should be documented in the source record (e.g., spilled tubes, preparation error, and instrument failure) and disclosed in the validation report. The rejection or exclusion of failing validation results without justification is not acceptable and does not provide a forthright description of the true assay performance.

12.2.5 Sample Analysis

In our experience, laboratories use various approaches for documenting the conduct of routine sample analysis. Laboratories can successfully use notebooks, worksheets, electronic input, or combinations thereof. Some laboratories use checklists that are specific to the individual bioanalytical method. Such standardized templates can streamline the documentation process and provide multiple analysts working on the same project with clear direction about the type and extent of record keeping needed to adequately document the various aspects of sample analysis. Although checklists might facilitate the processing of samples in accordance with the established method and SOPs, it is recognized that unexpected problems can crop up. In this regard, analysts must receive appropriate training to understand their responsibility in documenting issues that occur outside the routine aspects of sample analysis.

Regardless of the format of the source record (e.g., worksheet or notebook, paper or electronic), essential documentation must include all information critical to study reconstruction. All details must be recorded contemporaneously with the actual study events and the individual performing each task must sign and date the source record. For critical steps, verification at a second level with documentation is highly recommended. To reconstruct study conduct from source records, the following information, at a minimum, should be documented.

12.2.5.1 *Sample Accountability*

Source records should identify the source and number of subject samples[2] received by the bioanalytical laboratory, the date of sample receipt, the condition of the samples upon receipt, and the storage location (e.g., equipment identifiers) and temperature conditions for the duration of storage. Courier receipts of the sample shipment should be maintained in the study file.

12.2.5.2 *Reference Standard and Critical Reagents*

Source records should document lot numbers, date of receipt or preparation (as appropriate), the identity, purity, and stability at the time of use, expiration date (as applicable), storage location (e.g., equipment identifiers), and temperature conditions.

12.2.5.3 *Reference Standard Stock Solution*

Proper documentation should include the lot number of the reference standard, a weighing record for the reference standard with a second level of verification, solvent used, concentration prepared, date of preparation, expiration date, storage location (e.g., equipment identifiers), and temperature conditions.

12.2.5.4 *Calibration Standards and Quality Control Samples*

Documentation to confirm the accurate preparation of the calibration standards and QCs is essential and should include the type and source of matrix, the identity of the reference standard stock solution, the calibration range, concentrations of the individual calibration standards and QCs, regression type and weighting factor (if any), the storage location (e.g., equipment identifiers), and temperature conditions for duration of storage.

12.2.5.5 *Batch Records*

Batch records typically contain many elements that are critical to reconstruction of the study conduct. These records should include details such as the batch identification number (run ID) and a list of the samples in the batch (e.g., calibration standards, QCs, diluted QCs (as applicable), blanks, subject samples). Appropriate documentation also includes the date/time when samples were removed from the storage location for processing, the date/time when samples were returned to the storage location after processing, the date of sample processing, reagents used, storage conditions of processed samples prior to analysis, and the date of analysis. The sequence of sample analysis should be documented and the sequence verified to unequivocally associate individual samples with the resulting concentrations.

Instrumentation details such as the identification numbers of the equipment used and the instrument settings should be recorded. System suitability checks that demonstrate optimal operating conditions at the time of sample analysis (as applicable) are also essential records.

---

[2]In the case of GLP studies, specimens are derived from animals.

Proper documentation of the batch records also includes the responsibilities of all analysts involved with the batch, including details that describe the specific steps executed by each analyst. Confirmation that the analyst followed the approved bioanalytical method is critical, as is documentation to indicate whether any changes from routine method procedures were used (e.g., use of allowable variations in sample processing).

The results of instrumental analysis should include the raw data and calculated results for all samples in each batch. The basis for accepting or rejecting batches, reprocessing original results, and modifying the standard curve should reflect written procedures established *a priori*. If original results are reprocessed, both original and reprocessed results should be maintained. If the standard curve is modified, for example, by extending the standard curve range or deleting individual standard points that exceed predefined acceptance limits, the basis for the change should be documented. If the QC levels are modified, for example, by adding QCs or shifting QC levels, the basis must be clearly recorded in the source document. The documentation of such changes should be contemporaneous with the study conduct. The raw data should also include a list of samples targeted for repeat analysis and a description of the basis for repeating the samples. Unexpected problems, including instrument malfunction, sample processing errors, SOP deviations, repeated run failures, and highly anomalous results, should be recorded. Remedial actions to address the problems and the evaluation of the impact of the problems on the integrity of the data are also relevant source records.

12.2.5.6 *Supporting Documentation*   Supporting documentation should address related procedural and operational needs that must be in place to conduct a well-controlled study and produce high-quality data. Critical elements include standard operating procedures for laboratory operations, records of calibration and routine maintenance of laboratory equipment, storage units, and instrumentation, and a description of all circumstances that have the potential to affect sample integrity (e.g., freezer malfunction, instrument failure, etc.).

It is also necessary to maintain an audit trail of changes made to source data for both paper and electronic records. Changes should be made without obscuring the original entry and the reason for the change should be documented with sufficient details. Changes should be signed and dated by the individual responsible for making the change.

Records of correspondence are useful for study reconstruction and should be archived with the study data. For example, communications within the bioanalytical laboratory and external communications with the sponsor, clinical site, pharmacokineticist, and others are all relevant memoranda that should be retained.

The preceding descriptions are not all-inclusive and any detail critical to study conduct and necessary to demonstrate the integrity of the data must be recorded.

12.2.6 Bioanalytical Study Reports

As in the method validation report, the bioanalytical report should include sufficient details to allow an evaluation of the method and its performance under the actual conditions of sample analysis. It is understood that most bioanalytical methods are developed rigorously and their expected performance is well characterized by prestudy validation testing. However, it is not uncommon that issues sometimes arise during routine sample analysis that could potentially impact the integrity of the resulting concentration data. Of course, such issues must be thoroughly investigated, rectified, and described with sufficient details in both the source records and the bioanalytical study report. Narrative descriptions of problems in the bioanalytical study report should facilitate an independent evaluation of impact on the study data.

Although not an exhaustive list, reports that describe the bioanalysis of subject samples should provide the following information.

12.2.6.1 *Bioanalytical Method*   The bioanalytical method should be described with sufficient details to facilitate a clear understanding of sample processing, conditions of instrumental analysis, and the computerized systems used for data collection and reporting. The calibration range, regression type, and weighting factor (if applicable) should be reported. The bioanalytical method protocol/SOP should be included as a report appendix.

12.2.6.2 *Sample Accountability*   Records of sample accountability should document the source and number of subject samples,[3] the date of sample receipt, the condition of the samples upon receipt, the storage location, and the temperature conditions for the duration of storage.

12.2.6.3 *Reference Standard and Critical Reagents*   The report should include details related to the reference standard and critical reagents such as the source, purity, stability, and other pertinent characteristics, lot number, and stock solutions. Pertinent information about the preparation of the stock solutions (e.g., concentration, solvent, storage conditions, etc.) should also be reported.

12.2.6.4 *Calibration Standards and QC Samples*   The date of preparation and storage conditions of calibration standards and QC samples should be reported, as well as the matrix type and source used for the preparation. In cases where the matrix for calibration standards and QCs differs from the subject study samples, the impact of using a different matrix should be investigated during validation testing.

12.2.6.5 *Standard Operating Procedures*   The bioanalytical report should include a brief description of critical SOPs (e.g., acceptance criteria for batches and repeat analysis). As appropriate, SOPs should be included as report appendixes. SOP deviations and their impact on the integrity of the study results should be described.

12.2.6.6 *Tabular Data*   Bioanalytical study report tables should incorporate numerous details of study conduct, including but not limited to the information described in Table 12.2.

---

[3]In the case of GLP studies, specimens are derived from animals.

TABLE 12.2   Bioanalytical Study Report Tables: Recommended Contents

Table Contents	Additional Details
Study runs identified by batch name (run ID)	Date of sample preparation and instrumental analysis, subject samples included in the batch
Back-calculated results of calibration standards	Calculation of precision and accuracy
Standard curve parameters	For all accepted batches
Results of QCs for accepted batches	Calculation of precision and accuracy, report all results (even those outside predefined acceptance limits)
Results of subject samples	Include appropriate sample identification
Rejected batches	Include the reason for the rejection
Repeated samples	Both analytical and nonanalytical repeats, the list should include the original, repeat, and reported results
Incurred sample reproducibility	As appropriate for selected studies

All batches initiated during subject sample analysis should be included in the bioanalytical study report; an overall listing of all study batches and their status (i.e., accepted, rejected, and other) or separate tables prepared for accepted and rejected batches can be provided. Reporting the existence of rejected batches permits a greater understanding of the actual assay performance and completes the overall report. Although it is not necessary to report the data (i.e., concentration results) from rejected batches, the bioanalytical laboratory should maintain the records of all batches in the study file. In cases of repeated run failure, the bioanalytical laboratory should investigate the cause of such failures and include a description of the investigation and the conclusions made in the bioanalytical study report. If the investigation reveals that the bioanalytical method requires modification, the bioanalytical laboratory must determine if the method requires additional validation testing. In this situation, the validation report should be amended to include the results of the additional testing.

In cases where a failing calibration standard or QC result is deemed an outlier based on a statistical test, the actual result should be reported. Precision and accuracy calculations can be presented both with and without the outlier results to facilitate an assessment of the overall impact of the anomalous value. When anomalous results are numerous, the bioanalytical investigator should determine if the results are indicative of a pervasive method problem.

12.2.6.7   *Other Information*

Final reports should address unexpected results, including a description of problems that occurred before and during sample analysis. The impact of such problems on the integrity of the study should be discussed. A listing of critical individuals involved in sample analysis and reporting is essential to understand the duties and responsibilities of the various scientists, experts, and analysts. A description of QAU oversight, as applicable, is pertinent and required for GLP studies. The archive location of the study file and source data should be specified. In the case of chromatographic assays, representative chromatograms[4] should be included as a report appendix.

Bioanalytical reports should be signed and dated by the responsible analytical investigator. For GLP studies, Part 58 specifically requires that contributing scientist reports (e.g., toxicokinetic assessments), signed and dated by the scientist, be appended to the overall study report for a nonclinical safety study.

12.2.7 Repeat Testing

During the course of routine sample analysis, it is recognized that some samples will be reassayed for analytical (e.g., processing error, instrument malfunction, etc.) or nonanalytical (e.g., to check the pharmacokinetic profile, measurable analyte in predose samples, etc.) reasons. Regardless of the reason, the repeat analysis of any sample must be justified and documented. It is expected that written procedures, established in advance of sample analysis, will provide an objective, unbiased approach for the selection of samples for repeat analysis, the reassay scheme (e.g., number of replicates), and the results to report. In our experience, many laboratories use decision trees for comparing and reporting the original and repeat results. When a sample is repeated as a pharmacokinetic outlier, reassay procedures should consider repeating the analysis of samples that surround the time point with the undesirable result.

Bioanalytical study reports should describe the reason of repetition for each repeated sample. A table that lists each type of repeat is useful and facilitates straightforward and clear reporting. The table should include the original, repeat, and accepted result for use in pharmacokinetic calculations. To facilitate an understanding of the repeats as part of the overall study conduct, it is desirable to include the source of each result by listing the run ID for both the original and repeat results. Samples repeated in error (e.g., the analyst did not intend to repeat the sample) should also be reported. Furthermore, if no samples are repeated, the bioanalytical study report should include a statement in this regard.

In cases where the study sponsor or pharmacokineticist[5] assumes responsibility for selecting samples for repeat analysis, the bioanalytical laboratory should require and maintain written documentation of the request in the study file. The written documentation should identify the samples selected by the sponsor or pharmacokineticist, along with the basis for the selection. Ideally, the selection criteria used by the sponsor or pharmacokineticist should be provided to the bioanalytical laboratory in advance of sample analysis and maintained in the study file. Similarly, if the sponsor or pharmacokineticist assumes responsibility for determining the value reported for pharmacokinetic calculations, the SOP followed by the sponsor or pharmacokineticist in this regard should also be provided to the bioanalytical laboratory to facilitate a complete record for reconstructing the study conduct.

---

[4]Refer to the May 2006 conference report for recommendations regarding the chromatograms to be submitted [2].

[5]The pharmacokineticist might be either external or internal to the bioanalytical laboratory.

12.2.8 Incurred Sample Reproducibility

In addition to analytical and nonanalytical repeats, some samples in certain studies need to be reassayed to demonstrate incurred sample reproducibility (ISR). This type of testing is a critical step for demonstrating the reproducibility of the bioanalytical method with samples from dosed subjects (as distinct from precision demonstrated with QCs, i.e., blank matrix spiked with drug). Written procedures in this regard should include a description of how the samples are selected for reanalysis, the comparison and reporting of the original and repeat results, and the acceptance criteria for variability between results.

The repeat results from this type of testing are used to confirm the reproducibility of the assay and should be presented in the bioanalytical study report as a separate data table. In cases where repeat testing of incurred samples does not confirm that the method is reproducible, the bioanalytical laboratory should investigate the cause of the nonreproducibility before continuing its use of the method or reporting results from samples previously assayed.

Although there are many issues to consider in the conduct of appropriate and relevant ISR assessments, particular attention should be paid to the number of samples selected for reassay. To provide adequate coverage across a study in its entirety, 5–10% of the total sample size should be reassayed, with the 5% minimum limited to larger studies. It is also important to note that acceptance limits for ISR comparisons should be commensurate with the methodology (e.g., chromatographic vs. ligand binding assays) and demonstrated assay performance; wide acceptance limits are not recommended. Further details for these issues and other considerations pertinent to ISR can be found in the 2009 workshop report and follow-up publication from the February 2008 AAPS Workshop on assay reproducibility for incurred samples [8].

12.3 CONCLUSIONS

A critical step for assuring data integrity is the complete and contemporaneous documentation of source data. Such records provide the basis for reports that detail bioanalytical results, from method development through routine sample analysis. The lack of comprehensive information in source records and reports is likely to reduce the acceptance of bioanalytical data by regulatory agencies. Therefore, laboratories collecting bioanalytical data should strive to achieve good documentation and reporting practices to assure reliable results for regulatory review decisions. Valid bioanalytical data in pharmacokinetic and toxicokinetic studies benefit the bioanalytical laboratories and sponsors in their quest for successful drug applications.

REFERENCES

1. Guidance for Industry: Bioanalytical Method Validation. U.S. Department of Health and Human Services, Food and Drug Administration, Center for Drug Evaluation and Research (CDER), Center for Veterinary Medicine (CVM), 2001.

2. Viswanathan, C.T., Bansal, S., Booth, B., DeStefano, A., Rose, M., Sailstad, J., Shah, V.P., Skelly, J.P., Swann, P.G., and Weiner, R. (2007) Quantitative bioanalytical methods validation and implementation: best practices for chromatographic and ligand binding assays. *The AAPS Journal*, **9**, E30–E42.

3. Kelley, M., and DeSilva, B. (2007) Key elements of bioanalytical method validation for macromolecules. *The AAPS Journal*, **9**, E156–E163.

4. International Conference on Harmonisation of Technical Requirements for Registration of Pharmaceuticals for Human Use (ICH) (1995) ICH Guideline S3A. Toxicokinetics: the assessment of systemic exposure in toxicity studies. *Federal Register*, **60**(40), 11264–11268.

5. DeSilva, B., Smith, W., Weiner, R., Kelley, M., Smolec, J., Lee, B., Khan, M., Tacey, R., Hill, H., and Celniker, A. (2003) Recommendations for the bioanalytical method validation of ligand-binding assays to support pharmacokinetic assessments of macromolecules. *Pharmaceutical Research*, **20**, 1885–1900.

6. Findlay, J.W.A., Smith, W.C., Lee, J.W., Nordblom, G.D., Das, I., DeSilva, B.S., Khan, M.N., and Bowsher, R.R. (2000) Validation of immunoassays for bioanalysis: a pharmaceutical industry perspective. *Journal of Pharmaceutical and Biomedical Analysis*, **21**, 1249–1273.

7. Smolec, J., DeSilva, B., Smith, W., Weiner, R., Kelley, M., Lee, B., Khan, M., Tacey, R., Hill, H., and Celniker, A. (2005) Bioanalytical method validation for macromolecules in support of pharmacokinetic studies. *Pharmaceutical Research*, **22**, 1425–1431.

8. Fast, D.M., Kelley, M., Viswanathan, CT., O'Shaughnessy, J., King, S.P., Chaudhary, A., Weiner, R., DeStefano, A.J., and Tang, D. (2009) Workshop report and follow-up—AAPS Workshop on current topics in GLP bioanalysis: Assay reproducibility for incurred samples—implications of Crystal City recommendations. *The AAPS Journal*, **11**, 238–241.

CHAPTER 13

Alternative and Emerging Methodologies in Ligand-Binding Assays

HUIFEN F. WANG

Pfizer Inc., New London, CT, USA

JOHN W.A. FINDLAY

Gilead Sciences, Inc., Durham, NC, USA

13.1 INTRODUCTION

Ligand-binding assays (LBAs) have evolved from the use of radiolabeled ligands or antibodies as measures of the end point of the binding reaction, as in radioimmunoassays (RIAs) and immunoradiometric assays (IRMAs), to a range of other end points. The most common of these incorporate an enzyme activity readout, commonly leading to the formation of a colored product that is then quantified by absorbance measurement. This type of assay, implemented in different formats such as enzyme-linked immunosorbent assay (ELISA) or enzyme-multiplied immunoassay techniques (EMITs), not only provides sufficient sensitivity to meet a specific need but also allows the analyst to avoid the hazards of handling and disposal of radioactive materials. Several other methodologies have been developed and found applications in recent years, ranging from time-resolved fluorescence (TRF) and electrochemiluminescence (ECL) techniques to more exploratory-stage methodologies, such as the use of molecularly imprinted polymers (MIPs; "synthetic antibodies"), enzyme-linked immunospot (ELISPOT) assay, surface plasmon resonance (SPR), and online immunoassay techniques. The combination of affinity extraction and mass spectrometry so-called immunoaffinity mass spectrometry) also appears to be of renewed interest. In this chapter, a number of these alternative and emerging technologies are briefly

Ligand-Binding Assays: Development, Validation, and Implementation in the Drug Development Arena. Edited by Masood N. Khan and John W.A. Findlay
Copyright © 2010 John Wiley & Sons, Inc.

reviewed and relevant references provided, so that the reader may consider the potential applications of these techniques to their own experimental work.

13.2 DISSOCIATION-ENHANCED LANTHANIDE FLUOROIMMUNOASSAY

13.2.1 History and Principle of DELFIA Assays

The dissociation-enhanced lanthanide fluoroimmunoassay (DELFIA) technique is based on the principle of TRF. This theoretical concept was reduced to practice in the early 1970s [1–3] and was subsequently commercialized by the scientific equipment manufacturer, LKB/Wallac, as time-resolved fluorometric immunoassay methodology in the early 1980s [4–6]. DELFIA represents the first "ultrasensitive" nonisotopic immunoassay. This technology was reviewed in detail by Soini and Lovgren [7].

DELFIA is typically implemented as a heterogeneous assay either in a noncompetitive or competitive assay format. This analytical method is generally similar to an ELISA. In DELFIA, the enzyme label used is a lanthanide-labeled derivative that, by itself, is essentially nonfluorescent. Following antigen–antibody reaction and removal of unbound fractions, the lanthanide ion is dissociated from the labeled molecule during an enhancement step to form a highly fluorescent lanthanide chelate in solution [7]. The concentration of lanthanide chelate in the solution is measured using time-resolved fluorometry. The enhancement step is a unique feature of DELFIA technology in which the fluorescence of a lanthanide chelate can be amplified many times, which offers greater assay sensitivity. Four lanthanide metals, europium (Eu^{3+}), samarium (Sm^{3+}), terbium (Tb^{3+}), and dysprosium (Dy^{3+}), are commonly used as the chelate labels for antibodies or other reagents involved in the binding reaction step in the assay. Among these, europium has high specific fluorescence activity and offers the best sensitivity [6]. The lanthanide chelate labels have a number of unique fluorescence properties that contribute to high sensitivity, as summarized by Soini and Lovgren [7]. First, they have a long fluorescence lifetime, ranging from 10 to 1000 µs after excitation, which allows the label to be measured at a time when the background fluorescence has already decayed. Second, they display a large Stoke's shift, resulting in a large separation between excitation and emission spectra to minimize cross talk between excitation and emission signals and increase signal-to-noise ratios. Third, they have narrow emission peaks that also contribute to the increased signal-to-noise ratio. Besides providing high sensitivity, the lanthanide concentration can be measured over a wide dynamic range that often translates into a wider calibration range for DELFIA assays than for ELISAs or other conventional immunoassays [7,8].

13.2.2 Applications of DELFIA Assays

DELFIA has been used for the detection of a wide variety of analytes, including proteins, peptides, antibodies, microorganisms, oligonucleotides (ODNs), and other therapeutic agents in different matrices, such as plasma, serum, urine, and feces [9–14]. Numerous examples have shown that DELFIA assays can offer enhanced sensitivity compared to traditional ELISA, mainly due to the unique fluorescence properties of lanthanide chelates [8,15–17]. Compared to colorimetric ELISA, DELFIA increased the sensitivity of a mouse IL-2 assay 8- to 27-fold and a human GM–CSF assay 10-fold [18]. This increase in sensitivity allows the use of small sample volumes and the detection of low levels of analytes of interest. In other studies, DELFIA showed higher sensitivity for detection of both the respiratory syncytial virus antigen and the parainfluenza viruses, but similar sensitivity for detection of adenovirus antigen, compared to enzyme immunoassays [9,10]. Systematic comparisons between DELFIA and ELISA were conducted by Smith and coworkers [19] for the detection of microorganism antigens. In this comparison, three DELFIA methods were developed to mimic the previously developed ELISAs using the same common reagents for the detection of staphylococcal enterotoxin B, *Yersinia pestis*-specific F1 antigen, and Venezuelan equine encephalitis virus. The sensitivity and specificity of each assay were then determined by using a small panel of blinded spiked and nonspiked samples. All three DELFIA assays demonstrated at least 1 log greater sensitivity than corresponding ELISAs using the same reagents, and showed an increase in dynamic range of at least 2 $\log_{10}$ concentrations. The main benefit of a wider assay dynamic range compared to ELISA is that it allows the detection of a wide range of variable unknown concentrations of analyte with fewer dilutions, which could potentially improve assay throughput and minimize dilution errors.

Fluorescent lanthanides are also suitable for quantitative multianalyte assays by using different lanthanide ions as labels due to their narrow emission peaks at different wavelengths and different fluorescence lifetimes. Sm^{3+} and Tb^{3+} labels are often used for multiplexing assays as the second label in a dual-label assay for measuring analytes that require greater sensitivity [20–22]. A dual-label DELFIA immunoassay was developed by Kimura et al. [23] to measure methamphetamine (MA) and chlorpromazine (CPZ) or desipramine (DSP) simultaneously using Eu^{3+} and Sm^{3+} chelates as labels. The fluorescent intensities of Eu^{3+} and Sm^{3+} labels were quantified at 615 and 643 nm, respectively. Since the two lanthanide ions have distinguishable fluorescence peaks, both analytes can be simultaneously determined from a single sample. The lower limit of detection for MA, CPZ, and DSP was 1, 10, and 10 ng/mL, respectively, with a quantification range from 1 ng/mL to 10 µg/mL. Triple- and quadruple-labeled analytical methods have also been reported to measure up to four fluorescent labels simultaneously from one study sample using the same time-resolved fluorometric detection system and enhancement solution [24,25].

Despite the high detection sensitivity reported for DELFIA in general, equivalent sensitivity to ELISA was reported in some evaluations [9,26–28]. To achieve high assay sensitivity, reproducibility and wide dynamic range, coating capacity and quality, and washing steps are critical. Similar to ELISA, the DELFIA method also requires sequential addition of reagents, incubation, and wash steps that are, generally, labor-intensive and time consuming. The main disadvantage of DELFIA is sensitivity to exogenous lanthanide ion contamination [29]. Special washing buffer and rigorous decontamination procedures are required to reduce the background and improve assay reproducibility [19]. In addition, the DELFIA method is relatively more expensive than ELISA, due to the requirement for a time-resolved fluorescence detection counter and special reagents (lanthanide label, special buffer, enhancing reagents, etc.).

These requirements may have limited the broader application of this technology in many research and clinical labs, compared to ELISA.

13.3   ENZYME-LINKED IMMUNOSPOT ASSAY

13.3.1   History and Principle of ELISPOT Assays

The enzyme-linked immunospot technique was originally reported by Sedgwick's and Czerkinsky's groups almost simultaneously in 1983 [30,31] for enumeration of specific antibody-secreting cells. This technology was first applied to the detection of the distribution of IgE secreting cells during a primary immune response [32] and identification of heat-labile enterotoxin-producing *Escherichia coli* [33] by these two groups, respectively, and was then subsequently adapted for the detection of cytokine-secreting cells [34]. During the past 20 years, the ELISPOT method has emerged as one of the most important and widely used tools for monitoring immune responses in preclinical species and humans in the presence of infectious, neoplastic, and autoimmune diseases, as well as during immunotherapy [35–39].

The ELISPOT assay is based on the same principles as the traditional sandwich ELISA technique, using either antigen or antibody to capture the analyte (e.g., antibody, cytokine, or other soluble mediators secreted from a variety of different cell types) of interest and a secondary antibody for detection [30,34]. The basic principle and detailed procedures have been reviewed and outlined [40]. In this assay, the capture antibodies against the analyte of interest are immobilized on specially designed microtiter plates that have membranes of high protein-binding capacity in the bottom. Analyte-releasing cells and stimulating antigen are added to the coated wells. The released analyte binds to the capture antibodies on the membrane in the immediate vicinity of the cells, and the bound analyte is detected by a specific enzyme-labeled secondary antibody. With the addition of an insoluble enzyme-specific substrate, color is developed around the analyte-releasing cells to form a spot, as outlined in Fig. 13.1 [40]. Each individual spot represents a single cell releasing analyte in response to antigen stimulation. The number of spots provides an estimate of the frequency of analyte-producing cells responding to a specific antigen within the test cell population, and the size of a spot correlates with the amount of analyte released [41,42].

13.3.2   Applications of ELISPOT Assays

Although both ELISA and ELISPOT methods are based on the same immunologic principle, they assess immune responses at different stages and address different questions. For cytokine release and production, ELISPOT allows assessment of the frequency of cytokine production, while ELISA measures the total levels of cytokine released into blood or other biological fluids. Since cytokines generally have short half-lives and are often bound to soluble cytokine receptors or other binding proteins, the total concentration of cytokine may not always reflect the changes in relative rates or amounts of cytokine production and/or secretion [43,44]. Thus, ELISA cannot differentiate between the vigorous secretion activity of a few cells

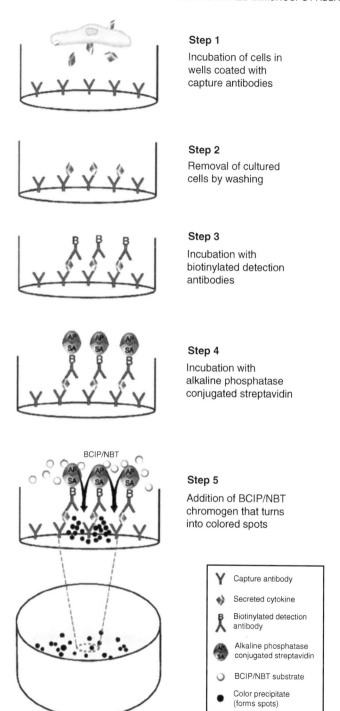

FIGURE 13.1 Principle of ELISPOT assay. *Source*: Reprinted with kind permission of Springer Science + Business Media from Ref. [40].

and the weak response of a large number of cells [41]. In contrast, ELISPOT allows the detection of low frequencies of cells [45], or a single cell [46], secreting a small amount of cytokine by allowing direct visualization of each analyte-secreting cell as a spot [47]. Therefore, ELISPOT has demonstrated greater sensitivity compared to ELISA in the detection of immune responses. Direct comparisons between ELISPOT and ELISA in their ability to detect cytokine secretion by cells were made by Tanguay and Killion [48]. Their results have shown that ELISPOT can detect cytokine secretion from a single cell, which was 10–200-fold more sensitive than ELISA [48]. It is not uncommon that low levels of cytokines or low frequencies of cells secreting cytokines can be detected by ELISPOT but not by ELISA [44,49].

Since ELISPOT combines immunoassay with bioassay, it shares similar challenges to both immunoassays and bioassays in requiring high-quality capture and detection reagents and good quality and reproducibility of cells. In addition, the ELISPOT method requires multiple laboratory steps, such as separation of cells and counting of cells and spots. Performing the ELISPOT assay requires specialized knowledge and technical skills. A recently published *Handbook of ELISPOT* provides a comprehensive review of assay design and performance, data analysis, and troubleshooting for ELISPOT assays [40]. In addition, due to the large number of spots and the variability in spot shape and density, manual assessment of ELISPOT is generally time-consuming, with low throughput, and the results may be subject to high operator-dependent variability in performing the assay and evaluating the results [50]. Introduction of automated systems may overcome this challenge, but increases the cost. In combination with ELISPOT, computer-assisted video image analysis (CVIA) has been reported to allow the objective enumeration of spots and determination of the spot area and has demonstrated increased consistency and precision compared to conventional microscopy [51].

ELISPOT methodology has also been employed for multiplex assays, as reviewed by Sachdeva and Asthana [52]. ELISPOT assay was reported to be able to simultaneously detect different types of cells secreting immunoglobulin G (IgG) and immunoglobulin A (IgA) antibodies [53] and differentiate three subtypes of Th cells producing different cytokines [54] using dual-color ELISPOT assays. A recent report has shown that ELISPOT assay can simultaneously detect four cytokines (hIFN-γ, hIL-2, hIL-4, and hTNF-α) released from the same cell by employing different capture antibodies [55]. Multiplexing of ELISPOT provides a useful tool to assess the combined effect of multiple cytokines or chemokines on the overall immune response.

13.4 IMMUNO-POLYMERASE CHAIN REACTION

13.4.1 History and Principle of IPCR Assays

The immuno-polymerase chain reaction (IPCR) technique was first described by Sano et al. as a highly sensitive method for antigen detection [56]. In this method, the enzyme label used in ELISA is substituted with a specific DNA molecule as a marker and the DNA marker is amplified by PCR to increase assay sensitivity. The production of specific PCR products indicates the presence of the antigen of

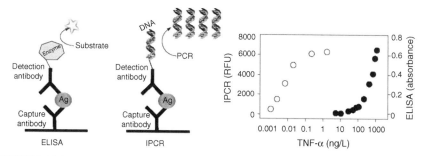

FIGURE 13.2   Principle of IPCR assay. *Source*: Reprinted with kind permission of Elsevier from Ref. [58].

interest by formation of an antigen–antibody complex with the attached DNA marker. Therefore, IPCR assays follow similar principles to those of the traditional ELISA method, requiring specific capture and/or detection antibodies; the IPCR assay can be performed in competitive or noncompetitive, direct, indirect, or sandwich formats. The main difference between ELISA and IPCR is that IPCR uses an antibody–DNA conjugate instead of an antibody–enzyme conjugate to generate assay end point signals for detection. The basic principle of a sandwich IPCR has been discussed and is presented graphically in Fig. 13.2 [57,58].

Efficient linking of a target-specific antibody with a DNA reporter molecule is critical for IPCR. Different approaches have been employed by different researchers to couple reporter DNA with specific antibodies. A recombinant streptavidin–protein A chimera with bispecific binding affinity for IgG and biotinylated DNA was initially used as a linker molecule [56]. Although the streptavidin–protein A chimera allows coupling biotinylated DNA with any unlabeled IgG, the protein A portion of the chimera could potentially cross-react with the Fc region of capture antibodies or other endogenous IgG in study samples, which has limited its broad applications, such as in sandwich IPCR assays. Commercially available avidin and streptavidin have become widely used as universal linker molecules for biotinylated secondary antibody and biotinlylated DNA markers [59–61]. Alternatively, the detection antibody can be labeled directly with a reporter DNA molecule via covalent linkage [62] to simplify the incubation procedures and improve the performance of IPCR [63,64].

Quantitation of amplified PCR products is another critical step that impacts the sensitivity and reproducibility of the method. Different separation and/or detection methods have been reviewed in detail by Niemeyer et al. [57,58], including direct staining, gel electrophoresis, and enzymatic reactions or real-time PCR (rt-PCR). Direct staining with intercalating fluorescent dye followed by fluorescence detection has shown low signal-to-noise ratio and provided the least sensitivity among the methods evaluated [57]. The gel electrophoresis method in which the PCR products are separated by electrophoresis and quantified following ethidium bromide staining has been widely used [56,60,65], although it is generally time-consuming and has low throughput. The enzyme-linked detection methods that employ either doubly labeled PCR amplification products for subsequent quantification by ELISA (PCR-ELISA) or singly labeled PCR amplification products for subsequent quantification by solid-phase hybridization assay or enzyme-linked oligonucleotide–sorbent assay (PCR-ELOSA) have demonstrated greater sensitivity and higher throughput than electrophoresis-based methods [57,66]. However, all of the aforementioned methods require additional sample-handling steps, resulting in high variability, low throughput, and the potential for false positive results due to contamination [58]. Real-time IPCR (rt-IPCR) has been developed during the last few years using fluorescent hybridization probes that allow direct and fast quantification of PCR amplification products [67–70]. The rt-IPCR method displayed improved assay performance over IPCR [71]. The reproducibility and robustness of IPCR have been further improved with the inclusion of an artificial DNA fragment as an internal standard that can be coamplified with the marker DNA during the PCR cycles [71]. This method enabled the sensitive quantitation of the anticancer drug, rViscumin (MW 57 kDa), in human plasma samples at a detection limit of 100 fg/mL, with a mean standard deviation of 14.2% from repeated analyses and a recovery ranging from 70% to 120% [66].

13.4.2 Applications of IPCR Assays

Since IPCR combines antibody specificity with the signal amplification power of PCR, this method provides enhanced detection sensitivity and broader quantitation ranges compared to conventional immunoassays. Direct comparisons between IPCR and ELISA were made by different groups and 10^5–10^6-fold increases of detection sensitivity over conventional ELISA were observed [56,60,72]. For example, this highly sensitive method allows the detection of pathologic prion protein in concentrations as low as 1 fg/mL (approximately 10–100 infectious units) [73] and the ribosome-inactivating proteins, dianthin and ricin, at a concentration of 10 fg/mL [72]. Use of presynthesized antibody–DNA conjugates has demonstrated greater assay sensitivity than assays in which this conjugate is formed during assay incubation [63,64]. The observed linear quantification ranges of IPCR assays were reported to be up to five to six orders of magnitude [64,66]. In addition, the extremely high specificity of PCR for a target sequence defined by a set of primers avoids generation of false signals from other nucleic acid molecules present in samples and allows simultaneous detection of multiple antigens [62] or generation of a competitive DNA sequence as internal standard [66,67] to improve assay sensitivity and reproducibility [58]. However, the relatively cumbersome procedures with prolonged experimental time, low throughput, and the need for special reagents and instrumentation have thus far limited applications of IPCR to situations in which ultrahigh sensitivity is needed.

13.5 ELECTROCHEMILUMINESCENCE-BASED LIGAND-BINDING ASSAYS

13.5.1 History and Principle of ECL Assays

Electrogenerated chemiluminescence, also known as electroluminescence or electrochemiluminescence, has been studied for many years and extensively reviewed by many researchers [74–78]. The applications of ECL detection to immunoassay and DNA probe analyses began to appear in the literature in the early 1990s [79–81] and this has now become a widely used technology for bioaffinity binding assays.

The most common application of ECL to bioaffinity binding assays involves labeling of biological molecules with an ECL-active species. Ruthenium bipyridyl derivatives such as $Ru(bpy)_3^{2+}$ have been widely used as the ECL label for bioaffinity assays coupled with tripropylamine (TPA) as coreactant [82]. The proposed mechanism of the ECL process using the $Ru(bpy)_3^{2+}$/TPA oxidation–reduction system has been discussed by Blackburn and coworkers and is illustrated in Fig. 13.3 [79]. Briefly, $Ru(bpy)_3^{2+}$ and TPA are oxidized at the surface of the electrode, forming $Ru(bpy)_3^{3+}$ and the excited-state molecule $TPA^{+\bullet}$, respectively. The $TPA^{+\bullet}$ molecule spontaneously loses a proton to form $TPA^{\bullet}$, a strong reductant that reacts with another strong oxidant $Ru(bpy)_3^{3+}$, to form the excited-state molecule $Ru(bpy)_3^{2+*}$ at the surface of the electrode. The excited form of the label decays to its ground state, emitting a photon at a wavelength of 620 nm [79,82]. The $Ru(bpy)_3^{3+}$/TPA reaction sequence allows regeneration of $Ru(bpy)_3^{2+}$ in its ground state near the electrode surface after emission of the photon. Therefore, a single molecule of label can generate many photons via multiple ECL reaction cycles to amplify the signal and enhance detection sensitivity [83].

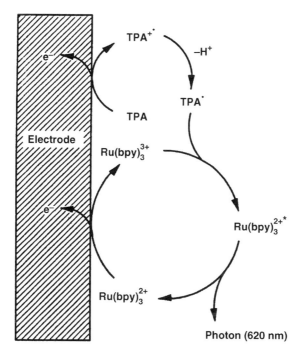

FIGURE 13.3   Mechanism of ECL excitation. *Source:* Reprinted with kind permission of American Association of Clinical Chemistry from Ref. [79].

ORIGEN-1 was the first commercially available ECL analyzer used for immunoassays and DNA probe analysis using a Ru(bpy)$_3^{2+}$-based label [79–81], marketed initially by IGEN International Inc. (later by Bioveris Corp., and now by Roche Diagnostics Corp.). A number of flow-based ECL systems using ORIGEN technology subsequently became available, including the second generation of ORIGEN-1, the M-SERIES, designed for higher throughput, and the Elecsys 1010 and Elecsys 2010 instruments for clinical immunoassay testing [82]. This technology employs magnetic beads as the solid-phase support to capture Ru (bpy)$_3^{2+}$-labeled immune complexes on an electrode surface for the detection of the ECL signal [84]. In recent years, a new class of imaging-based ECL device from Meso Scale Discovery (MSD), LLC has become commercially available. It uses the electrode surface instead of magnetic beads as the solid-phase capture support for bioaffinity binding assays. The electrodes are integrated into the bottom of disposable multiwell plates. The binding reagent is immobilized on the electrode surface; the ECL label is captured on the electrode surface via the binding complex and the light is collected by a charge-coupled device (CCD) camera [82,85]. Although the ORIGEN analyzers are no longer available commercially due to business reasons, the discussion of this technology and its applications in this chapter reflects the development of this technology and provides relevant information for other formats of ECL technologies.

13.5.2 Applications of ECL Assays

A variety of assay formats including sandwich, competitive, or bridging assays in homogenous or heterogeneous format can be implemented with ECL detection, as reviewed by Debad et al. [82] and Miao [85]. For a sandwich assay format, the capture antibody is biotinylated and captured by the streptavidin-coated solid phase. The analyte is then bound to the capture antibody and an ECL-labeled detection antibody to form a sandwich complex on the streptavidin-coated solid phase. For a competitive assay format, one antibody is biotinylated for capture by the streptavidin-coated solid phase, and an ECL-labeled analyte competes with the nonlabeled analyte for binding to the antibody [82,86]. Similar approaches have been employed for the detection and quantification of nucleic acid amplification products [87,88] via sandwich hybridization assay using an immobilized probe and a labeled probe, or via a direct binding assay using a labeled amplification product of nucleic acid [82].

ECL-based immunoassays combine the advantages of high sensitivity and broad dynamic range of ECL with the high specificity of the antibody capture reagent. Femtogram-level sensitivity for the detection of purified biotoxoids was reported [89] using a single-step sandwich reaction with the ORIGEN device. The detection limits were at least an order of magnitude lower than the results obtained with other common detection systems, except radioimmunoassay [89]. The flow-based assay offers significant advantages by eliminating incubation and wash steps for the convenience of rapid sample handling and higher throughput. Quantitation of lutenizing hormone (LH) using a sandwich ECL assay was 20–25-fold more sensitive than by RIA, while slightly improved sensitivity over RIA was observed for salmon calcitonin detection by the same group [83]. The high sensitivity of ECL detection made it possible to achieve a desired sensitivity using a competitive assay format when only one specific reagent is available [86]. The quantification ranges of ECL-based assays are generally greater than three orders of magnitude [79,83,86,90], which could dramatically reduce the required number of dilutions for study samples with a wide range of unknown concentrations, thus greatly increasing sample throughput.

ECL-based immunoassays offer a number of additional advantages over conventional immunoassays. The ECL label is extremely stable and can be stored for over a year at room temperature [76] or for 18 months at -10 to $-30°C$ [83]. This represents a significantly extended shelf life compared to radioisotope labels and improved reproducibility and convenience of the assay by reducing the number of times a switch to a new batch of this key reagent is required. In addition, because light is generated from an electrochemical reaction, biological substances do not contribute to, or alter, the background emission; therefore, matrix effects are generally minimized [84,90]. Good assay reproducibility and recovery were observed for neat (undiluted) normal human serum and serum from rheumatoid arthritis patients for quantitation of a fully human anti-TNF-α monoclonal antibody [86]. It has also been reported that excess therapeutic antibodies present in serum were tolerated better in an assay for the detection of antitherapeutic antibodies based on the MSD ECL device [91]. Furthermore, the ECL procedure has been reported to be stable over a broad range of magnetic bead concentrations, probe concentrations, and hybridization conditions for a nucleic acid binding assay, making these assays more versatile and easier to transfer from one laboratory to another [88].

The recently developed MSD ECL technology has also eliminated the challenging issues related to the flow-based ECL device, such as blockage of fluid-handling system components upon repeated assays, which requires stringent cleaning to refresh the electrode surface prior to and after each use, and the need for frequent decontamination [82,92,93]. This new technology also enables simultaneous detection and measurement of multiple analytes in the same sample using a Multi-Spot plate with multiple binding sites on the electrode surface of each well. A panel of 10 human cytokines (GM-CSF, IL-1-β, IL-2, IL-4, IL-5, IL-6, IL-8, IL-10, IL-12p70, and TNF-α) was able to be measured simultaneously in each well on a 96-well plate for proteomic analysis [94].

The high sensitivity and reproducibility, broad dynamic range, relative insensitivity to matrix effects, availability in a variety of assay formats, ease of use, and time-saving features make ECL-based bioaffinity assay an attractive alternative to conventional immunoassays. The application of ECL bioaffinity assays is growing rapidly and has been reviewed by several authors [77,78,82,85]. ECL-based bioaffinity assays offer great value in a wide range of biomedical research applications, such as in gene mutation detection [95,96], ligand–receptor interaction studies [97], enzyme–inhibitor interaction studies [98], drug discovery and development [86,90,99], clinical diagnostics [79,87,88], environmental assays such as food and water testing [100], and biowarfare agent detection [89].

13.6 HYBRIDIZATION-BASED LIGAND-BINDING ASSAYS

13.6.1 History and Principle of Hybridization Ligand-Binding Assays

Oligonucleotides, including antisense short-interfering RNA (siRNA), ribozymes, cytosine–guanosine (CpG) ODNs, aptamers, and spiegelmers [101] have recently emerged as potential therapeutics for the treatment of a variety of diseases, including cancer, viral and bacterial infections, autoimmune and inflammatory diseases, neurological disorders, and metabolic diseases [102–106]. Consequently, there is an increasing need to develop sensitive analytical methods for quantification of therapeutic ODNs in biological matrices and/or tissues to evaluate the pharmacokinetics (PK), toxicokinetics (TK), tissue distribution, and pharmacokinetic/pharmacodynamic (PK/PD) relationships of ODNs in support of their preclinical and clinical development.

Conventional approaches for quantitation of therapeutic ODNs in biological matrices have been previously reviewed [107,108], including the use of radiolabeled analogues, high-performance liquid chromatography (HPLC) methods, HPLC-MS (LC–MS), capillary gel electrophoresis (CGE), and matrix-assisted laser desorption–ionization time-of-flight mass spectrometry (MALDI-TOF MS). These approaches in general have limited sensitivity (ng/mL to μg/mL) and are often time-consuming, due in part to the requirement for sample extraction from biological matrix [109], and suffer from low throughput.

Over the last decade, different formats of hybridization-based analytical methods have been developed for quantitation of ODNs in biological matrices and/or tissues. These types of assays combined hybridization of nucleic acids with immunoassay principles by replacing an antigen–antibody interaction with a sense–antisense ODN reaction. A direct approach using a radiolabeled complementary ODN to detect oligodeoxynucleotide phosphorothioates in biological fluids and tissues was first described by Temsamani et al. [110]. This method requires extraction of analytes from biological samples prior to hybridization and this has apparently limited the throughput of the assay. Competitive hybridization-based assays using radiolabeled or nonradiolabeled analyte for detection have also been reported [111,112]. In these assays, sense ODNs were used as capture molecules and labeled analogues compete with unlabeled antisense analyte to form a double-stranded nucleic acid complex. The labeled analogues in the hybridization complex were detected either directly by radioactivity or via biotin–streptavidin–enzyme conjugate using a colorimetric detection. The general principle of a hybridization LBA with colorimetric readout is illustrated in Fig. 13.4. The reported detection limit of these assays ranged from 0.9 to ~5 nM (21 ng/mL) for phosphodiester or phosphorothioate ODNs [111,112]. Additional detection systems, for example, TRACE (time-resolved amplified cryptate emission), fluorescence, and time-resolved fluorescence, in conjunction with hybridization, for the detection of ODNs have also been reported by other researchers [113–115].

Following principles similar to those of immunoassays, noncompetitive hybridization assays in general demonstrate better sensitivity than competitive formats of

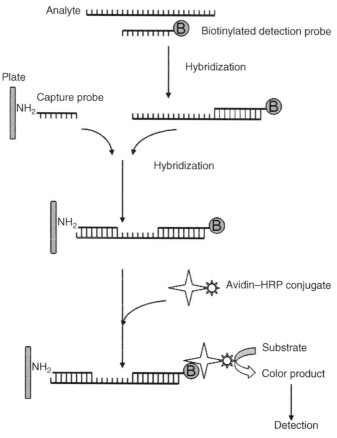

FIGURE 13.4   Scheme for hybridization ligand-binding assay.

these assays [116,117]. From a side-by-side comparison, a sandwich hybridization assay was reported to be about 30-fold more sensitive than a competitive hybridization assay to detect the DNA amplification product of tuberculosis from PCR [118]. In a recent report, a colorimetric sandwich hybridization assay using sequence-specific capture and detection ODN probes with locked nucleic acids achieved a detection limit of 2.8 pg/mL ($\sim$0.3 pM) for a 24-mer phosphorothioate ODN in human plasma [119].

13.6.2   Applications of Hybridization Ligand-Binding Assays

Hybridization-based methods in general demonstrated greater sensitivity compared to conventional methods for ODN detection [120], as well as requiring minimum sample cleanup, and being characterized by high-throughput and good accuracy and precision [107,119]. These methods have been used for quantitative analysis of ODNs from biological samples to support pharmacokinetic and toxicokinetic evaluations [109,111,119]. However, one of the limitations of hybridization assays is their lack of specificity for the full-length ODN relative to potential metabolites formed by loss of one or a few nucleotides from either the 3'- or 5'-end of the molecule [111,112]. Cross reactivity was reported generally to decrease with each base deletion, and was negligible after deletion of four bases from either the 3'- or 5'-terminus [112]. Similar results were observed for an antisense ODN where cross-reactivity of analogues with 3'- deletions from N-1 to N-4 was 55%, 36%, 27%, and 2% and with 5'-deletions from N-1 to N-4 was 33%, 62%, 11%, and 0%, respectively [111].

A noncompetitive hybridization–ligation ELISA was recently reported [121] to address this relative nonspecificity issue of hybridization assays. This assay is based on the principle of hybridization of both the analyte and a detection probe to a complementary sequence template, followed by ligation between the analyte and the detection probe. Only the full-length analyte can be ligated with the detection probe and subsequently detected via a digoxigenin–antidigoxigenin–alkaline phosphatase conjugate using fluorescence detection. Any metabolites with missing oligonucleotide(s) at the 3'-end cannot be ligated with the detection probe and unligated probe will be washed away. The method not only demonstrated excellent sensitivity with a dynamic range from 0.05 to 2 nM but also showed selectivity for the specific sequence tested. The cross-reactivity toward 3'-metabolites was confirmed to be minimal (<0.22%) [121]. Similar sensitivity (0.05 nM) and limited cross-reactivity with 3'-end deletion oligomers (<6%) have been reported by other researchers using hybridization–ligation methods [122]. With their demonstrated sensitivity, hybridization-based binding assays enable the detection of low concentrations of highly . potent therapeutic ODNs in biological samples following administration of low doses to support their preclinical and clinical development [119]. These assays can also be used as a powerful tool for clinical diagnosis by screening and identification of trace levels of bacterial or viral DNA or mRNA, gene mutation or infection, following DNA amplification by PCR [116].

13.7 MOLECULARLY IMPRINTED POLYMERS (SYNTHETIC ANTIBODIES)

13.7.1 History and Principle of MIP Development

Although characterized by high specificity, antibodies, particularly monoclonal antibodies, are time consuming and relatively resource intensive to produce, involving multiple immunizations of animals to stimulate a strong immune response and rounds of cloning to select a cell population expressing antibodies of the desired specificity. Given these challenges, it is not surprising that considerable efforts have been made to develop "synthetic" equivalents to antibodies that might be more rapidly and consistently available and less expensive to prepare. Considerable progress has been made in developing molecularly imprinted polymers retaining many of the specific recognition properties of antibodies [123–129]. The basis of this approach (Fig. 13.5) is the polymerization of functional and cross-linking monomers in the presence of the analytical molecule of interest (the imprint molecule); removal of the imprint molecule following polymerization leaves behind imprinted or memory sites

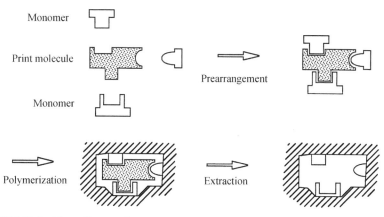

FIGURE 13.5 Flow diagram for preparation of molecularly imprinted polymers.
Source: Reprinted with permission of Elsevier from Ref. [123].

in the cross-linked polymer that are characteristic of some functional groups present in the imprint molecule. The imprint molecule is mixed with monomers and cross-linkers in a suitable solvent prior to initiation of the polymerization. Typical monomers include methacrylic acid, 2- and 4-vinylpyridines, trifluoromethacrylic acid, acrylamide, and hydroxyethylmethacrylate and cross-linkers include ethylene glycol dimethacrylate, divinylbenzene, and trimethylolpropane trimethacrylate. Following addition of an initiator, such as an azobisnitrile, the polymerization can be conducted either by elevation of the temperature or by irradiation with ultraviolet light. However, it has been shown [124] that MIPs prepared at lower temperatures (below 0°C), using photoinitiation, exhibit higher molecular recognition capabilities. Following polymerization, the imprint molecule is removed from the polymer by solvent washing, leaving cavities in the polymer matrix that are complementary to functional groups on the imprint molecule and are capable of binding the imprint molecule specifically and reversibly. For applications of MIPs in binding assays, it is important to remove the imprint molecule as completely as possible to avoid limiting sensitivity of the assay. Factors affecting the properties of MIPs and the physical basis of interactions between MIP and ligand are not completely understood and have been the subject of discussion in some detail by Nicholls et al. [129].

13.7.2 Applications of MIPs

Applications of MIPs have been wide ranging, from use as molecularly specific, solid-phase extraction media prior to chromatography [130] to antibody substitutes in "pseudo-immunoassays" [131]. The latter approach, sometimes referred to as "MIA" (molecularly imprinted sorbent assay), appears to be particularly suited to assay of low molecular weight organic molecules, since assay processes often include extraction of the molecules from the biological medium and incubation with the MIP in an organic solvent. Thus, Vlatakis et al. [132] developed MIA assays in organic media, using radiolabeled tracer, for theophylline and diazepam, demonstrating similar sensitivity and specificity to that of EMITs using biological antibodies. Ansell's review [131] covers recent developments in polymer formats, novel probes, and assay formats, including flow-through methods and flow-injection and scintillation proximity assays. Applications of MIPs to binding assays in organic solvents have included assays for morphine [133], cortisone and cortisol [134], and propranolol [135]. Although early studies were conducted in organic solvents, exploratory work in aqueous media led to an MIA for direct determination of propranolol in plasma [136]. These radioassays are similar in principle to competitive radioimmunoassay, with antibody being replaced in the MIA by imprinted binding polymers. Binding affinities of MIPs for their analytes were shown to be often in the nM range, and nM sensitivities were achievable in some cases. The ability of MIPs to distinguish between enantiomers was also shown for propranolol [135]. Nonradioactive end points have also been incorporated into binding assays using MIPs, including fluorescence [137] using a fluorescent tracer molecule with structural similarities to the analyte of interest, and chemiluminescence [138] through the use of an antigen conjugated to a peroxidase enzyme and luminol as substrate. The latter assay was demonstrated in 96- and 384-well formats. Other interesting applications of MIP-based binding assays include development of a flow-injection capillary chemiluminescent assay in a competitive format with sensitivities as low as the picomolar range [139] and a competitive-format scintillation proximity assay for (S)-propranolol that involved incorporation of an aromatic, cross-linking monomer (divinylbenzene) as a radiation-harvesting agent into the MIP [140]. The next application of MIPs to LBAs will likely be in the field of polypeptides and proteins, although no such assays appear to have been published to date. Clearly, creating molecular imprints of proteins is challenging, because of their three-dimensional structure and the greater difficulties of conducting polymerization reactions in the aqueous media needed to maintain protein solubility. However, an increasing number of papers are being published in this field, such as those for angiotensin II derivatives [141] and C-reactive protein [142]. Progress toward synthesis of protein MIPs has been reviewed by Bossi et al. [143], Janiak and Kofinas [144], and Bergmann and Peppas [145]. MIPs offer an interesting alternative to biologically derived antibodies and a potentially more secure source of key binding reagents at a lower cost than is the case for antibodies. Protein MIPs remain a challenge, but encouraging progress is being made, and successful application of these to LBAs for proteins is anticipated in the relatively near future.

13.8 SURFACE PLASMON RESONANCE METHODS

13.8.1 History and Principle of SPR Assays

The technique of SPR is based on a change in refractive index occurring in the close vicinity of a thin metal film surface upon binding of a ligand to a target molecule. Although observed earlier as a purely physical phenomenon, the application of SPR to biosensing was first reported by Liedberg and coworkers [146,147]. The underlying mechanism of the SPR technology has been discussed by many authors, including Mullett et al. [148] and Hsieh and coworkers [149], and in a brief historical review by

Liedberg et al. [150]. The SPR sensing mechanism exploits the properties of an evanescent field generated at the site of total internal reflection of an incident light beam. In the phenomenon of total internal reflection, light traveling through a medium of higher refractive index, such as a glass prism, is totally internally reflected at an oblique angle upon encountering a medium of lower refractive index such as a protein solution. The intensity of the reflected light is dampened by the presence of a metal film at the interface of the two media. As proteins adsorb onto the metal surface, the refractive index of the solution near the interface changes, resulting in a change in the angle at which the reflected light is dampened (Fig. 13.6). Detection of the change in this angle is the basis of a number of commercially available biosensor techniques, particularly the widely used BIAcore instrument. The metal typically used in the interface film is gold, and through the use of chemical conjugation to polymers coated on the gold surface, antibodies, receptors, target proteins, and others can be immobilized on the metal film. Changes in refractive index upon binding of appropriate species to these immobilized molecules in a flowing solution have allowed the SPR method to be used extensively in the study of association and dissociation kinetics of ligands, as well as to determine concentrations of analyte ligands in the solution flowing near the metal film. SPR immunoassays are capable of monitoring binding interactions in real time without the need for labeling of either the binding reagent or the ligand and have competitive sensitivity with ELISA or RIA.

13.8.2   Applications of SPR Assays

Comparisons of SPR immunoassays with commercially available conventional immunoassay kits (RIA or ELISA) for the detection of β-2-microglobulin, theophylline, and IgE [150] revealed good correlations. While good correlations were also obtained between SPR and ELISA assays for the detection of ractopamine, a β-adrenergic agonist animal food additive, comparison with HPLC suggested that the SPR immunoassay suffered from cross-reactivity of ractopamine metabolites, despite the fact that a monoclonal antibody was employed [151]. As for other LBAs, the accuracy of the data generated on incurred study samples depends on the specificity of the binding reagent employed in the assay for the analyte of interest. Other comparisons included that of the SPR immunoassay for the detection of antibody to porcine circovirus type 2 (PCV2) in swine serum [152], where the authors showed a strong positive correlation between SPR assay and ELISA, and a favorable comparison of ELISA and an SPR immunoassay for IGF-1 in cow's milk [153].

As regards sensitivity, the detection limit for a variety of molecules was stated to range between 10^{-9} and 10^{-13} mol/L using SPR detection [148]. Also, Masson and coworkers recently reported [154] sub-ng/mL detection limits for an SPR immunoassay for myoglobin and cardiac troponin in human serum, while Kreutzer and coworkers described an SPR assay for the steroid stanozolol with a detection limit of 6 ng/mL and a projected sensitivity, with assay improvements, in the pM range [155]. Femtomolar sensitivity has been described by Cao and Sim [156] for the detection of antiglutamic acid decarboxylase antibody using colloidal gold

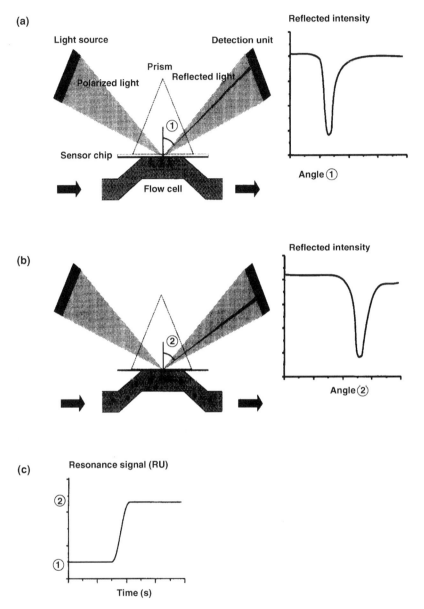

FIGURE 13.6 Principle of surface plasmon resonance assay. *Source*: Reprinted with kind permission of Elsevier from Ref. [149].

nanoparticles in conjunction with enzyme-mediated precipitation of an insoluble product on the chip surface.

The evolution of SPR methodology toward the commercially available BIAcore instrument line was outlined by Liedberg and coworkers [150]. Other commercially available systems have been reviewed by Mullet et al. [148] and Rich and Myszka [157]. Application of optical fibers, optical waveguide, or integrated optical waveguide for SPR has been reported for the development of miniature SPR sensors as well as multichannel detection [158].

Due to the widespread occurrence of biomolecular binding interactions, SPR has found broad applications in biomedical research, drug discovery, and clinical diagnosis in assessing the kinetics of ligand–receptor, ligand–antibody, sense–antisense, and enzyme–substrate interactions. This technology can also provide data on the specificity and affinity of such interactions, as well as data for epitope mapping and quantitation of analytes. In a recent survey, Rich and Myszka [159] report publication of 1219 articles on application of this technology in 2006 to a wide range of scientific applications. Examples of analytical applications as wide ranging as SPR immunoassays for the detection of fungal spores [160], the β-toxin of *Clostridium perfringens* [149], basic fibroblast growth factor [161], and a fluorescence-based SPR assay for prostate-specific antigen [162] have been reported. Several SPR immunoassays for small xenobiotics in agricultural applications have been reported, including methods for sulfonamide residues in tissues [163] and ivermectin [164] and progesterone [165] in bovine milk.

Of probable interest to the reader of this volume are the many applications of SPR to assays for the detection and characterization of antibodies elicited by therapeutic treatment with biologic macromolecules [166–169]. Given the current intense interest in the development of protein and ODN macromolecules as potential therapeutics, as well as the developing interest in "biosimilar protein products," immunogenicity of macromolecules will continue to be investigated for the foreseeable future. Further discussion of assay formats for the detection and characterization of antibodies elicited by treatment with macromolecular therapeutics is presented elsewhere in this volume.

Although SPR methods produce individual biomolecular interaction data in real time, overall throughput of the methods may still be relatively limited. Recent efforts have been targeted at higher throughput SPR methods [170]. Rich and Myszka [157] reviewed the evolution of SPR-based biomolecular interaction systems from handling one assay at a time to currently available high-throughput, parallel processing systems. One such new direction involves monitoring many interactions simultaneously by SPR imaging, made possible by merging the use of protein arrays with SPR microscopy [170]. This high-throughput approach to SPR analysis may have many important drug discovery applications, including in cell signaling pathway evaluation and therapeutic antibody development. In another direction, the SPR method has been extended to the detection of multiple analytes in a sample, as discussed by Homola et al. [171]. The SPR technique has also been coupled with the MIP approach in elegant work by Lotierzo and colleagues [172], including the generation of a 40 nm thin film of MIP as binding reagent on the gold surface of the sensor chip. Using this approach, an SPR MIP-based assay for the neurotoxic amino acid, domoic acid, with a limit of detection estimated to be 5 ng/mL was developed. Although the use of MIP gave somewhat lower assay sensitivity than an SPR immunoassay with a monoclonal antibody as immobilized binding reagent, the assay range was broader for the

MIP-based assay and the MIP sensor chip was able to be regenerated many more times than the antibody sensor chip. In another application reviewed by Nedelkov and Nelson [173], the detection and quantitation abilities of SPR technology were coupled with mass spectral identification of proteins captured, either directly on the sensor chip or following elution from the chip surface.

Although SPR technology has advanced significantly over the past 2 decades, it has remained, until recently, a relatively low-throughput technique with limited distribution of knowledge and skill and has required individual functionalized sensor chips for each assay application. Continuing advances are expected to improve further the sensitivity and throughput of SPR assays and reduce the size and cost of SPR devices, thus facilitating broader applications of these sensitive, label-free LBA methods.

13.9 CHROMATOGRAPHY–LIGAND-BINDING ASSAY COUPLED METHODS, IMMUNOAFFINITY SYSTEMS, AND ONLINE (FLOW-INJECTION) LIGAND-BINDING ASSAY METHODS

LBAs coupled with chromatographic systems have been used for many years to enhance assay specificity in situations in which mixtures of parent molecule and cross-reacting metabolites or coadministered medications are present in the biological sample under analysis.

13.9.1 Chromatography–Immunoassay Systems

Separation of parent drug prior to immunoassay may provide assay results that are specific for the parent molecule. The chromatographic separation provides specificity while the LBA (typically immunoassay) provides the required sensitivity. For example, HPLC followed by off-line immunoassay has been used for the specific analysis of digoxin in the presence of digoxin metabolites and endogenous digoxin-like factors [174]. However, because of relatively long run times on HPLC and collection and subsequent immunoassay of eluted fractions, these assays are cumbersome, labor-intensive, and low throughput and have largely been replaced by LC/MS-based methods. However, more recent advances in online chromatography–immunoassay systems, as reviewed by Tang and Karnes [175], provide more practical applications. These authors considered systems in two general categories—precolumn immunoassay and postcolumn immunoassay, coupled in each case to liquid chromatography. In the precolumn immunoassay system, an online immunoreaction occurs prior to HPLC. Antibodies are immobilized either covalently or noncovalently to a solid support. Following immunoadsorption, the immunoaffinity column is switched to be online with the HPLC column and the antibody-bound component(s) are dissociated with an elution buffer, concentrated on the HPLC precolumn and then subjected to HPLC separation with appropriately sensitive detection, such as by mass spectrometry. These methods offer advantages of specificity and increased sensitivity by concentration of analytes, and they avoid issues of compatibility of HPLC mobile phases with the immunoassay components, as may be the case with postcolumn immunoassay systems. Disadvantages include nonspecific binding of matrix components to the immunoaffinity column, which may then coelute with the desired analyte. The precolumn immunoassay adsorption technique has been applied to analysis of a wide range of compounds, including corticosteroids [176] and trace analysis of LSD analogues in human urine [177]. Protein applications include a dual microcolumn immunoassay with a reverse-phase capillary column for the determination of insulin secretion from single rat islet cells using a UV absorbance detector [178]. Tang and Karnes [175] also reviewed post-column immunoassay coupled to HPLC in formats of one-site, direct, sandwich, competitive, and heterogeneous or homogeneous immunoassays. Postcolumn immu-noassay systems generally have high specificity, but tend to suffer from nonspecific binding and issues of compatibility of aqueous-based immunoassay systems with organic mobile phases used in reversed-phase HPLC.

13.9.2 Immunosorbent Systems

Capillary electrophoresis–immunoassay (CEIA) combines the separating power of CE with the ligand-binding sensitivity of immunoassay either in competitive or noncompetitive assay formats. A "reversed" form of this approach has been reviewed in depth by Delaunay-Bertoncini and Hennion [179]. In this implementation, ligand binding in the form of immunoaffinity extraction with an immunosorbent (IS) has been described for a wide range of low molecular weight xenobiotics, with ISs designed to extract either a single compound or a group of related compounds, followed by further specific analysis, either off-line or online. Polyclonal or monoclonal antibodies are immobilized, either covalently or by simple adsorption, on inert support materials. Immunoaffinity often provides a cleaner extract for further analysis and offers the possibility of concentration of the sample prior to further analysis. Although the majority of applications have involved off-line analysis by such techniques as LC/MS, GC/MS, or CE following IS extraction, the authors also describe coupled online methods, again with HPLC, CE, and mass spectrometry for the separation or detection of the analyte(s). The concentration of analyte from a sample by immunoaffinity extraction is a benefit when CE is coupled with IS, since CE is a comparatively insensitive bioanalytical method. Application of an IS–CE system requires either adsorption [180] or covalent attachment [181] of antibodies to the capillary wall of the CE system. Since it is difficult to immobilize a large amount of antibodies onto a capillary column surface, this approach suffers from limited capacity and laborious construction. However, the approach has been applied successfully, for example, with neuropeptides, using laser-induced fluorescence for detection [182]. The IS approach has also been coupled with mass spectrometry, an example being the IS-MALDI-TOF MS detection of potato glycoalkaloids in serum [183]. This methodology has also been extended to IS extraction and separation of two enantiomers of diarylalkyltriazole using immobilized recombinant Fab fragments of monoclonal antibodies cloned to recognize either enantiomer [184].

13.9.3 Flow-Injection Immunoassays

Online (flow-injection) immunoassay methods have been of interest for a considerable time. In these methods, either all immunoassay steps take place in an online immunoreactor cell or the immunoreactor steps are preceded by an initial off-line incubation. One of the attractions of these approaches is that times for individual analyses are relatively short so that data may be obtained in shorter overall times than available from typical multiwell assay formats. The technique has been applied to immunoassays for both low molecular weight xenobiotics and macromolecules. A few examples to illustrate the range of applications investigated are given below. Fu and coworkers [185] reported a flow-injection chemiluminescent immunoassay for α-fetoprotein in noncompetitive format, involving an off-line incubation of the analyte with horseradish peroxidase-labeled α-fetoprotein antibody as tracer. This mixture was then passed through an immunoreactor containing immobilized α-fetoprotein and the trapped tracer molecule in the immunoreactor was detected by reaction with a p-iodophenol-luminol-H_2O_2 chemiluminescence system. The decrease in chemiluminescence signal was proportional to the α-fetoprotein concentration across the range 5–100 ng/mL. A similar assay was reported for carcinoembryonic antigen with a concentration range of 1–25 ng/mL and an online assay time of 5 min after an off-line incubation of 25 min [186]. Yang and colleagues [187] described a competitive-format flow-injection immunoassay for gentamicin that did not require a preincubation step and had a sample throughput time of only 10 min. This assay involved competition between gentamicin and fluorescein-labeled gentamicin for binding to immobilized antigentamicin antibody in an online immunoreactor. A competitive immunoassay for digoxin using the acridinium chemiluminescence system with femtomolar sensitivity by either continuous-flow or sequential-injection approaches has also been described [188]. Reinecke and Scheper [189] reported an automated flow-injection immunoassay for IgG applied to monitoring bioprocesses. In this simple assay, a cartridge containing protein G immobilized on a carrier was inserted online to bind IgG in the sample. Following washing steps, the IgG was eluted with a pH-adjusted buffer and the concentration monitored via fluorescence. An interesting online competitive immunoassay for insulin was reported by Tao and Kennedy [190]. Solutions of fluorescein-labeled insulin, monoclonal anti-insulin antibody, and insulin in a sample were pumped into a reaction vessel for mixing. The mixture flowed through a fused silica reactor capillary to a flow-gated interface. During this process, insulin and tracer-labeled insulin competed to form a complex with the antibody. At the interface, the mixture was injected into a separation capillary where bound and free insulin fractions were separated and detected by capillary electrophoresis with laser-induced fluorescence. Each separation took as little as 3 s and more than 1600 consecutive assays could be performed before there was need to rinse the separation column. The assay was applied for determination of the insulin content of single islets of Langerhans. Many more examples of online (flow-injection) assays are to be found in the scientific literature.

13.10   FUTURE TRENDS AND DIRECTIONS FOR LBA TECHNOLOGIES

Ligand-binding assay technologies continue to advance, as reviewed by Self and Cook [191]; these authors briefly discussed changes in signal detection methods, immunochemistry, and assay formats among other parameters. New binding reagents continue to be developed as alternatives to antibodies for LBA. In addition to MIPs, aptamers, which are ODNs composed of nucleic acid fragments possessing remarkably high affinity for binding to specific targets, have emerged as an alternative to antibodies in LBAs, particularly in clinical diagnostic applications [192,193]. The ability to chemically synthesize these molecules promises another alternative to shorten times for generation of key binding reagents and accelerate assay development times. New detection technologies will also continue to emerge for LBAs, including extensions of immunoaffinity extraction followed by mass spectrometric detection, as reviewed by Nedelkov [194]. In this paper useful applications in the protein analysis field are reviewed, using techniques of mass spectral analysis for antibody–protein conjugates or proteins eluted from antibody conjugates, as well as surface plasmon resonance or mass spectral analysis of protein bound to a microchip-adsorbed capture antibody. Ligand-binding assay technologies will continue to advance toward ultrasensitive, accurate, and high-throughput assays using simple, fast, and cost-effective procedures and/or automated devices. General themes for new and exciting research in LBAs will encompass the topics of biosensors, miniaturization, and microfluidics. Miniaturization offers potential benefits of sensitivity enhancement through concentration of analytes into very small reaction volumes, but faces challenges (mainly related to the physics and engineering issues involved in miniaturization), as discussed by Madou et al. [195]. Low picomolar sensitivities were reported for the quantification of antistreptavidin antibodies [(0.1–6.7 pM) [196]] and the immunosuppressant, tacrolimus [(10 pg/mL)[197]] using microfluidic ELISAs. The ultimate goal is the so-called lab-on-a-chip or lab-on-a-CD assay that combines procedures such as sample preparation, incubation, detection, and analysis into a single process. A CD-like microfluidic ELISA platform has been reported by Lai and coworkers [198]. Further review of progress on miniaturization and microfluidics systems, with a focus on immunoassays, is provided by Bange and colleagues [199]. They examine the possible advantages of combined microfluidics and miniaturization, including the possibility of providing point-of-care assays at the local site of sample collection.

Multiplexed immunoassays, which permit the simultaneous assay of several analytes in the same sample, are already available commercially. These systems typically depend on the use of reagent beads functionalized with different capture antibodies directed against the analytes of interest. Interest in multiplexed assays seems likely to continue to develop rapidly. The advantages and limitations of bead-based and microspot/microarray-based multiplexing approaches, as well as their application to the field of molecular diagnostics, have been discussed recently [200].

A recent interesting development has been the high-sensitivity flow-based immunoassay using single-molecule counting by fluorescence. This system has been applied to the development of an assay for cardiac troponin, with a limit of detection of 1.7 pg/mL [201]. The assay uses a fluorescent tracer to label the antibody–analyte complex that is then eluted from the plate and subjected to counting of fluorescence on a single-molecule basis. Since this is a new commercial diagnostic system (Singulex, Alameda, CA), extensive details of the methodology do not appear to have been published. However, this technology appears to hold substantial promise for broad application in the future.

13.11 CONCLUSIONS

Several LBA approaches have been developed as alternatives to the initially discovered radioimmunoassay and subsequent immunoassays with enzyme-based detection systems. These assays cover a wide range of formats and detection systems, ranging from IPCR to electrochemiluminescence to application of biosensor technologies, as reviewed in this chapter. A strong interest also continues in the further development of MIPs (a particular challenge for proteins and polypeptides) and aptamers as substitutes for antibodies as key binding reagents. Research into combined LBA–chromatography and LBA–mass spectrometry systems remains strong. We anticipate further development of a number of these technologies in the future, but with a particularly strong emphasis on miniaturization of assays, using microfluidics to develop "lab-on-a-chip or CD" systems suitable for high-throughput drug discovery support or development of point-of-care diagnostic systems.

ACKNOWLEDGMENT

The authors wish to thank Neel Neelkantan for his initial input to the section on IPCR.

REFERENCES

1. Sacchi, C.A., Svelto, O., and Prenna, G. (1974) Pulsed tunable lasers in cytofluorometry. *Histochemical Journal*, **6**, 251–258.
2. Lytle, F.E., and Kelsey, M.S. (1974) Cavity-dumped argon-ion laser as an excitation source in time-resolved fluorimetry. *Analytical Chemistry*, **46**, 855–860.
3. Leif, R.C., Thomas, R.A., Yopp, T.A., Watson, B.D., Guarino, V.R., Hindman, D.H.K., Lefkove, N., and Vallarino, L.M. (1977) Development of instrumentation and fluorochromes for automated multiparameter analysis of cells. *Clinical Chemistry*, **23**, 1492–1498.
4. Soini, E., and Kojola, H. (1983) Time-resolved fluorometer for lanthanide chelates: a new generation of non-isotopic immunoassays. *Clinical Chemistry*, **29**, 65–68.

5. Pettersson, K., Siitari, H., Hemmila, I., Soini, E., Lovgren, T., Hanninen, V., Tanner, P., and Stenman, U.H. (1983) Time-resolved fluoroimmunoassay of human choriogonadotropin. *Clinical Chemistry*, **29**, 60–64.

6. Hemmila, I., Dakubu, S., Mukkala, V.M., Siitari, H., and Lovgren, T. (1984) Europium as a label in time-resolved immunofluorometric assays. *Analytical Biochemistry*, **137**, 335–343.

7. Soini, E., and Lovgren, T. (1987) Time-resolved fluorescence of lanthanide probes and applications in biotechnology. *Critical Reviews in Analytical Chemistry*, **18**, 105–154.

8. Lovgren, T., Hemmila, I., Pettersson, K., Eskola, J.U., and Bertoft, E. (1984) Determination of hormones by time-resolved fluoroimmunoassay. *Talanta*, **31**, 909–916.

9. Hierholzer, J.C., Johansson, K.H., Anderson, L.J., Tsou, C.J., and Halonen, P.E. (1987) Comparison of monoclonal time-resolved fluoroimmunoassay with monoclonal capture-biotinylated detector enzyme immunoassay for adenovirus antigen detection. *Journal of Clinical Microbiology*, **25**, 1662–1667.

10. Hierholzer, J.C., Bingham, P.G., Coombs, R.A., Johansson, K.H., Anderson, L.J., and Halonen, P.E. (1989) Comparison of monoclonal antibody time-resolved fluoroimmunoassay with monoclonal antibody capture-biotinylated detector enzyme immunoassay for respiratory syncytial virus and parainfluenza virus antigen detection. *Journal of Clinical Microbiology*, **27**, 1243–1249.

11. Barnard, G., Helmick, B., Madden, S., Gilbourne, C., and Patel, R. (2000) The measurement of prion protein in bovine brain tissue using differential extraction and DELFIA® as a diagnostic test for BSE. *Luminescence*, **15**, 357–362.

12. Crooks, S.R., Ross, P., Thompson, C.S., Haggan, S.A., and Elliott, C.T. (2000) Detection of unwanted residues of ivermectin in bovine milk by dissociation-enhanced lanthanide fluoroimmunoassay. *Luminescence*, **15**, 371–376.

13. Knipping, G.B., Gogg-Fassolter, G., Frohnwieser, B., Krempler, F., Kostner, G.M., and Malle, E. (1997) Quantification of apolipoprotein D by an immunoassay with time-resolved fluorescence spectroscopy. *Journal of Immunological Methods*, **202**, 85–95.

14. Fahle, G.A., Parker, J.M., Fischer, S.H., and Gill, V.J. (1997) Rapid and sensitive detection of cytomegalovirus using PCR and the DELFIA time-resolved fluorescence hybridization assay. *Abstracts of the General Meeting of the American Society for Microbiology*, **97**, 153.

15. Ekins, R.P., and Chu, F.W. (1991) Multianalyte microspot immunoassay: microanalytical "compact disk" of the future. *Clinical Chemistry*, **37**, 1955–1967.

16. Minor, L.K. (2005) Assays for membrane tyrosine kinase receptors: methods for high-throughput screening and utility for diagnostics. *Expert Review of Molecular Diagnostics*, **5**, 561–571.

17. Bonin, E., Tiru, M., Hallander, H., and Bredberg-Raden, U. (1999) Evaluation of single- and dual-antigen delayed fluorescence immunoassay in comparison to an ELISA and the *in vivo* toxin neutralization test for detection of diphtheria toxin antibodies. *Journal of Immunological Methods*, **230**, 131–140.

18. Allicotti, G., Borras, E., and Pinilla, C. (2003) A time-resolved fluorescence immunoassay (DELFIA) increases the sensitivity of antigen-driven cytokine detection. *Journal of Immunoassay and Immunochemistry*, **24**, 345–358.

19. Smith, D.R., Rossi, C.A., Kijek, T.M., Henchal, E.A., and Ludwig, G.V. (2001) Comparison of dissociation-enhanced lanthanide fluorescent immunoassays to

enzyme-linked immunosorbent assays for detection of staphylococcal enterotoxin B, *Yersinia pestis*-specific F1 antigen, and Venezuelan equine encephalitis virus. *Clinical and Diagnostic Laboratory Immunology*, **8**, 1070–1075.

20. Hemmila, I., Holttinen, S., Pettersson, K., and Lovgren, T. (1987) Double-label time-resolved immunofluorometry of lutropin and follitropin in serum. *Clinical Chemistry*, **33**, 2281–2283.

21. Aggerbeck, H., Norgaard-Pedersen, B., and Heron, I. (1996) Simultaneous quantitation of diphtheria and tetanus antibodies by double antigen, time-resolved fluorescence immunoassay. *Journal of Immunological Methods*, **190**, 171–183.

22. Ito, K., Oda, M., Tsuji, A., and Maeda, M. (1999) Simultaneous determination of alpha-fetoprotein, human chorionic gonadotropin and estriol in serum of pregnant women by time-resolved fluoroimmunoassay. *Journal of Pharmaceutical and Biomedical Analysis*, **20**, 169–178.

23. Kimura, H., Mukaida, M., Wang, G., Yuan, J., and Matsumoto, K. (2000) Dual-label time-resolved fluoroimmunoassay of psychopharmaceuticals and stimulants in serum. *Forensic Science International*, **113**, 345–351.

24. Heinonen, P., Iitia, A., Torresani, T., and Lovgren, T. (1997) Simple triple-label detection of seven cystic fibrosis mutations by time-resolved fluorometry. *Clinical Chemistry*, **43**, 1142–1150.

25. Xu, Y.Y., Pettersson, K., Blomberg, K., Hemmila, I., Mikola, H., and Lovgren, T. (1992) Simultaneous quadruple-label fluorometric immunoassay of thyroid-stimulating hormone, 17 α-hydroxyprogesterone, immunoreactive trypsin, and creatine kinase MM isoenzyme in dried blood spots. *Clinical Chemistry*, **38**, 2038–2043.

26. Angeles, T.S., Lippy, J.S., and Yang, S.X. (2000) Quantitative, high-throughput cell-based assays for inhibitors of trkA receptor. *Analytical Biochemistry*, **278**, 93–98.

27. Meurman, O.H., Hemmila, I.A., Lovgren, T.N.E., and Halonen, P.E. (1982) Time-resolved fluoroimmunoassay: a new test for rubella antibodies. *Journal of Clinical Microbiology*, **16**, 920–925.

28. Schmidt, B., and Steinmetz, G. (1987) Time-resolved fluoroimmunoassay vs. ELISA for determination of α2-interferon. *Clinical Chemistry*, **33**, 1070.

29. Dickson, E.F.G., Pollak, A., and Diamandis, E.P. (1995) Time-resolved detection of lanthanide luminescence for ultrasensitive bioanalytical assays. *Journal of Photochemistry and Photobiology B*, **27**, 3–19.

30. Sedgwick, J.D., and Holt, P.G. (1983) A solid-phase immunoenzymatic technique for the enumeration of specific antibody secreting cells. *Journal of Immunological Methods*, **57**, 301–309.

31. Czerkinsky, C.C., Nilsson, L.A., Nygren, H., Ouchterlony, O., and Tarkowski, A. (1983) A solid-phase enzyme-linked immunospot (ELISPOT) assay for enumeration of specific antibody-secreting cells. *Journal of Immunological Methods*, **65**, 109–121.

32. Sedgwick, J.D., and Holt, P.G. (1983) Kinetics and distribution of antigen-specific IgE-secreting cells during the primary antibody response in the rat. *Journal of Experimental Medicine*, **157**, 2178–2183.

33. Czerkinsky, C.C., and Svennerholm, A.M. (1983) Ganglioside GM1 enzyme-linked immunospot assay for simple identification of heat-labile enterotoxin-producing *Escherichia coli*. *Journal of Clinical Microbiology*, **17**, 965–969.

34. Czerkinsky, C.C., Andersson, G., Ekre, H.P., Nilsson, L.A., Klareskog, L., and Ouchterlony, O. (1988) Reverse ELISPOT assay for clonal analysis of cytokine production. I. Enumeration of gamma-interferon secreting cells. *Journal of Immunological Methods*, **110**, 29–36.

35. Okamoto, Y., Murakami, H., and Nishida, M. (1997) Detection of interleukin 6-producing cells among various organs in normal mice with an improved enzyme-linked immunospot (ELISPOT) assay. *Endocrine Journal*, **44**, 349–355.

36. Pass, H.A., Schwarz, S.L., Wunderlich, J.R., and Rosenberg, S.A. (1998) Immunization of patients with melanoma peptide vaccines: immunologic assessment using the ELISPOT assay. *The Cancer Journal from Scientific American*, **4**, 316–323.

37. Goletti, D., Vincenti, D., Carrara, S., Butera, O., Bizzoni, F., Bernardini, G., Amicosante, M., and Girardi, E. (2005) Selected RD1 peptides for active tuberculosis diagnosis: comparison of a gamma-interferon whole-blood enzyme-linked immunosorbent assay and an enzyme-linked immunospot assay. *Clinical and Diagnostic Laboratory Immunology*, **12**, 1311–1316.

38. Eshofonie, A., van der Loeff, M.S., Whittle, H., and Jaye, A. (2006) An adaptation of recombinant vaccinia-based ELISPOT and intracellular cytokine staining for a comparative measurement of cellular immune responses in HIV-1 and HIV-2 infections in West Africa. *Clinical and Experimental Immunology*, **146**, 471–478.

39. Shata, M.T., Barrett, A., Shire, N.J., Abdelwahab, S.F., Sobhy, M., Daef, E., El-Kamary, S.S., Hashem, M., Engle, R.E., Purcell, R.H., Emerson, S.U., Strickland, G.T., and Sherman, K.E. (2007) Characterization of hepatitis E-specific cell-mediated immune response using IFN-γ ELISPOT assay. *Journal of Immunological Methods*, **328**, 152–161.

40. Kalyuzhny, A.E. (2005) Chemistry and biology of the ELISPOT assay. In: Kalyuzhny, A. E. (ed.), *Handbook of ELISPOT*, Methods in Molecular Biology™, Vol. **302**. Humana Press Inc., Totowa, NJ, pp. 15–31.

41. Meierhoff, G., Ott, P.A., Lehmann, P.V., and Schloot, N.C. (2002) Cytokine detection by ELISPOT: relevance for immunological studies in type 1 diabetes. *Diabetes/Metabolism Research and Reviews*, **18**, 367–380.

42. Cox, J.H., Ferrari, G., and Janetzki, S. (2006) Measurement of cytokine release at the single cell level using the ELISPOT assay. *Methods*, **38**, 274–282.

43. Samaras, V., Piperi, C., Korkolopoulou, P., Zisakis, A., Levidou, G., Themistocleous, M.S., Boviatsis, E.I., Sakas, D.E., Lea, R.W., Kalofoutis, A., and Patsouris, E. (2007) Application of the ELISPOT method for comparative analysis of interleukin (IL)-6 and IL-10 secretion in peripheral blood of patients with astroglial tumors. *Molecular and Cellular Biochemistry*, **304**, 343–351.

44. Díaz, I., and Mateu, E. (2005) Use of ELISPOT and ELISA to evaluate IFN-γ, IL-10 and IL-4 responses in conventional pigs. *Veterinary Immunology and Immunopathology*, **106**, 107–112.

45. McCutcheon, M., Wehner, N., Wensky, A., Kushner, M., Doan, S., Hsiao, L., Calabresi, P., Ha, T., Tran, T.V., Tate, K.M., Winkelhake, J., and Spack, E.G. (1997) A sensitive ELISPOT assay to detect low-frequency human T lymphocytes. *Journal of Immunological Methods*, **210**, 149–166.

46. Merville, P., Pouteil-Noble, C., Wijdenes, J., Potaux, L., Touraine, J.L., and Banchereau, J. (1993) Detection of single cells secreting IFN-gamma, IL-6, and IL-10 in irreversible

rejected human kidney allografts, and their modulation by IL-2 and IL-4. *Transplantation*, **55**, 639–646.

47. Helms, T., Boehm, B.O., Asaad, R.J., Trezza, R.P., Lehmann, P.V., and Tary-Lehmann, M. (2000) Direct visualization of cytokine-producing recall antigen-specific CD4 memory T cells in healthy individuals and HIV patients. *Journal of Immunology*, **164**, 3723–3732.

48. Tanguay, S., and Killion, J.J. (1994) Direct comparison of ELISPOT and ELISA-based assays for detection of individual cytokine-secreting cells. *Lymphokine and Cytokine Research*, **13**, 259–263.

49. Ekerfelt, C., Ernerudh, J., and Jenmalm, M.C. (2002) Detection of spontaneous and antigen-induced human interleukin-4 responses *in vitro*: comparison of ELISPOT, a novel ELISA and real-time RT-PCR. *Journal of Immunological Methods*, **260**, 55–67.

50. Janetzki, S., Schaed, S., Blachere, N.E.B., Ben-Porat, L., Houghton, A.N., and Panageas, K.S. (2004) Evaluation of ELISPOT assays: influence of method and operator on variability of results. *Journal of Immunological Methods*, **291**, 175–183.

51. Herr, W., Linn, B., Leister, N., Wandel, E., Meyer zum Buschenfelde, K.H., and Wolfel, T. (1997) The use of computer-assisted video image analysis for the quantification of CD8$^+$ T lymphocytes producing tumor necrosis factor α spots in response to peptide antigens. *Journal of Immunological Methods*, **203**, 141–152.

52. Sachdeva, N., and Asthana, D. (2007) Cytokine quantitation: technologies and applications. *Frontiers in Bioscience*, **12**, 4682–4695.

53. Czerkinsky, C., Moldoveanu, Z., Mestecky, J., Nilsson, L.A., and Ouchterlony, O. (1988) A novel two colour ELISPOT assay. I. Simultaneous detection of distinct types of antibody-secreting cells. *Journal of Immunological Methods*, **115**, 31–37.

54. Okamoto, Y., Abe, T., Niwa, T., Mizuhashi, S., and Nishida, M. (1998) Development of a dual color enzyme-linked immunospot assay for simultaneous detection of murine T helper type 1- and T helper type 2-cells. *Immunopharmacology*, **39**, 107–116.

55. Palzer, S., Bailey, T., Hartnett, C., Grant, A., Tsang, M., and Kalyuzhny, A.E. (2005) Simultaneous detection of multiple cytokines in ELISPOT assays. In: Kalyuzhny, A.E. (ed.), *Handbook of ELISPOT*, Methods in Molecular Biology™, Vol. **302**. Humana Press Inc., Totowa, NJ, pp. 273–288.

56. Sano, T., Smith, C.L., and Cantor, C.R. (1992) Immuno-PCR: very sensitive antigen detection by means of specific antibody–DNA conjugates. *Science*, **258**, 120–122.

57. Niemeyer, C.M., Adler, M., and Blohm, D. (1997) Fluorometric polymerase chain reaction (PCR) enzyme-linked immunosorbent assay for quantification of immuno-PCR products in microplates. *Analytical Biochemistry*, **246**, 140–145.

58. Niemeyer, C.M., Adler, M., and Wacker, R. (2005) Immuno-PCR: high sensitivity detection of proteins by nucleic acid amplification. *Trends in Biotechnology*, **23**, 208–216.

59. Ruzicka, V., Marz, W., Russ, A., and Gross, W. (1993) Immuno-PCR with a commercially available avidin system. *Science*, **260**, 698–699.

60. Zhou, H., Fisher, R.J., and Papas, T.S. (1993) Universal immuno-PCR for ultra-sensitive target protein detection. *Nucleic Acids Research*, **21**, 6038–6039.

61. Sanna, P.P., Weiss, F., Samson, M.E., Bloom, F.E., and Pich, E.M. (1995) Rapid induction of tumor necrosis factor α in the cerebrospinal fluid after intracerebroventricular

injection of lipopolysaccharide revealed by a sensitive capture immuno-PCR assay. *Proceedings of the National Academy of Sciences of the United States of America*, **92**, 272–275.

62. Hendrickson, E.R., Hatfield Truby, T.M., Joerger, R.D., Majarian, W.R., and Ebersole, R.C. (1995) High sensitivity multianalyte immunoassay using covalent DNA-labeled antibodies and polymerase chain reaction. *Nucleic Acids Research*, **23**, 522–529.

63. Sano, T., Smith, C.L., and Cantor, C.R. (1993) Response. *Science*, **260**, 699.

64. Niemeyer, C.M., Adler, M., Pignataro, B., Lenhert, S., Gao, S., Chi, L., Fuchs, H., and Blohm, D. (1999) Self-assembly of DNA–streptavidin nanostructures and their use as reagents in immuno-PCR. *Nucleic Acids Research*, **27**, 4553–4561.

65. Liang, H., Cordova, S.E., Kieft, T.L., and Rogelj, S. (2003) A highly sensitive immuno-PCR assay for detecting Group A *Streptococcus*. *Journal of Immunological Methods*, **279**, 101–110.

66. Adler, M., Langer, M., Witthohn, K., Eck, J., Blohm, D., and Niemeyer, C.M. (2003) Detection of rViscumin in plasma samples by immuno-PCR. *Biochemical and Biophysical Research Communications*, **300**, 757–763.

67. Adler, M., Schulz, S., Fisher, R., and Niemeyer, C.M. (2005) Detection of rotavirus from stool samples using a standardized immuno-PCR ("Imperacer") method with end-point and real-time detection. *Biochemical and Biophysical Research Communications*, **333**, 1289–1294.

68. Barletta, J.M., Edelman, D.C., and Constantine, N.T. (2004) Lowering the detection limits of HIV-1 viral load using real-time immuno-PCR for HIV-1 p24 antigen. *American Journal of Clinical Pathology*, **122**, 20–27.

69. Barletta, J. (2006) Applications of real-time immuno-polymerase chain reaction (rt-PCR) for the rapid diagnoses of viral antigens and pathologic proteins. *Molecular Aspects of Medicine*, **27**, 224–253.

70. Mackay, I.M. (2004) Real-time PCR in the microbiology laboratory. *Clinical Microbiology and Infection*, **10**, 190–212.

71. Adler, M., Wacker, R., and Niemeyer, C.M. (2003) A real-time immuno-PCR assay for routine ultrasensitive quantitation of proteins. *Biochemical and Biophysical Research Communications*, **308**, 240–250.

72. Lubelli, C., Chatgilialoglu, A., Bolognesi, A., Strocchi, P., Colombatti, M., and Stirpe, F. (2006) Detection of ricin and other ribosome-inactivating proteins by an immuno-polymerase chain reaction assay. *Analytical Biochemistry*, **355**, 102–109.

73. Barletta, J.M., Edelman, D.C., Highsmith, W.E., and Constantine, N.T. (2005) Detection of ultra-low levels of pathologic prion protein in scrapie infected hamster brain homogenates using real-time immuno-PCR. *Journal of Virological Methods*, **127**, 154–164.

74. Greenway, G.M. (1990) Analytical applications of electrogenerated chemiluminescence. *Trends in Analytical Chemistry*, **9**, 200–203.

75. Knight, A.W., and Greenway, G.M. (1994) Occurrence, mechanisms and analytical applications of electrogenerated chemiluminescence. A review. *Analyst*, **119**, 879–890.

76. Knight, A.W. (1999) A review of recent trends in analytical applications of electrogenerated chemiluminescence. *Trends in Analytical Chemistry*, **18**, 47–62.

77. Fahnrich, K.A., Pravda, M., and Guilbault, G.G. (2001) Recent applications of electrogenerated chemiluminescence in chemical analysis. *Talanta*, **54**, 531–559.

78. Richter, M.M. (2004) Electrochemiluminescence (ECL). *Chemical Reviews*, **104**, 3003–3036.

79. Blackburn, G.F., Shah, H.P., Kenten, J.H., Leland, J., Kamin, R.A., Link, J., Peterman, J., Powell, M.J., Shah, A., Talley, D.B., Tyagi, S.K., Wilkins, E., Wu, T.G., and Massey, R.J. (1991) Electrochemiluminescence detection for development of immunoassays and DNA probe assays for clinical diagnostics. *Clinical Chemistry*, **37**, 1534–1539.

80. Kenten, J.H., Casadei, J., Link, J., Lupold, S., Willey, J., Powell, M., Rees, A., and Massey, R. (1991) Rapid electrochemiluminescence assays of polymerase chain reaction products. *Clinical Chemistry*, **37**, 1626–1632.

81. Kenten, J.H., Gudibande, S., Link, J., Willey, J.J., Curfman, B., Major, E.O., and Massey, R.J. (1992) Improved electrochemiluminescent label for DNA probe assays: rapid quantitative assays of HIV-1 polymerase chain reaction products. *Clinical Chemistry*, **38**, 873–879.

82. Debad, J.D., Glezer, E.N., Wohlstadter, J., Sigal, G.B., and Leland, J.K. (2004) Clinical and biological applications of ECL. In: Bard, A.J. (ed.), *Electrogenerated Chemiluminescence*, Marcel Dekker, Inc., New York, NY, pp. 359–396.

83. Deaver, D.R. (1995) A new non-isotopic detection system for immunoassays. *Nature*, **377**, 758–760.

84. Bard, A.J., Debad, J.D., Leland, J.K., Sigal, G.B., Wilbur, J.L., and Wohlstadter, J.N. (2000) Chemiluminescence, electrogenerated. *Electroanalytical Methods*, **11**, 9842–9849.

85. Miao, W. (2008) Electrogenerated chemiluminescence and its biorelated applications. *Chemical Reviews*, **108**, 2506–2553.

86. Horninger, D., Eirikis, E., Pendley, C., Giles-Komar, J., Davis, H.M., and Miller, B.E. (2005) A one-step, competitive electrochemiluminescence-based immunoassay method for the quantification of a fully human anti-TNFα antibody in human serum. *Journal of Pharmaceutical and Biomedical Analysis*, **38**, 703–708.

87. Motmans, K., Raus, J., and Vandevyver, C. (1996) Quantification of cytokine messenger RNA in transfected human T cells by RT-PCR and an automated electrochemiluminescence-based post-PCR detection system. *Journal of Immunological Methods*, **190**, 107–116.

88. O'Connell, C.D., Juhasz, A., Kuo, C., Reeder, D.J., and Hoon, D.S.B. (1998) Detection of tyrosinase mRNA in melanoma by reverse transcription-PCR and electrochemiluminescence. *Clinical Chemistry*, **44**, 1161–1169.

89. Gatto-Menking, D.L., Yu, H., Bruno, J.G., Goode, M.T., Miller, M., and Zulich, A.W. (1996) Preliminary testing and assay development for biotoxoids, viruses and bacterial spores using the ORIGEN immunomagnetic electrochemiluminescence sensor. In: Berg, D.A. (ed.), *Proceedings of the ERDEC Scientific Conference on Chemical and Biological Defense Research*, National Technical Information Service, Springfield, VA, pp. 229–236.

90. Grimshaw, C., Gleason, C., Chojnicki, E., and Young, J. (1997) Development of an equilibrium immunoassay using electrochemiluminescent detection for a novel recombinant protein product and its application to pre-clinical product development. *Journal of Pharmaceutical and Biomedical Analysis*, **16**, 605–612.

91. Moxness, M., Tatarewicz, S., Weeraratne, D., Murakami, N., Wullner, D., Mytych, D., Jawa, V., Koren, E., and Swanson, S.J. (2005) Immunogenicity testing by

electrochemiluminescent detection for antibodies directed against therapeutic human monoclonal antibodies. *Clinical Chemistry*, **51**, 1983–1985.

92. Wang, P., Yang, Y., Zu, G., and Zhang, M. (1999) Progress in electrochemiluminescent analysis. *Fenxi Huaxua*, **27**, 1219–1225.

93. Richter, M.M. (2002) Electrochemiluminescence (ECL). In: Ligler, F.S., and Rowe Taitt, C.A. (eds), *Optical Biosensors: Present and Future*. Elsevier Science BV, Amsterdam, Netherlands, pp. 173–205.

94. Freebern, W.J., Haggerty, C.M., Montano, I., McNutt, M.C., Collins, I., Graham, A., Chandramouli, G.V.R., Stewart, D.H., Biebuyck, H.A., Taub, D.D., and Gardner, K. (2005) Pharmacologic profiling of transcriptional targets deciphers promoter logic. *The Pharmacogenomics Journal*, **5**, 305–323.

95. Gudibande, S.R., Kenten, J.H., Link, J., Friedman, K., and Massey, R.J. (1992) Rapid, non-separation electrochemiluminescent DNA hybridization assays for PCR products, using 3′-labelled oligonucleotide probes. *Molecular and Cellular Probes*, **6**, 495–503.

96. Tang, Y.B., and Tang, Y.H. (2005) Application of electrochemiluminescence in gene detection. *Jiguang Shengwu Xuebao*, **14**, 461–465.

97. Weinreb, P.H., Yang, W.J., Violette, S.M., Couture, M., Kimball, K., Pepinsky, R.B., Lobb, R.R., and Josiah, S. (2002) A cell-free electrochemiluminescence assay for measuring β1-integrin–ligand interactions. *Analytical Biochemistry*, **306**, 305–313.

98. Zhang, L., Schwartz, G., O'Donnell, M., and Harrison, R.K. (2001) Development of a novel helicase assay using electrochemiluminescence. *Analytical Biochemistry*, **293**, 31–37.

99. Li, Y., Qi, H.L., and Zhang, C.X. (2005) Electrochemiluminescence progress in nucleic acid hybridization detection and drug screening. *Shengming De Huaxue*, **25**, 336–339.

100. Rivera, V.R., Gamez, F.J., Keener, W.K., White, J.A., and Poli, M.A. (2006) Rapid detection of *Clostridium botulinum* toxins A, B, E, and F in clinical samples, selected food matrices, and buffer using paramagnetic bead-based electrochemiluminescence detection. *Analytical Biochemistry*, **353**, 248–256.

101. Kaur, G., and Roy, I. (2008) Therapeutic applications of aptamers. *Expert Opinion on Investigational Drugs*, **17**, 43–60.

102. Pirollo, K.F., Rait, A., Sleer, L.S., and Chang, E.H. (2003) Antisense therapeutics: from theory to clinical practice. *Pharmacology and Therapeutics*, **99**, 55–77.

103. Simons, C., Wu, Q., and Htar, T.T. (2005) Recent advances in antiviral nucleoside and nucleotide therapeutics. *Current Topics in Medicinal Chemistry*, **5**, 1191–1203.

104. Yacyshyn, B.R., Barish, C., Goff, J., Dalke, D., Gaspari, M., Yu, R., Tami, J., Dorr, F.A., and Sewell, K.L. (2002) Dose ranging pharmacokinetic trial of high-dose alicaforsen (intercellular adhesion molecule-1 antisense oligodeoxynucleotide) (ISIS 2302) in active Crohn's disease. *Alimentary Pharmacology and Therapeutics*, **16**, 1761–1770.

105. Khoury, M., Jorgensen, C., and Apparailly, F. (2007) RNAi in arthritis: prospects of a future antisense therapy in inflammation. *Current Opinion in Molecular Therapeutics*, **9**, 483–489.

106. Bhanot, S. (2008) Developing antisense drugs for metabolic diseases: a novel therapeutic approach. In: Crooke, S.T. (ed.), *Antisense Drug Technology*, 2nd edition. CRC Press LLC, Boca Raton, FL, pp. 641–663.

107. Yu, R.Z., Geary, R.S., and Levin, A.A. (2004) Application of novel quantitative bioanalytical methods for pharmacokinetic and pharmacokinetic/pharmacodynamic assessments of antisense oligonucleotides. *Current Opinion in Drug Discovery and Development*, **7**, 195–203.

108. Lin, Z.J., Li, W., and Dai, G. (2007) Application of LC–MS for quantitative analysis and metabolite identification of therapeutic oligonucleotides. *Journal of Pharmaceutical and Biomedical Analysis*, **44**, 330–341.

109. Brown-Augsburger, P., Yue, X.M., Lockridge, J.A., McSwiggen, J.A., Kamboj, D., and Hillgren, K.M. (2004) Development and validation of a sensitive, specific, and rapid hybridization-ELISA assay for determination of concentrations of a ribozyme in biological matrices. *Journal of Pharmaceutical and Biomedical Analysis*, **34**, 129–139.

110. Temsamani, J., Kubert, M., and Agrawal, S. (1993) A rapid method for quantitation of oligodeoxynucleotide phosphorothioates in biological fluids and tissues. *Analytical Biochemistry*, **215**, 54–58.

111. de Serres, M., McNulty, M.J., Christensen, L., Zon, G., and Findlay, J.W.A. (1996) Development of a novel scintillation proximity competitive hybridization assay for the determination of phosphorothioate antisense oligonucleotide plasma concentrations in a toxicokinetic study. *Analytical Biochemistry*, **233**, 228–233.

112. Deverre, J.R., Boutet, V., Boquet, D., Ezan, E., Grassi, J., and Grognet, J.-M. (1997) A competitive enzyme hybridization assay for plasma determination of phosphodiester and phosphorothioate antisense oligonucleotides. *Nucleic Acids Research*, **25**, 3584–3589.

113. Boutet, V., Delaunay, V., De Oliveira, M.C., Boquet, D., Grognet, J.-M., Grassi, J., and Deverre, J.-R. (2000) Real-time monitoring of the hybridization reaction: application to the quantification of oligonucleotides in biological samples. *Biochemical and Biophysical Research Communications*, **268**, 92–98.

114. Kandimalla, E.R., Pandey, R.K., and Agrawal, S. (2004) Hybridization-based fluorescence assay allows quantitation of single-stranded oligodeoxynucleotides in low nanomolar range. *Analytical Biochemistry*, **323**, 93–95.

115. Hakala, H., and Lonnberg, H. (1997) Time-resolved fluorescence detection of oligonucleotide hybridization on a single microparticle: covalent immobilization of oligonucleotides and quantitation of a model system. *Bioconjugate Chemistry*, **8**, 232–237.

116. Chevrier, D., Popoff, M.Y., Dion, M.P., Hermant, D., and Guesdon, J.-L. (1995) Rapid detection of *Salmonella* subspecies I by PCR combined with non-radioactive hybridisation using covalently immobilised oligonucleotide on a microplate. *FEMS Immunology and Medical Microbiology*, **10**, 245–251.

117. Chevrier, D., Rasmussen, S.R., and Guesdon, J.-L. (1993) PCR product quantification by non-radioactive hybridization procedures using an oligonucleotide covalently bound to microwells. *Molecular and Cellular Probes*, **7**, 187–197.

118. Jin, J., Peng, Y., and Lu, J. (2003) An enzyme-linked sandwich hybridization on microplate for quantification of hIL-18 mRNA. *Zhongguo Mianyixue Zazhi*, **19**, 499–501.

119. Efler, S.M., Zhang, L., Noll, B.O., Uhlmann, E., and Davis, H.L. (2005) Quantification of oligodeoxynucleotides in human plasma with a novel hybridization assay offers greatly enhanced sensitivity over capillary gel electrophoresis. *Oligonucleotides*, **15**, 119–131.

120. Edwards, K.A., and Beaumner, A.J. (2006) Sequential injection analysis system for the sandwich hybridization-based detection of nucleic acids. *Analytical Chemistry*, **78**, 1958–1966.

121. Yu, R.Z., Baker, B., Chappell, A., Geary, R.S., Cheung, E., and Levin, A.A. (2002) Development of an ultrasensitive noncompetitive hybridization–ligation enzyme-linked immunosorbent assay for the determination of phosphorothioate oligodeoxynucleotide in plasma. *Analytical Biochemistry*, **304**, 19–25.

122. Wei, X., Dai, G., Marcucci, G., Liu, Z., Hoyt, D., Blum, W., and Chan, K.K. (2006) A specific picomolar hybridization-based ELISA assay for the determination of phosphorothioate oligonucleotides in plasma and cellular matrices. *Pharmaceutical Research*, **23**, 1251–1264.

123. Andersson, L.I. (2000) Molecular imprinting for drug bioanalysis. A review on the application of imprinted polymers to solid-phase extraction and binding assay. *Journal of Chromatography B*, **739**, 163–173.

124. Wulff, G. (1995) Molecular imprinting in cross-linked materials with the aid of molecular templates: a way towards artificial antibodies. *Angewandte Chemie (International Edition in English)*, **34**, 1812–1832.

125. Mosbach, K., and Ramstrom, O. (1996) The emerging technique of molecular imprinting and its future impact on biotechnology. *Biotechnology*, **14**, 163–170.

126. Ansell, R.J., Ramstrom, O., and Mosbach, K. (1996) Towards artificial antibodies prepared by molecular imprinting. *Clinical Chemistry*, **42**, 1506–1512.

127. Steinke, J., Sherrington, D.C., and Dunkin, I.R. (1995) Imprinting of synthetic polymers using molecular templates. *Advances in Polymer Science*, **123**, 81–125.

128. Mallik, S., Plunkett, S.D., Dhal, P.K., Johnson, R.D., Pack, D., Shnek, D., and Arnold, F. H. (1994) Towards materials for the specific recognition and separation of proteins. *New Journal of Chemistry*, **18**, 299–304.

129. Nicholls, I.A., Abdo, K., Andersson, H.S., Andersson, P.O., Ankarloo, J., Hedin-Dahlstrom, J., Jokela, P., Karlsson, J.G., Olofsson, L., Rosengren, J., Shoravi, S., Svenson, J., and Wikman, S. (2001) Can we rationally design molecularly imprinted polymers? *Analytica Chimica Acta*, **435**, 9–18.

130. Olsen, J., Martin, P., and Wilson, I.D. (1998) Molecular imprints as sorbents for solid phase extraction. *Analytical Communications*, **35**, 13H–14H.

131. Ansell, R.J. (2004) Molecularly imprinted polymers in pseudoimmunoassay. *Journal of Chromatography B*, **804**, 151–165.

132. Vlatakis, G., Andersson, L.I., Muller, R., and Mosbach, K. (1993) Drug assay using antibody mimics made by molecular imprinting. *Nature*, **361**, 645–647.

133. Andersson, L.I., Muller, R., Vlatakis, G., and Mosbach, K. (1995) Mimics of the binding sites of opiod receptors obtained by molecular imprinting of enkephalin and morphine. *Proceedings of the National Academy of Sciences of the United States of America*, **92**, 4788–4792.

134. Ramstrom, O., Ye, L., and Mosbach, K. (1996) Artificial antibodies to corticosteroids prepared by molecular imprinting. *Chemistry and Biology*, **3**, 471–477.

135. Andersson, L.I. (1996) Application of molecular imprinting to the development of aqueous buffer and organic solvent based radioligand binding assays for (*S*)-propranolol. *Analytical Chemistry*, **68**, 111–117.

136. Bengtsson, H., Roos, U., and Andersson, L.I. (1997) Molecular imprint based radioassay for direct determination of S-propranolol in human plasma. *Analytical Communications*, **34**, 233–235.

137. Haupt, K., Mayes, A.G., and Mosbach, K. (1998) Herbicide assay using an imprinted polymer-based system analogous to competitive fluoroimmunoassays. *Analytical Chemistry*, **70**, 3936–3989.

138. Surugiu, I., Danielsson, B., Ye, L., Mosbach, K., and Haupt, K. (2001) Chemiluminescence imaging ELISA using an imprinted polymer as the recognition element instead of an antibody. *Analytical Chemistry*, **73**, 487–491.

139. Surugiu, I., Svitel, J., Ye, L., Haupt, K., and Danielsson, B. (2001) Development of a flow injection capillary chemiluminescent ELISA using an imprinted polymer instead of the antibody. *Analytical Chemistry*, **73**, 4388–4392.

140. Ye, L., Surugiu, I., and Haupt, K. (2002) Scintillation proximity assay using molecularly imprinted microspheres. *Analytical Chemistry*, **74**, 959–964.

141. Rachkov, A., Hu, M., Bulgarevich, E., Matsumoto, T., and Minoura, N. (2004) Molecularly imprinted polymers prepared in aqueous solution selective for [Sar^1,Ala^8] angiotensin II. *Analytica Chimica Acta*, **504**, 191–197.

142. Chou, P.-C., Rick, J., and Chou, T.-C. (2005) C-reactive protein thin-film molecularly imprinted polymers formed using a micro-contact approach. *Analytica Chimica Acta*, **542**, 20–25.

143. Bossi, A., Bonini, F., Turner, A.P.F., and Piletsky, S.A. (2007) Molecularly imprinted polymers for the recognition of proteins: the state of the art. *Biosensors and Bioelectronics*, **22**, 1131–1137.

144. Janiak, D.S., and Kofinas, P. (2007) Molecular imprinting of peptides and proteins in aqueous media. *Analytical and Bioanalytical Chemistry*, **389**, 399–404.

145. Bergmann, N.M., and Peppas, N.A. (2008) Molecularly imprinted polymers with specific recognition for macromolecules and proteins. *Progress in Polymer Science*, **33**, 271–288.

146. Nylander, C., Liedberg, B., and Lind, T. (1982) Gas detection by means of surface plasmon resonance. *Sensors and Actuators*, **3**, 79–84.

147. Liedberg, B., Nylander, C., and Lundstrom, I. (1983) Surface plasmon resonance for gas detection and biosensing. *Sensors and Actuators*, **4**, 299–304.

148. Mullett, W.M., Lai, E.P.C., and Yeung, J.M. (2000) Surface plasmon resonance-based immunoassays. *Methods*, **22**, 77–91.

149. Hsieh, H.V., Stewart, B., Hauer, P., Haaland, P., and Campbell, R. (1998) Measurement of *Clostridium perfringens* β-toxin production by surface plasmon resonance immunoassay. *Vaccine*, **16**, 997–1003.

150. Liedberg, B., Nylander, C., and Lundstrom, I. (1995) Biosensing with surface plasmon resonance: how it all started. *Biosensors and Bioelectronics*, **10**, i–ix.

151. Shelver, W.L., and Smith, D.J. (2003) Determination of ractopamine in cattle and sheep urine samples using an optical biosensor analysis: comparative study with HPLC and ELISA. *Journal of Agriculture and Food Chemistry*, **51**, 3715–3721.

152. Cho, H.-S., Kim, T.-J., Lee, J.-L., and Park, N.-Y. (2006) Serodiagnostic comparison of enzyme-linked immunosorbent assay and surface plasmon resonance for the detection

of antibody to *porcine circovirus type 2. The Canadian Journal of Veterinary Research,* **70**, 263–268.

153. Guidi, A., Laricchia-Robbio, L., Gianfaldoni, D., Revoltella, R., and Del Bono, G. (2001) Comparison of a conventional immunoassay (ELISA) with a surface plasmon resonance-based biosensor for IGF-1 detection in cows' milk. *Biosensors and Bioelectronics,* **16**, 971–977.

154. Masson, J.-F., Battaglia, T.M., Khairallah, P., Beaudoin, S., and Booksh, K.S. (2007) Quantitative measurement of cardiac markers in undiluted serum. *Analytical Chemistry,* **79**, 612–619.

155. Kreutzer, M.P., Quidant, R., Badenes, G., and Marco, M.-P. (2005) Quantitative detection of doping substances by a localised surface plasmon sensor. *Biosensors and Bioelectronics,* **21**, 1345–1349.

156. Cao, C., and Sim, S.J. (2007) Signal enhancement of surface plasmon resonance immunoassay using enzyme precipitation-functionalized gold nanoparticles: a femtomolar level measurement of anti-glutamic acid decarboxylase antibody. *Biosensors and Bioelectronics,* **22**, 1874–1880.

157. Rich, R.L., and Myszka, D.G. (2007) Higher-throughput, label-free, real-time molecular interaction analysis. *Analytical Biochemistry,* **361**, 1–6.

158. Hoa, X.D., Kirk, A.G., and Tabrizian, M. (2007) Towards integrated and sensitive surface plasmon resonance biosensors: a review of recent progress. *Biosensors and Bioelectronics,* **23**, 151–160.

159. Rich, R.L., and Myszka, D.G. (2007) Survey of the year 2006 commercial optical biosensor literature. *Journal of Molecular Recognition,* **20**, 300–366.

160. Skottrup, P., Hearty, S., Frokiaer, H., Leonard, P., Hejgaard, J., Kennedy, R.O., Nicolaisen, M., and Justesen, A.F. (2007) Detection of fungal spores using a generic surface plasmon resonance immunoassay. *Biosensors and Bioelectronics,* **22**, 2724–2729.

161. Zhu, G., Yang, B., and Jennings, R.N. (2000) Quantitation of basic fibroblast growth factor by immunoassay using BIAcore 2000. *Journal of Pharmaceutical and Biomedical Analysis,* **24**, 281–290.

162. Yu, F., Persson, B., Loras, S., and Knoll, W. (2004) Surface plasmon fluorescescence immunoassay of free prostate-specific antigen in human plasma at the femtomolar level. *Analytical Chemistry,* **76**, 6765–6770.

163. Crooks, S.R.H., Baxter, G.A., O'Connor, M.C., and Elliot, C.T. (1998) Immunobiosensor: an alternative to enzyme immunoassay screening for residues of two sulfonamides in pigs. *Analyst,* **123**, 2755–2757.

164. Samsonova, J.V., Baxter, G.A., Crooks, S.R.H., and Elliot, C.T. (2002) Biosensor immunoassay of ivermectin in bovine milk. *Journal of AOAC International,* **85**, 879–882.

165. Gillis, E.H., Gosling, J.P., Sreenan, J.M., and Kane, M. (2002) Development and validation of a biosensor-based immunoassay for progesterone in bovine milk. *Journal of Immunological Methods,* **267**, 131–138.

166. Mason, S., La, S., Mytych, D., Swanson, S.J., and Ferbas, J. (2003) Validation of the BIACORE 3000 platform for detection of antibodies against erythropoietic agents in human plasma samples. *Current Medical Research and Opinion,* **19**, 651–659.

167. Koren, E., Mytych, D., Koscec, M., Ferbas, J., Gupta, S., Moxness, M., and Swanson, S. (2005) Strategies for the preclinical and clinical characterization of immunogenicity. *Developments in Biologicals (Basel)*, **122**, 195–200.

168. Thorpe, R., and Swanson, S.J. (2005) Current methods for detecting antibodies against erythropoietin and other recombinant proteins. *Clinical and Diagnostic Laboratory Immunology*, **12**, 28–39.

169. Wadwa, M., Gaines-Das, R., Thorpe, R., and Mire-Sluis, A. (2005) Detection, measurement and characterization of unwanted antibodies induced by therapeutic biologicals. *Developments in Biologicals* (Basel), **122**, 155–170.

170. Boozer, C., Kim, G., Cong, S., Guan, H., and Londergan, T. (2006) Looking towards label-free biomolecular interaction analysis in a high-throughput format: a review of new surface plasmon resonance technologies. *Current Opinion in Biotechnology*, **17**, 400–405.

171. Homola, J., Vaisocherova, H., Dostalek, J., and Piliarik, M. (2005) Multi-analyte surface plasmon resonance biosensing. *Methods*, **37**, 26–36.

172. Lotierzo, M., Henry, O.Y.F., Piletsky, S., Tothill, I., Cullen, D., Kania, M., Hock, B., and Turner, A.P.F. (2004) Surface plasmon resonance sensor for domoic acid based on grafted imprinted polymer. *Biosensors and Bioelectronics*, **20**, 145–152.

173. Nedelkov, D., and Nelson, R.W. (2003) Surface plasmon resonance mass spectrometry: recent progress and outlooks. *Trends in Biotechnology*, **21**, 301–305.

174. Stone, J.A., and Soldin, S.J. (1988) Improved liquid chromatographic/immunoassay of digoxin in serum. *Clinical Chemistry*, **34**, 2547–2551.

175. Tang, Z., and Karnes, H.T. (2000) Coupling immunoassays with chromatographic separation techniques. *Biomedical Chromatography*, **14**, 442–449.

176. Creaser, C.S., Feely, S.J., Houghton, E., and Seymour, M. (1998) Immunoaffinity chromatography combined on-line with high-performance liquid chromatography–mass spectrometry for the determination of corticosteroids. *Journal of Chromatography A*, **794**, 37–43.

177. Cai, J., and Henion, J. (1996) On-line immunoaffinity extraction-coupled column capillary liquid chromatography/tandem mass spectrometry: trace analysis of LSD analogs and metabolites in human urine. *Analytical Chemistry*, **68**, 72–78.

178. Shen, H., Aspinall, C.A., and Kennedy, R.T. (1997) Dual microcolumn immunoassay applied to determination of insulin secretion from single islets of Langerhans and insulin in serum. *Journal of Chromatography B*, **689**, 295–303.

179. Delaunay-Bertoncini, N., and Hennion, M.-C. (2004) Immunoaffinity solid-phase extraction for pharmaceutical and biomedical trace-analysis: coupling with HPLC and CE—perspectives. *Journal of Pharmaceutical and Biomedical Analysis*, **34**, 717–736.

180. Ensing, K., and Paulus, A. (1996) Immobilization of antibodies as a versatile tool in hybridized capillary electrophoresis. *Journal of Pharmaceutical and Biomedical Analysis*, **14**, 305–315.

181. Phillips, T.M., Kennedy, L.M., and De Fabo, E.C. (1997) Microdialysis–immunoaffinity capillary electrophoresis studies on neuropeptide-induced lymphocyte secretion. *Journal of Chromatography B*, **697**, 101–109.

182. Phillips, T.M. (1998) Determination of *in situ* tissue neuropeptides by capillary immuno-electrophoresis. *Analytica Chimica Acta*, **372**, 209–218.

183. Driedger, D.R., and Sporns, P. (2001) Immunoaffinity sample purification and MALDI-TOF MS analysis of α-solanine and α-chaconine in serum. *Journal of Agricultural and Food Chemistry*, **49**, 543–548.

184. Nevanen, T.K., Soderholm, L., Kukkonen, K., Suortti, T., Teerinen, T., Lindner, M., Soderlund, H., and Teeri, T.T. (2001) Efficient enantioselective separation of drug enantiomers by immobilized antibody fragments. *Journal of Chromatography A*, **925**, 89–97.

185. Fu, Z., Hao, C., Fei, X., and Ju, H. (2006) Flow-injection chemiluminescent immunoassay for alpha-fetoprotein based on epoxysilane modified glass microbeads. *Journal of Immunological Methods*, **312**, 61–67.

186. Lin, J., Yan, F., and Ju, H. (2004) Noncompetitive enzyme immunoassay for carcinoembryonic antigen by flow injection chemiluminescence. *Clinica Chimica Acta*, **341**, 109–115.

187. Yang, H.-H., Zhu, Q.-Z., Qu, H.-Y., Chen, X.-L., Ding, M.-T., and Xu, J.-G. (2002) Flow injection fluorescence immunoassay for gentamicin using sol–gel-derived mesoporous biomaterial. *Analytical Biochemistry*, **308**, 71–76.

188. Dreveny, D., Seidl, R., Gubitz, G., and Michalowski, J. (1998) Development of solid-phase chemiluminescence immunoassay for digoxin comparing flow injection and sequential injection techniques. *Analyst*, **123**, 2271–2276.

189. Reinecke, M., and Scheper, T. (1997) Fast on-line flow injection analysis system for IgG monitoring in bioprocesses. *Journal of Biotechnology*, **59**, 145–153.

190. Tao, L., and Kennedy, R.T. (1996) On-line competitive immunoassay for insulin based on capillary electrophoresis with laser-induced fluorescence detection. *Analytical Chemistry*, **68**, 3899–3906.

191. Self, C.H., and Cook, D.B. (1996) Advances in immunoassay technology. *Current Opinion in Biotechnology*, **7**, 60–65.

192. Jayasena, S.D. (1999) Aptamers: an emerging class of molecules that rival antibodies in diagnostics. *Clinical Chemistry*, **45**, 1628–1650.

193. Liss, M., Petersen, B., Wolf, H., and Prohaska, E. (2002) An aptamer-based quartz crystal protein biosensor. *Analytical Chemistry*, **74**, 4488–4495.

194. Nedelkov, D. (2006) Mass spectrometry-based immunoassays for the next phase of clinical applications. *Expert Reviews in Proteomics*, **3**, 631–640.

195. Madou, M., Zoval, J., Jia, G., Kido, H., Kim, J., and Kim, N. (2006) Lab on a CD. *Annual Reviews of Biomedical Engineering*, **8**, 601–628.

196. Herrmann, M., Veres, T., and Tabrizian, M. (2006) Enzymatically-generated fluorescent detection in micro-channels with internal magnetic mixing for the development of parallel microfluidic ELISA. *Lab on a Chip*, **6**, 555–560.

197. Murakami, Y., Endo, T., Yamamura, S., Nagatani, N., Takamura, Y., and Tamiya, E. (2004) On-chip micro-flow polystyrene bead-based immunoassay for quantitative detection of tacrolimus (FK506). *Analytical Biochemistry*, **334**, 111–116.

198. Lai, S., Wang, S., Luo, J., Lee, L.J., Yang, S.-T., and Madou, M.J. (2004) Design of a compact disk-like microfluidic platform for enzyme-linked immunosorbent assay. *Analytical Chemistry*, **76**, 1832–1837.

199. Bange, A., Halsall, H.B., and Heineman, W.R. (2005) Microfluidic immunosensor systems. *Biosensors and Bioelectronics*, **20**, 2488–2503.

200. Ling, M.M., Ricks, C., and Lea, P. (2007) Multiplexing molecular diagnostics and immunoassays using emerging microarray technologies. *Expert Reviews of Molecular Diagnostics*, **7**, 87–98.

201. Wu, A.H.B., Fukushima, N., Puskas, R., Todd, J., and Goix, P. (2006) Development and preliminary clinical validation of a high sensitivity assay for cardiac troponin using a capillary flow (single molecule) fluorescence detector. *Clinical Chemistry*, **52**, 2157–2159.

Ligand-Binding Assays: Development, Validation, and Implementation in the Drug Development Arena. Edited by Masood N. Khan and John W.A. Findlay
Copyright © 2010 John Wiley & Sons, Inc.